IN HER HANDS

IN HER HANDS

Women's Fight against AIDS in the
United States

EMMA DAY

UNIVERSITY OF CALIFORNIA PRESS

University of California Press
Oakland, California

© 2023 by Emma Day

Library of Congress Cataloging-in-Publication Data

Names: Day, Emma, 1993- author.
Title: In her hands : women's fight against AIDS in the United States / Emma Day.
Description: Oakland, California : University of California Press, [2023] |
    Includes bibliographical references and index.
Identifiers: LCCN 2022057643 (print) | LCCN 2022057644 (ebook) | ISBN 9780520389052
    (cloth) | ISBN 9780520389069 (paperback) | ISBN 9780520389076 (ebook)
Subjects: LCSH: AIDS (Disease) in women—Social aspects—United States—20th
    century. | Social movements—United States—20th century.
Classification: LCC RA643.83 .D39 2023 (print) | LCC RA643.83 (ebook) |
    DDC 362.19697/920082—dc23/eng/20221223
LC record available at https://lccn.loc.gov/2022057643
LC ebook record available at https://lccn.loc.gov/2022057644

Manufactured in the United States of America

32 31 30 29 28 27 26 25 24 23
10 9 8 7 6 5 4 3 2 1

To Mum,
You are in every word.

Contents

Illustrations

Acknowledgments

ᴉ FINISHED WRITING this book during the most difficult period of my life, as my Mum was dying of secondary breast cancer. My writing partner and closest friend, you taught me to persevere through the toughest times and have the courage to follow my dreams. It has been so hard to finish this book without your daily messages of encouragement, and it breaks my heart that you won't see it in print. But I know you are raising a glass to me now, wherever you are. I love you, Mum. This book is dedicated to you.

I could not have completed *In Her Hands* without the love of my family. My amazing partner, Jamie, has supported me through every stage of the process, joining me on research trips, listening to conference papers, reading chapter drafts, and generally sharing in every high and low. I am grateful every day to have such a generous, kind, and brilliant partner. My wonderful Dad is my rock—a true advocate whose unwavering support over the years has taken many forms, including reading so much of my work and always being on the other end of the phone. Thank you for everything, Dad. My incredible brother and sister, Helena and Richard, are the best role models a little sister could ask for. They have taught me the value of hard work and to never take anything too seriously. They have also brought into my life their partners, Jodie and Francis, and my niece and nephews, Amelie, Henri, and Remy, all of whom I love dearly. Thanks to all my family and friends who have supported me along the way.

In Her Hands began as a masters' thesis at the University of Oxford, where I was incredibly fortunate to have been supervised by Mara Keire. It is hard to summarize all that Mara has taught me since I began graduate study. She has made me a sharper writer, a clearer thinker, and, perhaps most of all, given me confidence in myself and my ideas. She has always helped me to prioritize what is important in life when the road ahead hasn't seemed clear. I am lucky to consider her not only a mentor but a friend for life. As the project developed into a doctoral thesis, I was also lucky to be co-supervised by Stephen Tuck, whose advice and ongoing support has helped get me to this stage. Always pushing me to think about the bigger picture, Stephen's involvement has made this book infinitely better.

The University of Oxford and the Rothermere American Institute provided the perfect academic home to undertake this project. There, I found friendship as well as a supportive community in which to develop my ideas. A special shout out to the Coven—Nonie Kubie, Sage Goodwin, Grace Mallon, Lynne Foote, and Mara Keire—and other dear friends at Oxford, Kiran Mehta, Tim Wade, Drew Holland, Mitch Robertson, and Dan Rowe. I am also immensely grateful to colleagues at the RAI for their professional and intellectual support and guidance, especially Halbert Jones, Adam Smith, Stephen Tuffnell, Pekka Hämäläinen, Uta Balbier, Stephen Tuck, and Mara Keire. My thanks to colleagues at St. Mary's University, as well as students who helped me place the book's themes within the larger framework of US history.

In Her Hands benefited immensely from the feedback of others who read, commented on, and helped me develop the manuscript at different stages. As my doctoral examiners, Jonathan Bell and Gareth Davies set me on the path to turning the dissertation into a book. Jon was one of the earliest advocates of the project, and I thank him for all his advice and input over the years. Thanks also to Nick Witham, David Sim, Alex Goodall, Jesse Milan, Sarah Phillips, Manon Parry, Giles Scott-Smith, Damian Pargas, Dario Fazzi, Mara Keire, and Stephen Tuck, and participants of workshops and conferences at the Institute of Historical Research, Roosevelt Institute for American Studies, University of Edinburgh American History Workshop, John W. Kluge Center at the Library of Congress, Organization of American Historians, Historians of the Twentieth Century United States, British Academy for American Studies, Centre for Gender Identity and Subjectivity at Oxford University, Queer Studies Research Network at Oxford University, Society for the History of Women in the Americas, Rothermere American Institute American History Graduate Seminar, Pembroke College, Oxford, and the Queen's College, Oxford. Thanks to my editors at the University of California Press, Niels Hooper and Naja Pulliam Collins, for all their guidance, and for the kindness they have shown me in more difficult recent times. Thanks also to the peer reviewers for their expert insights.

I am grateful to the funding bodies that provided the financial support that made the research and writing of *In Her Hands* possible. These include the British Arts and Humanities Research Council, the John Kluge Center at the Library of Congress, the Organization of American Historians, Harvard University, Pembroke College, Oxford, the Queens College, Oxford, Oxford History Faculty, Santander, the Rothermere American Institute, American Politics Group, and Roosevelt Institute for American Studies. My thanks, also, to Chris McKenna and the Global History of Capitalism Project at Oxford for giving me the time and space to revise the manuscript.

Finally, I would like to thank the librarians and archivists who helped me access and granted me permission to reproduce materials, especially the Arthur & Elizabeth Schlesinger Library on the History of Women in America at Harvard University, GLBT Historical Society Archives and Special Collections, the Lesbian Herstory Archives, LGBT Community Center National Archive, the Library of Congress, National Library of Medicine Archives & Modern Manuscripts, New York Public Library Manuscripts and Archives Division, New York University Library Tamiment Library & Robert F. Wagner Labor Archives, Ronald Reagan Presidential Library and Museum, San Francisco Public Library, University of California San Francisco Archives and Special Collections, and the Rothermere American Institute. A special thanks to the Gay Men's Health Crisis, Ann P. Meredith and the Ann P. Meredith Collection at the Schlesinger Library on the History of Women, and Cathy Guisewite, who also kindly granted permission to reproduce material.

Portions of chapter 4 were previously published as "The Fire Inside: Women Protesting AIDS in Prison since 1980," *Modern American History* 5, no. 1 (2022): 79–100.

Abbreviations

AAP	AIDS Action Pledge
ACA	Affordable Care Act
ACE	AIDS Counseling and Education
ACLU	American Civil Liberties Union
ACT UP	AIDS Coalition to Unleash Power
ACTG	AIDS Clinical Trials Group
AIA	Abandoned Infants Assistance Act
AIDS	acquired immunodeficiency syndrome
APHA	American Public Health Association
ART	antiretroviral therapy
AZT	azidothymidine
BWHBC	Boston Women's Health Book Collective
CCWF	Central California Women's Facility
CCWP	California Coalition for Women Prisoners
CDC	Centers for Disease Control and Prevention
CDCR	California Department of Corrections and Rehabilitation

CIW	California Institution for Women
COYOTE	Call Off Your Old Tired Ethics
CSWPC	Coalition to Support Women Prisoners at Chowchilla
DOJ	Department of Justice
DPC	Domestic Policy Council
ERA	Equal Rights Amendment
FDA	Food and Drug Administration
GCM	Global Campaign for Microbicides
GMHC	Gay Men's Health Crisis
GRID	gay-related immunodeficiency
HHS	Department of Health and Human Services
HIV	human immunodeficiency virus
HLP	HIV Law Project
HRT	hormone replacement therapy
IPC	in-patient care unit
IPM	International Partnership for Microbicides
IUD	intrauterine device
KS	Kaposi's sarcoma
LAP	Lesbian AIDS Project
LSPC	Legal Services for Prisoners with Children
MDA	Microbicide Development Act
MMWR	*Morbidity and Mortality Weekly Report*
MSM	men who have sex with men
MTA	Medical Technician Assistant
MTN	Microbicide Trials Network
N-9	nonoxynol-9
NBWHP	National Black Women's Health Project
NGO	nongovernmental organization
NIAID	National Institute of Allergy and Infectious Diseases
NIH	National Institutes of Health
NOW	National Organization for Women
PAS	post-abortion syndrome

PCP	Pneumocystis carinii pneumonia
PEPFAR	President's Emergency Plan for AIDS Relief
PHS	Public Health Service
PrEP	pre-exposure prophylaxis
RRPL	Ronald Reagan Presidential Library
SHIPP	Sustainable Health Center Implementation PrEP Pilot Study
SOC	Save Our Children
SSA	Social Security Administration
SSI	Supplementary Security Income
STD	sexually transmitted disease
T&D	Treatment & Data Committee
TAG	Treatment Action Group
VA	Veterans Administration
VSPW	Valley State Prison for Women
WAC	Women's Action Coalition
WARN	Women and AIDS Resource Network
WHAM!	Women's Health Action Mobilization
WSW	women who have sex with women

INTRODUCTION

IN HER HANDS tells the story of women who fought the state neglect of their health-care needs alongside the state intervention into their lives during the HIV/AIDS epidemic. When the health crisis of AIDS (acquired immunodeficiency syndrome) first emerged in the United States in the early 1980s, doctors, scientists, and public health professionals overlooked women in the response to a novel disease that they first associated with white, gay men. Throughout the decade, as the acknowledgment that women could contract the human immunodeficiency virus (HIV), the virus that causes AIDS, and die from it grew, women became vulnerable not only to a fatal new disease but government policies that threatened their health and rights. Women living with HIV/AIDS constantly navigated the tension between needing to access state-funded services and needing to protect themselves from state interference, as state recognition easily tipped to state coercion. State interference always coexisted with state neglect to shape the experiences of women with HIV/AIDS.

In 1979, scientists discovered cases of immunodeficiency disorders in men.[1] Nearly three years passed before physicians began noticing similar symptoms in women, often after the infants and children of these women began getting sick.[2] As the US Centers for Disease Control and Prevention (CDC)—the federal public health agency responsible for addressing disease outbreaks—began receiving reports of the disease among groups who did not report male homosexuality, scientists expanded their conception of who AIDS affected, sorting the reported cases into four "at risk" groups: homosexual and bisexual males, heroin users, Haitians, and hemophiliacs.[3] What became known as the "4-H" club largely attributed a person's vulnerability to infection to their sexual identity or, if Haitian, their perceived foreignness. Attributing risk to racial and sexual identity and associated behaviors, the 4-H categories gave the impression that the differing rates of AIDS among diverse racial, ethnic, sexual, and social groups arose not from the systemic factors that impact a person's health but—in line with the advancing neoliberal politics of the period that shifted responsibility for addressing social problems from the state to private citizens—an individual's supposedly "deviant" behavior.[4]

Women scholars mobilized to critique the resulting coverage that rendered some women invisible and others hyper-visible in the epidemic and which perpetuated existing sexist and racist tropes of certain women as the "carriers" of disease to men and children. Evelynn Hammonds, a Black lesbian feminist and historian of science, explained that the media's association of Black women's risk with sex work and drug use continued the stereotyping of all Black women as inherently immoral that dated back to slavery.[5] As the cultural theorists Paula Treichler and Cindy Patton similarly observed, the vilification of Black and Latina women as the "vectors" of HIV, rather than as individuals requiring treatment and care for themselves, contrasted with the sympathetic portrayal of white, middle-class women as "inefficient" and "incompetent" transmitters of the virus who became sick through circumstances seemingly beyond their control.[6] Treating AIDS as a disease predominantly among those in stigmatized "risk groups," the Reagan administration, which came to power as the epidemic began devastating communities across the United States in the early 1980s, intervened to regulate the lives of marginalized groups already vulnerable to attack from the new government without mounting the robust, systematic, and egalitarian political and public health response required to meet the crisis. Racism, sexism, homophobia, and classism coalesced to blunt the government response to HIV/AIDS.

Like other scholars who have examined the discriminatory effects of diseases, Hammonds predicted that society's understanding of HIV/AIDS would determine "who lives and who dies."[7] Just as Ronald Reagan and other conservative lawmakers maligned Black women who used state aid as "welfare queens" and those requiring state support as the crack mothers of crack babies to justify their anti-welfare, tough-on-crime agenda, the assumption that AIDS mostly affected apparently deviant women similarly legitimized simultaneously neglectful and discriminatory AIDS policy.[8] The media's simultaneous objectification and marginalization of women dovetailed with the CDC's initial refusal to acknowledge women's symptoms as indicators of HIV, which led to misdiagnosis and early death, and denied women access to lifesaving housing, disability, and medical services and benefits. At the same time, the designation of multiply marginalized HIV-positive women—those whose identities and social status placed them at the intersection of more than one form of discrimination with limited access to traditional power structures, and who therefore experienced HIV as what Celeste Watkins-Hayes described as an "injury of inequality"—as unfit mothers by some lawmakers, journalists, and public health officials, fueled the assumption that HIV-positive women should not have children, which led to interventions that undermined their health and rights.[9]

As the early work of Hammonds and other feminist intellectuals attest, women did not accept mistreatment passively. They rejected and subverted harmful stereotypes and demanded that officials and communities center their collective needs and demands within the multifaceted response to AIDS. Women employed various strategies and tactics, from media campaigns and direct-action protests to class-action lawsuits, and organized across multiple settings, from prison cells to the courts. *In Her Hands* tells the story of women who, in the life and death context of the new epidemic, fought to save each other's lives. The question of how, when, and on what terms they succeeded in securing state recognition for the sake of accessing nondiscriminatory state support animates this book.

Focusing on the underappreciated impact of AIDS on women and their role in framing the fight against the disease, *In Her Hands* centers women in both the history of the AIDS epidemic and the broader history of the twentieth- and twenty-first-century United States. Shifting the focus of the history of HIV/AIDS in the US both chronologically and thematically, it chronicles women's struggle against the disease from the early 1980s to the present day and explores five distinct, yet overlapping, arenas of women's activism related to the epidemic: transmission and recognition, reproductive justice, safer sex campaigns for women who have sex with women (WSW), the carceral state, and the economics of health-care access around HIV prevention and treatment.[10] Centering women within the AIDS epidemic and concurrent political debates, *In Her Hands* opens avenues to explore the relationship between the state and women's status in modern America.

The examples of activism by multiply marginalized women unable to leverage race and class privilege to access health and social services in the same way as some white, gay men highlight the numerous, mutually reinforcing forms of discrimination in US politics. The privilege of whiteness failed to protect women like Joan Baker, a lesbian woman who died of AIDS in 1993, from experiencing government neglect on account of her gender and sexual identity. While men with relative class and race privilege also encountered debilitating discrimination as a result of the deepening homophobia of this period, the women whose stories are the subject of this book often came second to men in terms of setting AIDS policy, receiving health care, and accessing new health technologies.[11] Women like Baker found it even more difficult to access equal treatment and care when they rejected the politics of respectability that demanded they adhere to strict standards of normative social and sexual behavior to win sympathy and support.

The historian Evelyn Brooks Higginbotham coined the term "respectability politics" in 1993 to signify how Black women in the Progressive era modified their behavior to counter harmful stereotypes of them as hypersexual and uncivilized. Instead, they presented themselves as polite and pure, seeking to conform to ideals of middle-class whiteness, heterosexuality, and femininity to win acceptance from, and assimilation into, mainstream society.[12] Throughout the twentieth century, people on the margins of society similarly adhered to and manipulated dominant notions of respectable behavior in their fight for equality, freedom, and rights, including—with the outbreak of AIDS in the 1980s—women with HIV. Nonetheless, unlike singly oppressed groups that sometimes downplayed aspects of their identities to win legitimacy in and beyond the AIDS crisis, multiply marginalized women often chose not to place their arguments in a framework of racialized and gendered respectability politics out of the necessity of their interventions and political choice.[13] For instance, the safer sex materials of the Lesbian AIDS Project (LAP), which outlined in explicit detail nonnormative sexual practices between women, reflected the group's dual agenda to save lives and promote pro-sex lesbian erotics. Like Black feminist scholars such as Hammonds and Cathy Cohen, who critiqued discriminatory representations of Black women with HIV in the 1980s and 1990s, multiply marginalized women were alert to the impact of inequality that informed their demand for political change and justice.[14] In challenging the terms on which those in power considered their lives worthy of sympathy and state support, women's AIDS activism often embodied Cohen's theory of transformative queer politics—one in which those on the margins of state-sanctioned, white, middle-class heterosexual society rejected dominant sexual norms.[15] While this book primarily focuses on women's experiences of and resistance to HIV/AIDS, it also acknowledges that women and men on the margins of respectability often worked in coalition to challenge the power structures fueling the discriminatory effects of HIV/AIDS.

Race, class, gender, health status, and positionality to power therefore shaped whether people fought for specific gains to tackle HIV/AIDS or petitioned for transformative justice. Like men who experienced AIDS alongside the structural oppressions with which it converged, multiply marginalized women fought for transformative changes that both addressed the roots of inequality, such as universal health care and prison abolition, and treated AIDS as one health crisis among many. As the prisoner-rights advocate Judy Greenspan articulated, women AIDS activists in prison fought not for more money to fund "unworkable prison medical systems" but to end mass incarceration.[16] Moreover, with limited access to elite power structures, they struggled to not only access existing services but change the terms of that access, free from prescription and risk. Activists' ability to secure distinct wins, such as expanding the CDC's AIDS definition and gaining access to experimental research, underscores Beatrix Hoffman's conclusion about different health-care movements throughout the twentieth century, namely, that people found it easier to win changes that did not challenge the governing principle in America that health care is a privilege and not a right.[17] The challenges they faced in realizing an alternative, more just, and humane vision of society also reflected the political moment that saw public health become increasingly privatized and politicized at the onset of the AIDS crisis.

AIDS emerged at a moment of political backlash to women's rights, including the right to plan for, terminate, or bring a pregnancy to term. After the US Supreme Court upheld a woman's constitutional right to abortion in the 1973 case *Roe v. Wade*, conservatives immediately mobilized to overturn the decision. Establishing that a fetus is a human being with moral and legal rights equal to a woman became central to their strategy. Immediately after the *Roe* decision, conservative members of Congress began introducing statutes and amendments to the constitution declaring that life began at conception, thereby equating abortion with murder.[18] As attempts at a national ban on abortion failed, antiabortion activists pursued other options, passing in 1976 the Hyde Amendment, which banned the use of Medicaid to fund abortions.[19] As Congress succeeded in making abortion less accessible to low-income women, the language of fetal rights began informing abortion restrictions at the state level.[20] The fight to establish fetal personhood also advanced with the "war" on drug use, which in the 1980s disproportionately impacted communities of color, as medics began testing and reporting to law enforcement mostly pregnant Black and Native American women suspected of using substances that allegedly harmed their fetuses.[21] The same argument that the state should intervene to protect fetuses from the behaviors of supposedly "irresponsible" women, and society from the financial and social costs of providing for the care of sick and apparently "undesirable" children, similarly legitimized and overlapped with the testing, reporting, and punishment of HIV-positive women in connection with their pregnancies. *In Her Hands* adds AIDS to the battle over reproductive justice, which centers on the right to both have and to not have children.

The assault on reproductive justice symbolized the punitive turn that accompanied the advance of neoliberalism in American politics at the end of the twentieth century. In the 1970s, lawmakers proposed competing visions of the causes of and solutions to the challenges facing the country following the social, economic, and political upheavals of the previous decades. Those calling to cut welfare support for the supposedly "nonworking" poor tapped into deep-seated racial and gender prejudices that attributed poverty and social unrest in certain racial communities to their perceived pathology, especially the apparent shortcomings of single, non-white women. Instead of addressing the deep-seated inequalities that underpinned social disparities by, for example, investing in public health care, conservative policy makers shifted the responsibility of supporting marginalized communities from state agencies to private organizations and the white, heterosexual, middle-class, male-headed nuclear family that they framed as the regulator of acceptable private behavior. The shrinking of the welfare state, and emphasis on the family and private sector as the guarantors of public order, did not signal a reduction in government size, capacity, or will. Instead, the state "mutated" and "redeployed" its administrative power, increasing funding to law-enforcement agencies and building new prisons to survey and punish those seen to have violated the strict standards of normative behavior prescribed by the rising "family values politics" of the period.[22] With the retrenchment of the welfare state and expansion of the carceral state that underpinned the development of neoliberalism in the late twentieth century, conservative lawmakers framed the state as the "protector" of "innocent" citizens from the supposedly "immoral" lifestyles of those who fell outside the bounds of normative society, including—from the 1980s onward—marginalized women with HIV.[23] *In Her Hands* reveals the contradictory nature of neoliberalism, with its proponents advocating for nongovernmental action while implementing laws and policies that reach into the most intimate parts of people's lives. It joins a body of scholarship that uses HIV/AIDS as a lens to explore how, when, why, and to what effect the state decided to flex its administrative power at the close of the twentieth and onset of the twenty-first century.[24]

With the power to direct where money goes and how it is spent, successive Republican governments since the 1980s have used federal funding as a wedge to advance a health agenda that undermines women's sexual rights and reproductive freedoms both at home and abroad, keeping the health of women—especially those reliant on state aid—precarious in the process.[25] The fact that women of color disproportionately rely on public coverage means that the persistent political assault on public health care and women's nonprofit treatment spaces, as detailed in this book—seen recently in the actions of President Donald Trump to limit the scope of the Affordable Care Act (ACA) of 2010 and reform Title X of the Public Health Service Act—impacts women of color particularly negatively.[26] Affording medications is also more difficult without health coverage. The ability of the pharmaceutical industry to set and raise drug prices free from government regulation has also put lifesaving HIV prevention and treatment medicine beyond the reach of many.[27] Just as Keeanga-Yamahtta Taylor showed that housing policies aimed at profit reproduced and reinforced racial discrimination in the postwar period, the profiteering of the pharmaceutical industry that became increasingly politically protected with the advance of neoliberalism in the 1980s and 1990s has similarly compounded existing health inequalities, resulting in disproportionately adverse health outcomes for women of color.[28] While this book is primarily concerned with examining the underexplored story of how women confronting HIV/AIDS in the US accepted, navigated, resisted, and subverted state power, it also acknowledges that many of these struggles transcended national borders and places them in a global context. The neoliberal response to HIV/AIDS that put profit before public good threw into sharp relief whose life the state valued and considered worthy of support.

Speaking to the politicization of fetuses and children in the 1980s, the state responded more readily to women's needs and demands when they involved infants and children. The pattern of the state responding proactively to women as mothers played out in the early medical and political response to HIV, as many diagnosticians and doctors first realized that women could contract the virus after their children became sick, and subsequently that women required access to clinical trials to prevent mother-to-child transmission of the disease. Furthermore, state authorities moved quickly to support residential programs that advocacy groups set up for infants considered "abandoned" by their mothers. The debates over the medical viability of abortion, the focus on preventing HIV in children, and the discussion of how to care for infants neither prevented nor aborted but born to women with HIV in the 1980s effectively erased HIV-positive women from the story.[29]

In contrast, government authorities overlooked the needs of childless women and interfered in the lives of women who foregrounded actual sexual activity and practice instead of their childbearing potential. In the 1990s, amid the political realignment that saw the increasingly extreme right-wing faction of the Republic Party gain prominence, politicians in conservative states, such as Representative Mel Hancock (R-MO), worked to censor the explicit, nonnormative sex education materials of women who had sex with women.[30] Women who had sex with women also struggled for recognition as a group that required inclusion in the surveillance, research, and treatment of AIDS. Women, such as those in prison, deemed unwilling or incapable of fulfilling their civic obligations by virtue of their incarceration and seen to have forfeited their right to make claims on the state, also suffered from a lack of financial support.[31]

Women's ability to gain political traction often depended on them leveraging their childbearing capacity as opposed to their own sexual agency. This pattern speaks to a longer history of the state responding more proactively to white, heterosexual, middle- and upper-class women as mothers, while devaluing women of color's childbearing, ignoring the non-childbearing claims of women of all races, and regulating women's nonnormative and nonprocreative sex acts. Although the social justice movements of the twentieth century succeeded in expanding women's civil rights, including granting Black women access to the welfare benefits originally denied to them, *In Her Hands* demonstrates that reproduction, and a concern for the health and well-being of children, still informed women's ability to make a set of collective claims and demands on the political process at the end of the twentieth and into the twenty-first century.[32] While the social movements of the mid-twentieth century equipped activists with a vocabulary to articulate their rights, the state continued to deal with women through the abstract identity of sexless mother rather than people with multiple lived experiences that transcended rigid categories and labels.

Women's relative ability to achieve their goals also depended on the different types of activism available to them based on their legal status, race, sexuality, and class. Activist success was often tied to the power of the people being targeted. As Sarah Schulman, an AIDS Coalition to Unleash Power (ACT UP) New York member and writer, astutely observed, "People who must have change choose the playbook their social position demands."[33] For women in prison with limited resources, connecting to groups with existing activist networks and deep fundraising histories, and therefore greater means to take up their cause, helped them to launch a class-action lawsuit against the state of California. Equally, their inability to fundamentally improve the health services at their facilities spoke to the stark power imbalance that existed between women in prison suffering from HIV and a host of other severe health complications and a carceral state that was expanding in increasingly punitive and misogynistic ways in this period.[34]

While the egregious conditions of incarceration brought many women in prison into activism for the first time, others—such as those involved in the Boston Women's Health Book Collective, the Lesbian Avengers, LAP, ACT UP, and the AIDS Counseling and Education (ACE) program at Bedford Hills—used the skills and knowledge learned from other progressive causes to mobilize effectively against the health crisis of AIDS. As Jennifer Nelson noted, "Political frameworks do not emerge wholly formed without connections to previous movements."[35]

Many who fought to center women in AIDS policy and education and broaden women's access to health care continued the work of the feminist, racial justice, and LGBTQ health movements of the 1960s and 1970s, which challenged the discrimination diverse groups of women experienced within white, male-led, male-dominated, heteronormative medical institutions. Earlier feminist organizing related to reproductive justice, birthing, and motherhood, as well as nonreproductive, specialist health care, set a precedent for self-advocacy upon which these activists built. The health networks forged and the experience gained in creating health manuals and LGBTQ guides, coupled with the sentiment that communities should become experts in their health and be their own health advocates, provided a model for addressing AIDS from the 1980s onward.[36] Women's previous experiences with civil rights, feminist, and LGBTQ health care put them at the center of the fight against HIV/AIDS in the following decades, bridging the alternative health-care movements of the 1960s and 1970s with the health activism of the present day.

The diverse and intersectional efforts of women to protest the co-occurring neglect of their health-care needs and intervention into their lives was such that it does not lend itself to the study of an individual biography or even a single grassroots organization. Instead, *In Her Hands* traces the reach of women's activism in locations with high incidences of HIV/AIDS and deep histories of progressive organizing across the United States, from Boston to San Francisco. It also adds a gendered perspective to well- and lesser-studied sites of HIV/AIDS activism, such as prisons, reproductive health centers, and schools.

In Her Hands combines a diverse range of sources—from activist records to government papers, newspapers and periodicals, scientific literature, and digital collections—that not only highlight the scale and scope of women's untiring efforts to address HIV/AIDS across different levels of society but also reveal how women interacted with state regulation and political discourse in their efforts to frame the fight against the disease. In so doing, it moves the historical understanding of the impact of HIV/AIDS on women beyond their exclusion from the initial medical response and the important role women played in the epidemic as the supporters and carers of gay men, and contributes to the burgeoning historical scholarship that builds on the work of feminist sociologists and ethnographers to bring more fully the voices, perspectives, and protest of a diverse coalition of HIV-positive women and their advocates who organized across identity categories to fight AIDS into accounts of the US epidemic.[37] It also historicizes a series of other gender-based issues that women have struggled against since the onset of AIDS in the 1980s and which remain largely understudied, namely, motherhood and the threats HIV/AIDS posed to women's reproductive freedoms; the persistent underrepresentation of women in biomedical research; the challenge of navigating health-delivery systems made by and for men; gender-based violence; and sexual silencing in the public sphere. These issues not only reflected the historical moment in which AIDS emerged but also a set of racist, sexist, classist, ableist, and heteronormative assumptions governing women's treatment throughout the twentieth century. *In Her Hands* uses HIV/AIDS as a lens through which to analyze women's experiences of, and resistance to, these deep-seated gendered and racialized citizenship issues at the close of the twentieth and beginning of the twenty-first century.

In Her Hands also joins AIDS scholarship that has foregrounded the ongoing resistance of those navigating the discriminatory effects of HIV/AIDS to acknowledge that the epidemic persisted beyond the groundbreaking introduction of drugs called protease inhibitors in 1996 that facilitated the experiential shift from dying of AIDS to living with HIV.[38] Since then, women, and all those living at the intersection of multiple and mutually reinforcing forms of discrimination, have continued to fight to access care and battle the ongoing stigma associated with AIDS that keeps them from getting tested and securing treatment within a changed treatment environment, prompting historians to extend the chronology of the history of the HIV/AIDS crisis beyond this landmark medical development. Their experiences, in turn, challenge historians more broadly to resist neat endings following scientific discoveries. Chronicling women's struggle against HIV/AIDS from the 1980s into the twenty-first century subverts such easy closure.

ORGANIZATION

In Her Hands is a thematic study that moves chronologically through the epidemic's forty-year history. It charts five distinct yet interrelated themes: transmission and recognition; motherhood, AIDS, and reproductive rights; lesbian organizing; incarceration; and gender, economics, and health care. Each of these five themes maps onto five chronological, yet overlapping, chapters, examining how they intersected with developments in the history of AIDS in women. Looking through the forty-year history, each chapter focuses on a particular gender-specific issue related to women and AIDS. I do this to show how women responded to the epidemic as they navigated four, interconnected historical developments that symbolized the advancing neoliberal, family values, and law and order politics from the late twentieth century onward that stymied the government's political and public health response to AIDS: the anti-abortion politics of the Reagan era, the homophobic and misogynistic agenda of political conservatism in the 1990s, the simultaneous expansion of the carceral state, and the profiteering of the pharmaceutical industry in the twenty-first century.

Chapter one shows that the discovery that AIDS could pass sexually between men and women and between women and infants increased doctors' and public health agencies' urgency to diagnose and treat AIDS in women, with motherhood becoming a major crux of women's inclusion in the official epidemic response. When public health officials began recognizing AIDS in women, they also made individual women responsible for preventing HIV transmission both sexually and reproductively. In response, a diverse coalition of feminist activists fought to broaden the scope of how women counted in public health. By the mid-1990s, HIV-positive women and activists succeeded in expanding the official public health response to include them as subjects requiring treatment and services for themselves and not just on behalf of infants.

But securing state recognition always brought the risk of state interference. The discovery of AIDS in women sparked political and public health debates over how best to prevent the birth of HIV-positive children, which included punitive measures that threatened women's reproductive freedoms and overlapped with existing efforts to police pregnancy along the lines of race and class in the 1980s and into the 1990s. Chapter two explores how the state not only burdened women with the responsibility of preventing perinatal transmission, but also passed legislation that made possible the punishment of women who fell short. Focusing on the actions of US Surgeon General Charles Everett Koop and the interrelated debates over abortion politics and AIDS in and beyond the Reagan administration, the chapter examines the impact of AIDS on the advance of the antiabortion and fetal rights movements since the 1980s.

Chapter three explores how debates over women and AIDS shifted to lesbian women in the 1990s, as Republican lawmakers who felt that the Reagan administration had not gone far enough to restore American "family values" pushed national politics further to the right, and as the sharp drop-off in cases of perinatal HIV following the approval of the use of the AZT drug in pregnancy in 1994 eased much of the moral panic over prevention, abortion, and motherhood.[39] Focusing on the activism of the pro-sex radical Amber Hollibaugh and her organization LAP, the chapter examines the impact that AIDS had on conceptions of what it meant to be a lesbian woman, especially as it related to sexual practice, and the impact of AIDS on shaping the relationship between sexual minority women and the state at the end of the twentieth century.

The battles over safer sex during the 1990s coincided with the rise of the carceral state. Conservatives evoking family values politics not only silenced women's expressions of nonnormative sexuality in the public sphere but also removed from it altogether the women deemed to have forfeited their right to make claims on the state because they broke the law. Chapter four explores what the punishment of women judged to have violated prescribed social norms in the era of heightened criminalization looked like in practice. As an engine of systemic misogyny, the ramped-up carceral state of the late twentieth century not only neglected women's basic health needs but also actively obstructed their fight to survive, keeping women incarcerated and sick based on the assumption that society needed "protecting" from them. The chapter explores how women responded to this situation and petitioned for transformational justice, drawing on the consciousness raising and self-advocacy tradition of intersectional feminist health-care movements and culminating in the 1995 *Shumate v. Wilson* court case.

In and out of prison, women with HIV and their advocates have continued to confront the systemic obstacles to securing lifesaving treatment and care in the twenty-first century, addressed in chapter five. This includes bringing to market a woman-controlled tool to prevent new cases of HIV, as the high cost of antiretroviral medicines, which resulted from lawmakers allowing pharmaceutical companies to set and raise drug prices as high as they wanted, limited their effectiveness in curbing the virus. At the same time, the extreme misogynistic agenda of the Trump administration intensified the conservative assault on abortion, restricting women's access to the nonprofit spaces where they receive treatment for a host of health issues. In the twenty-first century, in a new treatment era, the censorship of women's sexual bodies and neglect of their sexual and reproductive health needs that is the culmination of a forty-year political campaign against women's health on the part of conservative politicians and activists continues to perpetuate gender inequities and thwart efforts to end the HIV/AIDS epidemic.

The structure of *In Her Hands* highlights the outcomes won and inequities sustained in women's fight against HIV/AIDS over the past forty years. Since the 1980s, women have challenged officials, the media, and communities to acknowledge AIDS as a woman's disease that includes their reproductive capacity but in ways that do not violate their reproductive rights. They also petitioned officials to address AIDS as a disease in women who used their bodies not to have children but for sexual pleasure. Rejecting prescriptive labels believed to determine a woman's "risk," their interventions focused on the structural inequalities that made women vulnerable to and shaped their ability to address the virus. Women's fight to dismantle the systemic barriers that kept them from accessing nondiscriminatory treatment came up against the political agenda of lawmakers seeking to reinscribe hierarchies of sex and gender as well as class and race through the obliteration of state support and expansion of state surveillance. The battles between women seeking to expand and lawmakers seeking to contract women's access to lifesaving health care documented throughout speaks to the overall trajectory of the four decades that this book chronicles, one in which the state increasingly approached women's health through coercion and punishment with devastating consequences for women's already fragile rights. As explored in the epilogue, the view of women's bodies as a threat of HIV in children as seen in the response to AIDS in the 1980s has become more institutionally entrenched in the decades since. At the same time, deep-seated assumptions about who is deserving of government-funded support that are rooted in heteronormative whiteness, maleness, and middle-classness continue to marginalize women in the latest efforts to "end" the epidemic.

While this book seeks to find patterns in women's responses to the AIDS epidemic, women are not a homogenous group, and neither is their activism. No single study can encapsulate the entirety of women's subjective experiences of and response to HIV/AIDS in the US. The category of "women" applies to both cisgender and transgender women. While some of the issues addressed in this book affected both cis and trans women, trans women also have a distinct set of political needs and demands that often go beyond its scope. Focusing on both cis and trans activism reveals how women whose multiple lived experiences do not fit neatly into prescriptive identity categories engage with the state. As transgender rights have become increasingly visible within the media and political debate in recent years, so too has the transgender community become subject to political attack. Future studies might examine whether the pattern of vulnerability assisting visibility, and the tension between needing state recognition for services but resisting state regulation that the women AIDS activists of this book have navigated, also applies to trans activism.

History has the power to shape not only what we remember but what we forget. The initial conceptualization of AIDS as a white, gay, male disease; the persistently high rates of HIV/AIDS among men who have sex with men; the vibrant mobilization of gay men to resist the devastation of the new epidemic, coupled with the institutionalized sexism and racism entrenched within medicine, shaped women's marginalization within the official and community responses to HIV/AIDS in the US at different historical moments, as well as their underrepresentation in the historiography and cultural depictions of the epidemic.[40] Yet, the stories of the women chronicled here, often spoken out of institutionally enforced silences, and navigating the political and interpersonal risks that came with mobilizing around their HIV status, provide insight into the relationship between the state and women's status in modern America. They illuminate how and under what circumstances policy makers, state regulators, prison administrators, health-care providers, and others in positions of authority ignore or discriminate against women, and how and when they become more accommodating or responsive to women's collective claims and demands. Women with HIV protesting the state neglect of their health-care needs always risked encountering discriminatory state intervention into their bodies and lives on behalf of the symbolic needs of fetuses and children—as well as wider society—deemed to need protecting from them. Despite setbacks, their activism speaks to the power of women organizing to secure the right to decide for themselves about their bodies. The need to tackle systemic barriers to decent health and social services—whether in the form of economics, politics, racism, sexism, classism, ableism, homophobia, or interpersonal relationships—is imperative to this goal. As the women AIDS activists of this book remind us, equality requires not only freedom from punitive state interference but also the right to humane and compassionate care available to all via the state.

1

AIDS IS A DISASTER, WOMEN DIE FASTER

IN OCTOBER 1983, Sonia (Sunnye) Sherman from Washington, DC, received an AIDS diagnosis. She had experienced regular bouts of the rare Pneumocystis carinii pneumonia, and died, aged thirty-five, in August 1986 of AIDS-related brain damage. Journalists covering Sherman's story described it as unusual. As a heterosexual, middle-class woman without a history of intravenous drug use, she was an "anomaly" among people with AIDS.[1]

Sherman's case only seemed unusual because of how the government first responded to the epidemic in the early 1980s. In September 1982, the CDC defined AIDS based on how the disease developed in the young, white gay men first discovered with the virus. It also identified four groups at increased risk for contracting the disease, creating the misconception, as these journalists articulated, that women either rarely got AIDS or, if they did, it was because of their perceived foreignness, if Haitian, or their engagement in seemingly deviant acts, like drug use.[2] Although the media usually associated Black women like Sherman with such supposedly "bad" behavior, her sexual and class status shaped journalists' presentation of her as "low risk." Sherman's story challenged conventional assumptions about women and AIDS in the early 1980s.

The government responded more quickly to women as mothers. Reports in the early 1980s that people could transmit HIV not only during sex but also in pregnancy increased the public health urgency to study AIDS in pregnant women.[3] Throughout the epidemic's first decade, the initial medical response to AIDS neglected women not only because doctors and diagnosticians first focused on the disease in young, previously healthy, white gay men, but also because medical professionals, federal agencies, and pharmaceutical companies saw them as reproductive agents. The bias toward seeing women as mothers in the epidemic continued the historic treatment of pregnant women as the vectors of disease in men and children.[4] It also reflected the larger monitoring of women's reproductive lives, and especially that of Black, single women who used state aid, during the Reagan era, a period during which deeply racialized ideas of who deserved state welfare and support topped the political agenda.[5]

As diagnosticians began diagnosing AIDS in increasing numbers of women, and increasing numbers of women began qualifying for clinical research, researchers first enrolled them in a major way in drug trials as mothers. In response, a dynamic coalition of activists from around the country mobilized not only to expand the official definition of AIDS to include symptoms of women but also ensure that the design of clinical trials did not compromise the rights of women or their infants.

Moreover, not only did women shoulder the responsibility of getting themselves recognized as people vulnerable to HIV, but they also became responsible for preventing HIV transmission both sexually and reproductively, as public health officials began counting women as sexual as well as reproductive agents.

This chapter explores the underacknowledged risks that came with women's inclusion in the early response to AIDS, especially as it related to their reproductive rights. As activists fought for the diagnosis of AIDS in women, motherhood became a major crux of women's inclusion in the epidemic. A series of systemic attempts on the part of right-wing politicians and political commentators to address the discovery of AIDS in women and their role in its transmission followed. Several of these proposals, such as mandatory premarital testing, failed, proving unworkable in the post–sex revolution era. In contrast, the statewide, public health initiatives that put the onus of prevention on individual women aligned more closely with the neoliberal politics of the period that promoted personal responsibility over government action, and which had greater reach.[6] Feminist campaigners challenged this burden of prevention, creating alternative public health publicity that emphasized the need to recognize women for treatment, provide women with accurate information, and protect their sexual and reproductive rights. In the 1980s, feminist activists took this message to the largest international platform on AIDS. After 1989, women succeeded in widening the CDC's AIDS definition to include women's symptoms and securing access to clinical trials. These important but discrete victories nevertheless illustrate that federal agencies responded more proactively to the collective needs and demands of women when they involved the symbolic needs of fetuses and infants. Winning immediate policy changes to keep them alive, women therefore struggled to change the terms on which the state responded to their health needs—for instance, by treating reproductive justice as part of women's holistic health care and committing to extending access to health care to all. Policies and messaging that shifted the responsibility of HIV prevention to women actually undermined their reproductive rights.

DISCOVERING AIDS IN WOMEN

In autumn 1979, Dr. Linda Laubenstein, a hematologist and oncologist at New York University Medical Center, began noticing increased cases of the rare cancer Kaposi's sarcoma (KS) in young, otherwise healthy men.[7] KS typically appeared as purple-colored lesions on the skin of elderly Mediterranean men.[8] Two years later, Dr. Alvin E. Friedman-Kien, professor of microbiology and dermatology at New York University Medical Center, also began seeing unusual cases of KS. The two doctors exchanged stories of their patients and identified at least three things they had in common: each was a man who engaged in sex with other men and did not survive his illness.[9]

On the other side of the country, the immunologist Michael Gottlieb and his colleagues at UCLA began reporting cases of another infection in previously healthy gay men, Pneumocystis carinii pneumonia (PCP), to the CDC in Atlanta. Like KS, PCP rarely appeared outside those with severely suppressed immune systems.[10] In June 1981, the CDC published a notice on five of the cases in its weekly journal, *Morbidity and Mortality Weekly Report (MMWR)*.[11] The report failed to mention the races of the five men and excluded the two cases of PCP reported in Black male patients.[12] Instead, it emphasized their sexual histories, identifying "an association between some aspect of a homosexual lifestyle or disease acquired through sexual contact and *Pneumocystis* pneumonia in this population."[13] Four months later, the *Lancet* published Dr. Laubenstein and her colleagues' research on KS in a group of eight men in New York.[14] The first two major medical publications of what became known as AIDS, these reports strengthened the association between the new disease and young, otherwise healthy, white, gay men.

The men profiled in these reports had access to the physicians who reported AIDS cases to the CDC, so they became known to the agency first, a reality that shaped the racial, class, sexual, and gender profile of the epidemic from its outset.[15] Soon, physicians in other cities began reporting similar occurrences of immune deficiency among white gay men to the CDC.[16] In September 1982, the CDC defined AIDS as the presence of KS, PCP, and a series of other infections that suggested the failure of an otherwise healthy person's immune system.[17] In only counting formerly rare diseases as indicators of AIDS, the CDC established AIDS as a disease in the previously healthy and therefore failed to investigate how AIDS converged with existing health problems that tended to afflict women, as well as people of all genders living in poverty with compromised immune systems and limited access to the public health system—people who, due to long-standing racial inequities in access to health care, also tended to come from communities of color.[18] Studies published in the early 1980s suggested that before its official discovery, AIDS likely claimed the lives of an unknown number of poor women and men without medical establishments noticing.[19] Reflecting the strength of association between the new syndrome and gay men, the CDC first defined it as "gay-related immunodeficiency (GRID)."[20]

Reports of KS and other opportunistic infections—diseases that appear in people with weakened immune systems—among small numbers of women, as well as intravenous drug users who did not report male homosexuality, challenged CDC epidemiologists to rethink their original conceptualization of the syndrome as exclusively gay and male.[21] In its September 1982 notice, the CDC sorted reported cases into four groups apparently at greatest risk for contracting the disease: homosexual or bisexual males, heroin and other intravenous drug users, Haitians, and hemophiliacs, and a category for people whose risk fell outside the designated groups.[22] Dubbed the "4-H club," the risk group concept largely attributed a person's risk to their racial background or sexual identity, obscuring knowledge of how the virus passed between people and creating the perception that AIDS only affected limited, socially stigmatized groups whose perceived foreignness or engagement in certain behaviors put them into contact with the virus.[23]

The risk-group concept fueled the mistreatment and misdiagnosis of AIDS in women. CDC epidemiologists either placed women in the category of Haitian, drug user, hemophiliac, or "unknown."[24] As testament to how the reliance on categories undermined the credibility of women, one doctor accused a non-Haitian woman who claimed not to have engaged in any of the institutionally recognized risk factors of lying about her symptoms.[25]

Following reports of opportunistic infections in infants with no history of blood transfusion, women became visible to the CDC as mothers. On December 17, 1982, the CDC published a notice on KS and other opportunistic infections in four infants in New York, New Jersey, and California. Speculating on the cause of infection, the editor noted that "transmission of an 'AIDS agent' from mother to child, either in utero or shortly after birth, could account for the early onset of immunodeficiency in these infants."[26] The editor did not dwell on how the mothers became infected beyond noting histories of intravenous drug use, sex work, and Haitian nationality. Instead, the emphasis placed on vertical transmission of the virus from woman to infant presented women as the vectors of transmission. Reported cases of heterosexual transmission from men to women led to further conjecture in the January 1983 notice that the unknown "AIDS agent" may "occur among both heterosexual and male homosexual couples."[27] Four years after Dr. Laubenstein had noticed cases of KS in men in 1979, the CDC acknowledged that the unidentified "AIDS agent" causing illness in infants and men could also infect women.

The breakthrough discovery of the "AIDS agent" came in 1983, when scientists in Paris learned that HIV caused AIDS. The discovery of HIV led to a slight broadening of the official AIDS case definition in 1985, adding severe manifestations of HIV not included in the 1982 classification.[28] This expansion did not, however, cover symptoms in women.

Throughout the 1980s, the CDC's official AIDS surveillance case definition excluded women-specific conditions, resulting in the misdiagnosis and undercounting of women with AIDS. Receiving an AIDS diagnosis depended not only on a person having antibodies to HIV in their blood but also on how they became sick.[29] As the CDC based its original case definition on how the disease developed in young, white men, it failed to address whether and in what ways AIDS manifested differently in women.[30] Unlike the men whose advanced AIDS often developed as rare and severe diseases, such as KS, women tended to experience infections and diseases like cervical cancer and pelvic inflammatory disease.[31] Due to the historic failure of public health agencies to address sexually transmitted diseases in Black communities, Black women tended to experience these infections and diseases at higher rates, increasing their chances of contracting HIV without a doctor diagnosing it as AIDS.[32] An unknown number of women died from AIDS-related illnesses in the epidemic's first decade without ever having received an AIDS diagnosis.

Misdiagnosis led to early death. As physicians used the CDC's definition as a guideline to diagnose AIDS, the exclusion of women's symptoms meant that most physicians did not associate their patients' symptoms with HIV. Women, therefore, tended to receive an AIDS diagnosis later in the course of their illness, which limited the benefits of treatment. As a result, women, on average, died faster of AIDS than men.[33] Risa Denenberg, a family nurse practitioner at the Bronx Lebanon Hospital in New York City and a member of ACT UP, highlighted this disparity, noting that an HIV-positive woman from Newark, New Jersey, lived an average of 15.5 weeks after receiving an AIDS diagnosis, whereas an HIV-positive, white, gay man in a similar location lived an average of 20.8 months.[34]

The CDC's exclusion of AIDS symptoms specific to women also prevented them from accessing the social security, disability benefits, and other services to which they were entitled based on their illness. The

Social Security Administration (SSA), which administered the Disability Insurance Benefits and the Supplementary Security Income (SSI) programs, relied on the CDC's AIDS definition to administer disability benefits, only awarding them to people with CDC-defined AIDS.[35] The AIDS definition also served as a gateway to accessing local benefits and housing.[36] Moreover, as federal, state, and local agencies developed prevention, education, and research programs using the CDC's data, few adequately served women.[37] Men and women with limited incomes reliant on state aid bore the heaviest burden of this exclusion.[38]

As President Ronald Reagan worked to gut health-care funding in the early 1980s, the CDC cited austerity as an excuse to act as a gatekeeper for medical and social services.[39] In 1987, as the introduction of HIV antibody tests increased scientists' understanding of the virus, the CDC added wasting syndrome and dementia to the list of recognized AIDS symptoms, taking the total number to twenty-three.[40] The expansion of the AIDS definition resulted in a sixty percent increase in the number of reported AIDS cases in women after 1987. The CDC acknowledged that "a higher proportion of patients . . . with illnesses meeting only the 1987 case definition were female, black or Hispanic or heterosexual intravenous drug-users."[41] This rise in cases underscored how the CDC's original definition kept the number of reported AIDS cases artificially low to the detriment of those whose infections it did not cover. The CDC nevertheless remained steadfast in its refusal to recognize women-specific opportunistic infections. As agency officials admitted in consultations with women activists, the inclusion of diseases that occurred in HIV-negative women could double the official AIDS caseload and commit the government to spending a politically unpalatable amount on disability benefits and health care.[42] The CDC did not consider those cases, or the people they affected, serious or valuable enough to warrant defying the anti-welfare agenda of the Reagan administration.

Misleading articles in the mainstream press compounded women's struggle to acquire accurate information about the virus. In December

1985, overlooking women's susceptibility to other sexually transmitted diseases, the science writer John Langone published an article in the medical journal *Discover*, claiming that AIDS did not threaten women because the virus cannot penetrate "the rugged vagina," which, he implied (as Treichler noted), was "built to be abused by such blunt instruments as penises and small babies."[43] In the wake of rising alarm over the spread of HIV among heterosexuals that followed the death of the actor Rock Hudson in October 1985, as well as sensationalized, xenophobic accounts of the virus being transmitted heterosexually in Haiti and countries in Africa, commentators such as Langone wanted to reassure American women that they could not contract HIV through vaginal sex.[44]

Writers like Langone did not seek to reassure all women. Instead, they portrayed white, middle-class, heterosexual women as "incompetent" or "inefficient" transmitters of HIV who "passively" received HIV through contaminated blood or from their male sex partners. At the same time, they demonized sex workers and intravenous drug users, most often represented as Black, for supposedly "carrying" HIV from "the world of drug abuse to the larger community."[45] The representation of some women as deserving of sympathy while others of blame underscores how racialized and gendered respectability shaped discourses of AIDS in the 1980s, implying that only women of color who conformed to prescribed sexual and social norms could elicit sympathy, as their contracting of the disease was assumed not to come from their own, supposedly "deviant" actions but from those of their male partners who had sex with men on the "down low."[46] Similar to the media and medical responses to sexually transmitted diseases (STDs) like syphilis in the past, their arguments relied not on the latest scientific data but on racist, homophobic, classist, and patriarchal assumptions about the lives and sexual practices of different groups of women.[47]

In January 1988, the psychiatrist Dr. Robert Gould popularized Langone's arguments, publishing a misleading article on women's vulnerability not in a niche medical journal but in *Cosmopolitan*, a widely read, mainstream women's magazine. Gould reassured the magazine's 2.4 million readership that American women with "healthy" vaginas could safely engage in unprotected vaginal sex with men.[48] He attributed the high number of cases of heterosexual transmission in Africa to the "brutal way" in which "men in Africa take their women."[49] In attempting to differentiate between the threat HIV posed to women in African countries and those in the US, Gould perpetuated what Kimberly Christensen termed "the myth of 'first world uniqueness,'" in which US commentators sought to account for the high rates of HIV among heterosexual women in countries in Africa without acknowledging the possibility for any woman of contracting the virus.[50] Echoing the arguments of prominent demographers and journalists, Gould based his analysis of the epidemiology of HIV/AIDS in Africa on the perceived "otherness" of African sexuality and culture.[51] At the time of his article's publication, AIDS was the leading cause of death among women aged 25 to 34 in New York City, with the highest percentages among Black and Latina women.[52] Gould either did not know this statistic or did not think it undermined his argument that AIDS posed little threat to white women. In fixating on individual sexual practices, Gould gave the impression that a woman's "risk" derived solely from her engagement in sexual acts as opposed to the systemic problems that made all women vulnerable in the epidemic, such as poverty, sexual abuse, domestic violence, a lack of access to prevention tools, limited health insurance, and inadequate medical care.[53] In his attempt to reassure white, middle-class, heterosexual women, Gould fueled all women's confusion about their susceptibility to HIV and contributed to stigmatizing coverage that deterred women from getting tested and seeking treatment for the disease.[54]

The desire to correct Gould's article inspired ACT UP/New York Women's Caucus.[55] Founded by mostly white, lesbian women with experience in arts, politics, activism, and academia, the caucus drew on the resources, networks, and professional and organizational skills gained from other progressive causes to direct actions that centered women's needs.[56] Maxine Wolfe and Marion Banzhaf came to AIDS activism from the women's health and reproductive justice movements, bringing with them the theory of self-advocacy that empowered people to become experts in their health and challenge race, gender, class, and other biases in medicine.[57] Sarah Schulman attributes the ability for ACT UP—a predominantly white, male organization—to secure progressive change to this patient-centered politics learned from feminism.[58] The video and multimedia skills of others, like Jean Carlomusto and Maria Maggenti, ensured coverage of the demonstrations and any police violence.[59] As Schulman and Jim Hubbard's oral history project on ACT UP illustrates, a racially, socially, and culturally diverse constituency of women, including Iris De La Cruz, Katrina Haslip, and Phyllis Sharpe and others who lived with HIV, many of whom became involved with ACT UP after leaving the Bedford Hills Correctional Facility in Westchester County, New York, also played key leadership and rank-and-file roles within the organization.[60] In a city where the deep devastation of HIV/AIDS was matched by a powerful grassroots movement to overcome it, women with experience taking on state power mobilized to ensure that activist efforts did not leave women behind.[61]

The caucus chose *Cosmopolitan* as their first target. On January 15, 1988, a large group of women and men braved the new year cold and gathered outside the magazine's headquarters in Manhattan after Gould refused to retract his article. Guards blocked the protestors from entering the editorial offices to speak with Helen Gurley Brown, the magazine's editor and author of the 1962 bestseller *Sex and the Single Girl*. Undeterred, they sent Brown hundreds of condoms every day, stopping only after she had published the first article in the magazine's history urging women to use condoms for safer sex two months later.[62] They also handed out flyers that corrected Gould's false claims and urged women to not "Go to Bed with *Cosmo*."[63] The campaign helped shape popular knowledge of AIDS as a disease in women in the 1980s. Victorious, the caucus, along with others in ACT UP, joined a powerful interracial, regional, and professional coalition of men and women activists with diverse perspectives and skills, and took on the CDC and SSA.

Terry McGovern, a young, white, lesbian legal-aid lawyer and founder of the HIV Law Project (HLP), used her professional expertise to advocate on behalf of HIV-positive women and men in New York City, especially those with limited resources, including women recently released from prison. On October 1, 1990, eleven men, women, and children filed a class-action lawsuit, *S. P. v. Sullivan,* in the Southern District of New York against the Secretary of HHS, Louis W. Sullivan, M.D. The experiences of the lead plaintiff, S. P., a Latina woman from the Lower East Side of Manhattan, illustrated how the state neglect of women's health needs coexisted with state intervention into their lives on behalf of children. In January 1989, S. P. received a positive HIV test. That summer, aged twenty-one, she filed for SSI benefits, as the severity of her symptoms, including the chronic pelvic and abdominal pain she experienced because of her chronic pelvic inflammatory disease, prevented her from working. Despite the support of her physician, the SSA denied S. P.'s SSI claim, classifying her as HIV-positive but asymptomatic because her symptoms did not match those on CDC's list for AIDS. S. P. appealed the SSA's ruling, but an administrative law judge did not consider her testimony of disabling pain credible, and again denied her claim. S. P. persevered and, after two more years of advocacy, the judge eventually found her disabled based on the original evidence. S. P. nevertheless continued to suffer because of government interference. State agencies considered her financially unfit to care for her daughter, even as she fought for the benefits that would have helped to provide care for her child, and terminated her parental rights. She died in January 1994 before she could reunite with her daughter.[64] Using cases like S. P.'s, which exposed the interconnections among

HIV, poverty, and other vectors of discrimination, McGovern mounted a two-pronged attack against the SSA. First, she argued that by only carrying out research in young, white men, the CDC ignored the ways HIV converged with existing epidemics and illnesses that are more common in women, people living in poverty, and other disenfranchised groups. Moreover, in relying on the flawed definition to award disability benefits, McGovern accused the SSA of knowingly discriminating against women and other populations that the CDC understudied.[65]

The following day, as the *New York Times* brought news of the lawsuit to its readers, two hundred activists took the stories of women like S. P. to the streets.[66] Gathering outside the Department of Health and Human Services (HHS) in Washington, DC, the agency responsible for distributing social security benefits, crowds demanded, "How many more have to die before you say they qualify?"[67] HIV-positive women of color, including De La Cruz, and plaintiffs in *S. P. v. Sullivan*, such as Phyllis Sharpe, shared their experiences of medical and political discrimination and neglect. Sharpe, a thirty-nine-year-old mother of six, quit her job because the pain, exhaustion, and persistent vaginal yeast and urinary tract infections that she suffered from left her unable to work. She explained how the denial of disability benefits frequently forced her and her children to go hungry.[68] The art/activist collective Gran Fury designed posters emphasizing the disconnect between sickness and diagnosis, explaining "Women Don't Get AIDS, They Just Die From It."[69] Following protests at the CDC in early 1990, in which activists like Dixon Diallo of SisterLove, Atlanta, highlighted the particular harms the CDC definition posed to women of color in the South, protestors closed the year with a five-hundred-strong rally outside CDC headquarters in Atlanta on December 3.[70] White, middle-class women in ACT UP leveraged their race and class privilege during direct-action demonstrations, confronting law enforcement and risking arrest.[71] Police arrested ninety-two white protestors who broke into the CDC offices that day.[72]

What McGovern called the "joint strategy" of combining direct-action activism, media attention, and litigation forced the CDC back to the negotiating table.[73] In its December 1992 *MMWR* notice, the CDC announced its plans to expand the surveillance definition to include cervical cancer, recurrent bacterial pneumonia, and pulmonary tuberculosis, as well as a white blood cell count below two hundred, effective January 1, 1993.[74] The SSA amended its social security criteria, adding conditions common in women, in July 1993, granting more women access to critical federal programs Medicaid and Medicare, as well as disability benefits and other services.[75] The near doubling of AIDS cases in women, and the increase from 49,016 to 103,500 in the total number of AIDS cases reported to the CDC that year, underscored the inadequacy of the original definition.[76]

The slowness on the part of the CDC to recognize the gynecological symptoms of HIV contrasted with the willingness of federal agencies and pharmaceutical companies to include women in clinical trials for the sake of preventing mother-to-child HIV transmission. The focus on preventing perinatal transmission, and the ensuing debates around pregnant women's involvement in clinical research, perpetuated the false distinction between a woman's health and that of her fetus, and erased the deep concern that pregnant women both in the US and elsewhere expressed about also finding ways to protect the health of children.

Throughout the twentieth century, researchers often excluded women from clinical trials, fearing they may become pregnant during a trial of an experimental drug that harmed developing fetuses. Drug companies and medical institutions also wanted to avoid financial liability for potential fetal damage, a concern stemming from the thalidomide scandal of the 1960s, when a drug doctors prescribed for morning sickness caused malformation in the children.[77] The toxic effects of drugs, such as diethylstilbestrol (DES), and contraceptive devices, such as the Copper 7 and Dalkon Shield intrauterine devices (IUD), also

raised concerns over the safety of new medicines for women's reproduction.[78] The thalidomide incident shaped the view that pregnancies
harmed fetuses.[79] In 1977, the US Food and Drug Administration (FDA)
issued guidelines excluding women of childbearing age, which they
defined as a "premenopausal female capable of becoming pregnant,"
from drug trials until animal reproduction studies confirmed that the
drug was safe for fetuses.[80]

Fear of causing "reproductive damage" provided the same rationale
for women's exclusion from the early clinical trials for HIV. The
National Institutes of Health (NIH) excluded women of childbearing
age from trials until lifting the ban in response to protests in 1986.
Nonetheless, the agency regularly failed to enforce its guidelines, and
the FDA also continued its ban on women's participation in trials until
1993. Most trial participants, including those for azidothymidine (AZT),
the first antiretroviral drug to treat HIV, which the FDA approved for
sale in the US in 1987, were white, middle-class men with access to private health care.[81] Some trials for experimental drugs also barred
women who had undergone a hysterectomy or sterilization, even
though they had no possibility of becoming pregnant.[82] The requirement for women to prove they could not get pregnant also extended to
women who had no intention of becoming pregnant, including some
who self-identified as lesbian and those who did not have sex with men,
thereby reinforcing the heteronormative treatment of all women as
potential mothers. Pharmaceutical companies also lacked financial
incentives to include women in trials involving mostly men, as testing
medicines on a homogenous group cost less than having to account for
potential differences.[83]

The fact that research predominantly done in men determined the
safety and efficacy of HIV medicine spoke to a historic gender bias in
biomedical research. As women did not qualify for most clinical trials
to test new drugs, little data existed on how HIV and drugs to treat it
acted in women's bodies. Factors that might impact a woman's suscep-

tibility to HIV or tolerance of HIV medicine included body fat, size, and hormonal cycles. Women's exclusion not only hampered doctors' understanding of how treatments affected women, but according to men and women in ACT UP who early in the epidemic fought to get "drugs into bodies," it also denied them the only chance of legally accessing drugs that might prolong their lives.[84] With the discovery of mother-to-child transmission, the government and pharmaceutical companies shifted tactics. Originally excluded to protect fetuses from potentially harmful drugs, women now gained entry to trials for the sake of protecting fetuses from HIV. As more women qualified for clinical research, activists and advocates fought to ensure that the design of the trials did not undermine the rights of women or their infants.

In 1988, researchers such as Dr. Harold E. Fox, vice chairman of obstetrics at Columbia University's School of Physicians and Surgeons, proposed testing AZT on HIV-positive pregnant women to determine whether it reduced the chance of perinatal transmission.[85] One year later, the drug's manufacturer, Burroughs Wellcome, which was already facing criticism from organizations such as AIDS Action Pledge (AAP) and ACT UP over the drug's high price, reported that AZT caused cancer in the reproductive organs of animals.[86] This announcement did not deter Burroughs Wellcome or the FDA from starting a federally run clinical trial for AZT in pregnant women.

In 1991, the AIDS Clinical Trials Group (ACTG), an organization established in 1987 to develop AIDS research at the National Institute of Allergy and Infectious Diseases (NIAID), began recruiting women for a new treatment protocol, 076, funded through HHS, NIH, and NIAID. Researchers based at the University of Medicine and Dentistry of New Jersey—the state with the highest numbers of women with AIDS in the country—designed the trial to establish the efficacy of AZT in preventing perinatal transmission of HIV if given to women during pregnancy and to infants after birth.[87] The three-year trial began in 1993 and involved more than seven hundred pregnant women.[88]

Gaining entry to clinical trials did not signal a straightforward victory for women and other groups originally underrepresented in experimental AIDS research. The medical exploitation of Black, Latinx, and Native American communities in previous trials carried out in the name of objective science made many hesitant to participate in clinical research.[89] Particularly egregious cases of mistreatment, such as the Tuskegee Syphilis Study, in which government researchers tricked six hundred Black men in Alabama, four hundred of whom had syphilis, into participating in a study in which they received no available treatment, inspired mistrust in the mainstream medical establishment.[90] Other cases of medical exploitation, such as scientists' use of Puerto Rican women to test the first birth control pill in the mid-twentieth century, underscored the medical community's willingness to experiment on communities of color with little concern for the human cost.[91] With this history of racial violence in mind, activists from ACT UP, including New York's Treatment & Data (T&D) Committee, which worked to accelerate drug development, and which originally comprised mostly white gay men, and the Women's Caucus, which wanted to widen access to newly approved drugs through universal health care, as well as African American Women United Against AIDS and women doctors, such as Janet Mitchell, a Black physician based at Harlem Hospital, debated the ethics of trial 076, especially as it related to the question of how to define treatment access and protect the reproductive rights of women of color.[92]

Supporters of the trial, such as Mitchell, framed it as a positive step toward helping pregnant women block transmission of the virus and a way for women with little traditional access to health care to receive drugs. Marion Banzhaf, a founding member of the ACT UP Women's Caucus and the coordinator of the New Jersey Women and AIDS Network, agreed that many pregnant Black women with whom she spoke expressed their wish to help find an effective treatment. Nonetheless, Banzhaf also noted the concern community groups like African American Women United Against AIDS raised about enrolling Black women given the toxicity of AZT and the history of experimentation on Black people in the US. To maximize its benefits, she proposed reforming the trial—removing the placebo arm that denied women and infants access to treatment that might help them. She also suggested letting women decide for themselves whether to give their child the potentially toxic AZT. Coming to the debate with a different set of concerns and priorities, namely, to develop new treatment options as quickly as possible, T&D also supported the trial.[93]

In contrast, critics of the trial, including Carrie Wofford, an ACT UP member, likened it to the Tuskegee experiment, deeming it "unnecessary" because a number of HIV-positive women gave birth to HIV-negative children without intervention, and "unethical" because animal trials confirmed that AZT caused vaginal tumors in mice.[94] Members of the ACT UP Women's Caucus, including Maxine Wolfe, Tracy Morgan, and Heidi Dorow, objected to the trial on other grounds, including the unknown side effects women and their children might experience later in life and researchers' failure to guarantee women and their infants' continued access to potentially beneficial treatment once the study ended. They also rejected Mitchell's argument that experimental research equaled health care.[95] Morgan, Dorow, and other Women's Caucus members disrupted a meeting in which investigators of the trial discussed its design. According to Banzhaf, the protest prevented a productive conversation about the possibility of reforming aspects of the trial from taking place.[96] Mitchell and three other people of color involved in the study charged the mostly white women activists who failed to see its potential benefits for women of color as racist.[97] The debates over 076 highlighted the different stakes involved in clinical trial participation for different groups of women, which, in turn, shaped women and men's diverging and sometimes oppositional visions of how to protect women's rights and advance their health during research. These debates extended beyond the US, as follow-up trials of AZT in women in African countries, Thailand, and the Dominican Republic similarly raised concerns that researchers cared more about using pregnant women to prove the efficacy of AZT to prevent perinatal transmission than in guaranteeing women access to the drugs that they helped approve.[98]

The trial went ahead as planned, proving that the 076 regimen could reduce perinatal transmission by two-thirds—from twenty-five percent to less than eight percent.[99] Based on the results, the US Public Health Service (PHS) in 1994 issued recommendations for the use of AZT to reduce perinatal transmission of the virus.[100] The results eased much of the moral panic over the pregnancies of HIV-positive women.

The fact that pharmaceutical companies and federal agencies largely treated women as reproductive agents and not as individuals needing treatment for themselves did not pose the only concern for activists in this period. Illustrating Trevor Hoppe's concept of "punitive disease control," in which state authorities survey, control, and punish individuals blamed for spreading infectious diseases, several measures proposed by right-wing politicians and political commentators in the 1980s to "protect" the "general population"—designated as white, middle-class, heterosexual men and women excluded from the 4-H "high risk" groups—from HIV infection in the 1980s also raised concern over women's rights.[101]

THE COERCIVE STATE

The licensing in March 1985 of ELISA (enzyme-linked immunosorbent assay), the first commercial test to screen human blood for HIV, sparked political debate over the efficacy and ethics of different forms of HIV testing.[102] Many of the proposals for mandatory, mass testing mirrored the large-scale, institutional measures that the state had used in the past to tackle diseases that women could transmit perinatally, including mandatory blood testing for granting a marriage license.[103] In the post–sex revolution era, these proposals did not reflect how marriage functioned as an institution and largely failed. In July 1987, the AIDS scholar Cindy Patton described the media's message that people "should just stop having sex outside of marriage" to avoid contracting HIV as sexist and misguided.[104]

During the early years of the epidemic, several right-wing political figures called for mandatory HIV testing and contact tracing, as well as the tattooing, quarantining, and internment of people who tested positive for HIV.[105] Conservatives often made the gay community, as well as other marginalized groups associated with AIDS, such as drug users, the subject of rhetorical and legislative attack.[106] In 1986, the conservative commentator William Buckley remarked that "everyone detected with AIDS should be tattooed in the upper forearm, to protect common-needle users, and on the buttocks to prevent the victimization of other homosexuals."[107] Hostile commentators did not draw on the latest scientific information to justify these punitive proposals. Instead, they capitalized on the fear, confusion, and stigma surrounding AIDS, arguing that protecting the symbolic health of the nation warranted the penalization of vulnerable groups of individuals. Buckley and other right-wing commentators' calls for mandatory, identifiable HIV testing and other punitive measures alarmed both women and men in organizations like ACT UP, who expressed concern that the proposals would deter people from getting tested for fear of retribution.[108] The most extreme of these policy suggestions made the proposals that eventually passed—such as the 1987 ban on HIV-positive immigrants entering and legalizing in the US—seem more reasonable. HIV testing became a tool to exclude and confine in ways that solidified the perception of AIDS as a disease in the racialized foreign "other," despite the high cases in the US.[109]

Sex workers, and especially Black women, whom Karma R. Chávez identified as early targets of media frenzy and quarantine laws, also encountered hostile rhetoric and treatment.[110] As journalists fueled panic about the growing threat AIDS posed to the "general population," lawmakers called for greater powers to test and punish sex workers, singled out as the "carriers" of disease and "reservoirs" of infection.[111] Throughout the 1980s, several states debated or passed into law HIV-testing measures for the purposes of surveillance and control. In 1986, Nevada, a state with legal prostitution, required the testing of any person arrested for sex work. Those who tested positive faced felony charges if authorities discovered them selling sex again.[112] The media construction of sex workers as malicious actors intent on harming their male customers legitimized authorities' calls for such draconian legislation. The media rebuked Wendy Blakenship, a white sex worker from Florida, for not telling "her customers that she carried the AIDS virus." Blakenship's case inspired the Florida legislature to introduce a law in 1988 allowing health officials to "quarantine promiscuous AIDS carriers for up to four months."[113] She died aged twenty, with reports of her death lacking any compassion. By 1995, ten states passed felony HIV-specific penalties targeting sex workers, despite evidence of the low prevalence of HIV among that group.[114] The punishment of sex workers with HIV mirrored past initiatives to police women's sexual behavior in the name of public health, as well as the growing contemporary impetus to penalize those who engaged in nonnormative and anti-normative sexual and gender behavior during the era of advancing family values and tough-on-crime politics.[115] Other populations under the purview of state institutions also became targets of mandatory testing, including people in the military, those in prison or hospitals, applicants for residency and citizenship, and couples requesting a marriage license.[116]

Beginning in the Progressive era, many states required applicants for a marriage license to get a blood test to identify cases of venereal diseases, such as syphilis. By the end of 1938, twenty-six states denied marriage certificates to couples if either partner tested positive for a communicable infection. Proponents of premarital testing, such as

Thomas Parran, US surgeon general from 1936 to 1948, argued that it helped prevent the spread of disease, including perinatally. In practice, premarital testing cost a lot with little benefit. To avoid the expensive and invasive test, many couples chose to marry in states without the requirement or to forgo marriage altogether, a phenomenon bolstered by the mid-century, second-wave feminist critique of the institution.[117] The same arguments over the efficacy of premarital testing framed the debates over HIV testing with the onset of AIDS in the early 1980s.

Throughout the 1980s, politicians and public health officials argued at length over whether to encourage states to offer AIDS testing to couples for marriage licenses.[118] In his first speech devoted exclusively to the growing health crisis, at a gala for the American Medical Foundation for AIDS Research in the summer of 1987, Reagan called for a wide range of AIDS testing at the state and federal levels, including the routine testing of applicants for marriage licenses in order to stop "AIDS . . . surreptitiously spreading throughout our population" and prevent "at least some babies being born with AIDS."[119] Reagan's comments buoyed conservatives, such as the Republican governor of New Hampshire John H. Sununu, who embraced premarital testing to curb the spread of HIV among heterosexuals and prevent the birth of HIV-positive children.[120] Activists and public health professionals opposed proposals for compulsory premarital testing, framing it as an expensive, ineffective use of resources that did more to deter marriage than to stop the spread of HIV.[121] Moreover, as many conservatives viewed HIV/AIDS as punishment for nonnormative sex, including sex outside marriage, critics also viewed premarital testing as another ideologically driven proposal aimed at symbolically protecting the American family from infection. While several states debated requiring HIV testing for marriage licenses, only two, Illinois and Louisiana, adopted it into law in 1988. The high cost of the test, which ranged from $30 to $200; its failure to identify many cases of HIV; and the fact that couples unwilling to foot the bill married in neighboring states or decided not to marry at all led Louisiana and Illinois to repeal the requirement by 1989.[122] State legislatures took seriously proposals to test pregnant women and women considering pregnancy, as well as newborns. These groups were already accessible to doctors, so this interest reflected the moral panic over women with HIV giving birth to sick and disabled children.

Proposals to test pregnant women had particularly dangerous connotations for women of color disproportionately impacted in the epidemic and already vulnerable to state intervention into their reproductive lives. Throughout the twentieth century, scientists routinely experimented on Black, Latina, and Native American women's bodies to develop new reproductive tools that they hoped would tackle social issues such as poverty, overpopulation, and alcohol use, while states passed eugenics laws that legalized the compulsory sterilization of mostly poor, mentally and physically disabled, and non-white women in an effort to promote able-bodied, middle-class, white hegemony.[123] In 1973, the Southern Poverty Law Center, a civil rights organization, discovered that throughout the century, doctors had sterilized tens of thousands of women, half of whom were Black, using federal funds.[124] Scientists also developed the birth control pill that came to market in the US in the 1960s on Puerto Rican women and coerced Native American women into using long-acting hormonal contraceptives such as Depo-Provera and Norplant to address fetal alcohol syndrome.[125] During the 1960s and 1970s, the women's movement fought to restrict the widespread practice of coercion for the purposes of reproductive control. In 1974, HHS issued guidelines requiring informed consent and a minimum age of twenty-one for women undergoing sterilization.[126] In the wake of AIDS, women's rights advocates, such as Barbara Santee and Carol Leigh of the sex worker's rights organization Call Off Your Old Tired Ethics (COYOTE), worried that the federal efforts to reduce perinatal transmission might repeat past reproductive abuses disproportionately waged against women of color, warned that women "must be prepared to confront the challenges which will be thrown at reproductive freedom in the guise of 'protecting the public good from the threat of AIDS.'" Others feared doctors might coerce women into making unwanted decisions about their pregnancies following a non-anonymous positive test result, instead of educating them about the thirty to fifty percent chance of perinatal transmission.[127]

The federal proposal to reduce perinatal HIV transmission through marriage-license testing did not reflect the reality that, in the 1980s, sex and motherhood often happened outside of marriage. Instead, with the rise of neoliberal politics that shifted the responsibility of tackling social inequities from the federal government to the states, private citizens, and organizations under Reagan, the state-level, voluntary, and educational campaigns of different public health departments had greater reach.

Throughout the 1980s, women called for public health agencies to recognize them as whole, sexual, and reproductive beings. Such recognition brought prescriptions about motherhood and sexuality. Specifically, public health campaigns encouraged women to seek treatment and services on behalf of their fetuses before seeking treatment and services for their own condition, as well as to modify their sexual behavior through abstinence or insisting on male condom use. Signaling the gap between policy and ideology, agencies created advertisements that put the burden of prevention on women, while the Reagan administration attacked the services that helped them plan for a pregnancy and seek medical care.

FIGHTING FOR WOMEN'S SEXUAL RIGHTS

In the first decade of the AIDS epidemic, sexual HIV-prevention strategies available to women included abstinence, condom use, and limiting sexual partners. Proponents of these methods often failed to recognize

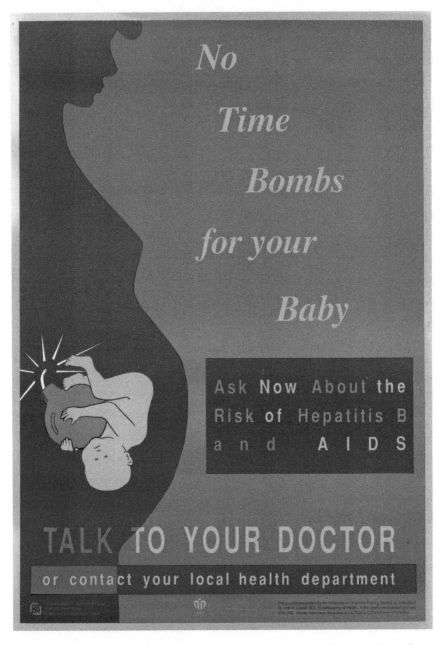

Fig. 1. Oklahoma Department of Public Health, No Time Bombs for Your Baby, 1990. Library of Congress Prints and Photographs Division.

that many women lacked control over matters related to sex. Although some scientists called for prevention options that gave women greater control in the epidemic during the 1980s, the FDA did not approve the female condom until 1993, and public health campaigns continued to place the emphasis of prevention on male condoms, the use of which women did not control.[128]

In the 1980s and early 1990s, various national and state public health departments ran sexist publicity campaigns that framed women as the vectors of disease in infants and perpetuated the neoliberal trope that individual women bore responsibility for preventing the transmission of HIV, absolving both the state, and men, of action.[129] A 1990 poster from the Oklahoma Department of Public Health entitled "No Time Bombs for Your Baby" displayed the body of a faceless pregnant woman whose fetus is hugging a bomb. The poster highlighted the threat that the woman's womb, framed as an explosive, posed to her own body. In encouraging the silhouetted woman who lacked an identity to seek medical treatment on behalf of her fetus, it perpetuated the false distinction between the health of a woman and that of a fetus of whose body it was a part and presented women's bodies as harmful to fetuses—messaging that echoed that of abortion opponents seeking to limit women's reproductive rights.[130]

In a CDC poster, a young Black woman looks concerned as she leans on a cot next to the caption, "I Didn't Know I had AIDS . . . Not Until my Baby was Born with it." The accompanying text reveals that the woman contracted AIDS from her "man," and that "had I known better, I would have made him use condoms, and if that didn't work, I'd have stopped being with him."[131] The woman in this poster not only bears the responsibility for protecting herself but also her child. Despite the necessity of raising awareness of the issue of HIV/AIDS among women and, similar to contemporaneous efforts to prevent perinatal transmission of rubella, the messaging urging women to modify their behavior assigned women the sole responsibility of preventing transmission of HIV.[132] This messaging not only absolved the state of its duty to improve the provision of health care and social services, while making women who fell short vulnerable to punishment, it also fed into homophobic and sexist tropes suggesting that Black women otherwise at "low risk" from contracting HIV needed protection from gay and bisexual Black men "on the down low."

Public health agencies ran similar campaigns encouraging women to take greater responsibility in preventing heterosexual transmission of the virus. On posters designed to give women verbal strategies to encourage men to engage in safer sex, the CDC told women "If he doesn't have a condom, you just have to take a deep breath and tell him to go and get one."[133] Corporate campaigns reinforced public messaging, as advertising agencies and condom manufacturers created adverts with similar themes. In *Sex, Drugs & AIDS*, a film made for the New York City Board of Education, three girls discuss where to buy male condoms and the importance of using them. The New York advertising executive Jerry Della Femina's campaign entitled "I enjoy sex, but I don't want to die for it" featured a woman debating the effectiveness of male condoms. Neither featured men nor discussed their role in prevention.[134]

Feminist commentators critiqued and, as seen in figure 2, satirized messages that put the onus of prevention on women. Created at a time of growing awareness about the phenomenon of acquaintance rape, these campaigns also failed to acknowledge women's vulnerability to sexual violence.[135] Women's inability to use male condoms or control men's use of them during heterosexual sex left Esther R. Rome of the Boston Women's Health Book Collective (BWHBC) wondering, "Is what started out as a beneficial increase of awareness and comfort for women turning into another areas [sic] of responsibility in which they have to convince a man to do something for his and her own good?"[136] Other women's health advocates similarly noted the limitations of such campaigns for women.[137] "Since men are the ones with the penises,

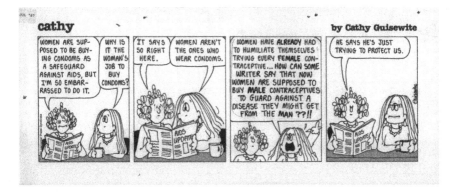

Fig. 2. *Cathy* for *Glamour*, 1987. © Cathy Guisewite, reprinted with permission.

wouldn't it make better sense to require johns to make sure condoms are worn during sex?" asked the ACT UP members Zoe Leonard and Polly Thistlethwaite.[138] Marie St. Cyr, director of the Women and AIDS Resource Network (WARN), noted that "heterosexual men aren't even asked to share responsibility. Over and over, the image projected is that it's a woman's own fault if she gets AIDS."[139] The physicians Kathryn Anastos and Carola Marte concurred, noting, "Discussions of heterosexual HIV transmission in the United States are also frequently permeated with sexist assumptions . . . . [L]ack of empowerment is a problem for all women, and especially poorer women, in protecting themselves against HIV infection. . . . [A] heterosexual woman is usually not an equal partner in the bedroom," thereby limiting her ability to insist on condom use.[140] Such campaigns failed to recognize the gender power imbalance in condom use.

The presentation of women as the carriers and preventers of HIV transmission both sexually and reproductively in public health campaigns, as well as commercial advertisements, inspired activists to create their own feminist public health publicity. In books, pamphlets, and journals, feminist activists offered women accurate information on HIV/AIDS. They also centered the need to protect the sexual and reproductive rights of multiply marginalized women most impacted in the epidemic, which included countering messaging that positioned fetuses as separate from the women of whom they were a part.

FEMINIST PUBLIC HEALTH ALTERNATIVES

In March 1989, members of the ACT UP Women's Caucus ran a Women and AIDS teach-in in New York that culminated in the publication of an anthology of essays exploring the structural oppressions shaping different women's experience of the epidemic one year later. Published as *Women, AIDS, and Activism*, edited by ACT UP/NY Women & AIDS Book Group with the progressive publisher South End Press, the anthology mirrored the BWHBC's 1971 feminist bestseller, *Our Bodies, Ourselves*. The authors' "primary objectives" were to provide "information about women's particular needs, analyze the impact of AIDS on women's lives from a feminist perspective, and promote grassroots activism."[141] Featuring essays from a racially, sexually, socially, and culturally diverse cohort of authors, the handbook covered a broad range of issues that addressed, among others, the obstacles of safer sex for women, including negotiation with men over condom use. In her essay "Demanding a Condom," the ACT UP member Kat Doud recalled her struggles to convince her male partner to use condoms as protection against HIV:

> Max (not his real name) was putting a lot of pressure on me to get birth control pills for protection, only the only protection pills would offer would be for pregnancy—not AIDS. During this time, my fear of AIDS was growing. I was getting really paranoid, so I called the hotline. They talked a lot about condoms and safer sex. I went immediately to Max to tell him how I was feeling and that I wouldn't have sex with him without condoms. His reaction was horrible. He got very angry and full of contempt and accused me of having AIDS, and angry that I insinuated he did.[142]

Doud's passage spoke of the hostile and sometimes violent reactions women encountered when confronting men about condom use.

Women artists similarly explored the relationship between HIV disclosure and gender-based violence. During the 1990s, to address the rising rates of HIV/AIDS among Black women and reflecting the leading role theater played in publicizing the experiences of women and other affected groups during the epidemic, the playwright Ntozake Shange updated her choreopoem, *for colored girls who have considered suicide/ when the rainbow is enuf*, adding a passage recounting the abuse a woman received when she told her boyfriend she tested positive for AIDS:

> i saw his left hand clench into something that was dangerous
> & i fell out on the floor . . .
> i was out & when i started to wake up I rubbed the blood streaming from
> my eyes.[143]

Doud's and Shange's interventions that centered women's lived experiences highlighted the dangerous consequences of insisting that women demand safer sex.

Mobilizing in Boston, a city with a rich history of women's and LGBTQ health organizing, the BWHBC that informed members of the Women's Caucus continued its interventions beyond the publication of their landmark text. Since the 1970s, the authors have published new editions that weave diverse perspectives, address new challenges in women's health, and have wide appeal—selling more than four million copies.[144] This has included incorporating the expertise of women whose backgrounds differ from the mostly white and middle-class founding members whose earlier work often overlooked the intersections among gender, race, sexuality, and class.[145]

For the 1992 edition, entitled the *New Our Bodies, Ourselves: A Book by and for Women*, original members of the BWHBC, such as Jamie Penney, collaborated with ACT UP members Marion Banzhaf and Risa Denenberg, as well as Black health practitioners such as Janet Mitchell and Patricia Loftman of the Harlem Hospital Center, both of whom worked on ACTG 076.[146] In the preface, the authors explained that they "added new topics such as AIDS, new birth control methods and special disorders that affect primarily women—subjects we did not cover in the 1984 edition."[147] Like other women activists and advocates, BWHBC tied AIDS to reproductive health. Both sections on "AIDS, HIV Infection and Women" and "Abortion" in the 1992 edition come under the section "Controlling Our Fertility." Similar to the *Women, AIDS, and Activism* handbook and other feminist books, articles, posters, and cartoons, the information on AIDS in the *New Our Bodies, Ourselves* also covers safer sex. "If a man refuses to use a condom and overpowers you into having intercourse, at least get some spermicide into your vagina, or use a female condom," the authors wrote.[148]

The collaborative work of the women in ACT UP and BWHBC demonstrate how the women's health movement of the 1960s and 1970s continued with the movement to address AIDS in women in the 1980s. Approaching health as a political issue, both argued that politics, economics, and interpersonal relationships shaped women's health outcomes as much as biology. Moreover, like the women organizing to equip women with knowledge of their bodies in the 1960s and 1970s, the authors wrote both guides to demystify medical expertise and provide women with basic information about HIV/AIDS that they found lacking in the available resources. Crucially, both books sought to empower women with the latest scientific information, education, and resources to help them make informed decisions about their bodies, including over reproduction.

Tying HIV to long histories of reproductive abuse and inadequate health care, the authors of the anthologies centered race in their analysis. As a teenager, the ACT UP member Risa Denenberg was pressured into having an illegal abortion by the man with whom she became pregnant, an experience that motivated her to become involved in the women's health movements and shaped her perspective on reproductive justice.[149] In *Women, AIDS, and Activism*, Denenberg wrote that, similar to past coercive measures that resulted in high sterilization rates among Native American and Puerto Rican women, the policies aimed at reducing mother-to-child transmission, such as pre- and post-pregnancy testing, threatened women's reproductive freedoms.[150] Such measures aimed at preventing the birth of HIV-positive infants violated what Marion Banzhaf, Tracy Morgan, and Karen Ramspacher of the ACT UP/Women and AIDS Book Group described as "HIV-positive women['s] . . . right to have children if they so desire."[151] In the chapter "AIDS, HIV Infection, and Women," the authors of the New Our Bodies, Ourselves similarly argued that the medical advice given to practitioners to actively discourage all women with HIV from becoming pregnant and encourage pregnant HIV-positive women to end their pregnancies "has greatly threatened the reproductive lives and choices of HIV+ women," putting a "HIV+ woman's right to decide whether to continue or terminate her pregnancy in serious jeopardy." They raised particular concern about the advice to delay or forgo pregnancy given that "the medical evidence regarding the effects of pregnancy on the health of HIV+ women and the rates, methods and risk factors for transmission to the fetus are inadequate and inconclusive."[152] Denenberg insisted that doctors counsel pregnant women on the available information and offer full medical and social support for a woman's decision: only a nondirective approach that championed women's wishes could prevent a repeat of past reproductive abuses against poor and non-white women.[153]

Throughout the 1980s, in publications, anthologies, articles, magazines, and on television, women's health advocates persistently articulated the need to educate women about HIV and to protect the rights of all HIV-positive women, including the reproductive freedoms of women who wanted to become pregnant, end a pregnancy, or have a child. In addition, women's health advocates used the largest international platform on AIDS to call attention to the policies proposed to reduce transmission that threatened women's rights. As a result, their fight for decent state services and against discriminatory state intervention during the epidemic's first decade also played out internationally. By the mid-1990s, their efforts synthesized into policy that recognized women as people requiring access to clinical research. Nonetheless, the artificial distinction that this policy made between a woman and a fetus blunted its progressive potential.

SHAPING AN INTERNATIONAL PLATFORM

Since the inaugural meeting in Arizona in 1985, women's health activists regularly attended the International Conference on AIDS—a major forum for exchanging scientific information about the disease that provides an index for AIDS campaigning throughout the epidemic's forty-year history.

The conference activism of ACT UP, the BWHBC, the International Working Group on Women and AIDS, and other organizations underscored women's desire to center reproductive justice within a holistic approach to AIDS. Their interventions contributed to what Emily K. Hobson has described as the multi-issue politics of conference protest that tackled AIDS alongside other social issues, such as poverty and criminal justice.[154] Moreover, the intersectional feminist scope of protestors' demands that framed the fight against AIDS as part of a larger, interconnected struggle for human, economic, reproductive, and immigrant rights reflected the growing intellectual influence of third-world feminism on AIDS activism in the early 1990s.[155] Women have used the conference since its inception as an international platform to counter the treatment of women in the political and public health response to AIDS, and of women as the vectors of transmission, either prenatally or through sex work. Until 1993, women also used the conferences—the CDC's most visible international platform—to object to women's exclusion from the AIDS surveillance definition.

At the third International Conference on AIDS in Washington, DC, in June 1987, activists from the International Working Group on

Women and AIDS wrote a two-page, open letter to the planning committee critiquing the treatment of women in the HIV/AIDS epidemic and underscoring the need for conference organizers to include women in conference organizing, steering, and program committees. Asserting that "AIDS is a woman's issue," the letter addressed the impact of AIDS in women in the US, Africa, and the Caribbean.[156] The working group expressed particular concern for "the paternalistic and cavalier disregard for the reproductive rights of the women at highest risk for HIV infection," including calls for the compulsory, mandatory, or routine testing of pregnant women on behalf of the CDC, President Reagan, and other public health organizations. Like the authors of *Women, AIDS, and Activism* and the *New Our Bodies, Ourselves*, the working group tied the urgency to protect the dignity of HIV-positive pregnant women of color to a long history of racist "forced sterilization and coerced family planning decisions." The group also linked reproductive justice to health and welfare, noting, "No meaningful reproductive options exist in the absence of adequate nutrition, prenatal and medical care, or without daycare, education and schooling for all children, including those born with disease or HIV positivity, and the availability of abortion on demand for women who chose it."[157] Women's health advocates therefore saw the threat AIDS posed to women's reproductive freedoms not only in terms of the reproductive abuses carried out against women of color in the past, but the new struggles that women faced following the attack on domestic welfare programs under Reagan.[158] They called for the greater representation of women at conferences to ensure that the meetings addressed these feminist concerns.

In June 1992, Jamie Penney of the BWHBC traveled to the fifth conference, held in Amsterdam, to again argue that "AIDS is directly related to community health" and "also to reproductive rights." Like Denenberg and others, Penney called for greater information about women, AIDS, and reproduction, because "a woman's decision to use a contraceptive or not, which contraceptive to use, whether or not to have a child and whether or not to breastfeed that child will depend on the information she has about AIDS." She encouraged women to "demand that resources and information be made available to women's groups all over the world, and that governments and international organizations make information about women and AIDS widely available to us."[159] Women could only make informed decisions about their health, including whether and when to have children, with access to accurate and unbiased information.

Penney's statement, like other conference ephemera, attests to women's health advocates' concern that a lack of sexual and reproductive health care, as well as accurate information, education, and resources on HIV/AIDS available to women, jeopardized their rights. As Penney astutely observed, in the absence of institutional support, women "are the ones who will have to do the work" in educating and empowering women in the epidemic.[160] This work included not only compelling the CDC to widen its AIDS case definition, which activists demanded at conferences, but creating their own public health publicity.[161] As the publication of *Women, AIDS, and Activism* and *New Our Bodies, Ourselves*, as well as women's numerous other public health initiatives illustrate, women did not wait for people in positions of power to meet their demands. Instead, they published their own information designed to reach women and educate them on the routes of transmission and the ways they might protect the health of themselves and their partners.

Women also continued to "do the work" back home. In the early 1990s, alongside the campaign to change the CDC definition, members of ACT UP and WHAM!, a reproductive rights organization based in New York City, "stormed the NIH" to demand the inclusion of women and people of color in experimental AIDS research, as McGovern's HLP filed a citizen petition charging the FDA with gender discrimination.[162] In 1993, the FDA announced its plan to lift the ban on women participating in clinical trials.[163] That same year, Congress passed the

NIH Revitalization Act, requiring all NIH-sponsored clinical trials to include women and racial and ethnic minorities, prohibiting cost as a reason for their exclusion. In 1994, Congress established at the FDA an Office of Women's Health, which is dedicated to advancing women's health and advocating for women's participation in clinical research.[164] These announcements signaled a partial victory for HIV-positive women, aiding in their access to experimental treatment and facilitating greater understanding of the gender-specific effects of drugs.

Nonetheless, the steps the FDA took to include women in clinical research, while important, failed to treat reproduction as part of women's holistic health care and thereby undermined reproductive rights. Under the new regulations, the FDA placed on individual women the responsibility of deciding whether to accept the reproductive risks involved in clinical trial participation and take the necessary steps to prevent becoming pregnant or exposing a fetus to a potentially dangerous drug during the study.[165] McGovern, who wanted the FDA to go further than simply lifting their ban on women, had called on researchers to complete all animal reproductive studies before Phase 1 testing to ensure that the drug posed no reproductive risk to any participants, thus acknowledging women's reproductive capacity without using it to discriminate against them. McGovern's proposal required the FDA to reform the structure of experimental drug design, a greater commitment than incorporating women into existing research models.[166] In shifting the burden of reproductive risk from federal agencies to individual women, the FDA, like public health agencies, positioned women as responsible for ensuring fetal health as the federal government worked to gut prenatal and maternal health care. Ultimately, the FDA's revision failed to acknowledge that women both in the US and abroad wanted to find ways to protect their health, whether pregnant or not. As explored in the next chapter, the notion that women posed a threat to their pregnancies informed government policy that not only placed the burden of prevention on women but punished those who fell short.

CONCLUSION

The first thirteen years of the AIDS epidemic saw HIV-positive women and advocates secure several limited, albeit significant, victories. After scientists began reporting on cases of opportunistic infections in men and infants in the early 1980s, the CDC's epidemiological categories and AIDS case definition hampered the diagnosis of the "AIDS agent" in women. The discovery that HIV passed not only through sex but also reproduction increased the urgency to diagnose and treat the disease especially in pregnant women. As doctors diagnosed increasing numbers of women with HIV and increasing numbers of women qualified for clinical trials, activists called for interventions that did not separate a woman's reproduction from their overall health, seeking to ensure that treatment programs did not threaten the rights of women in ways that repeated the racist medical abuses of the past.

The women in this chapter fought for inclusion in the early political and public health response to AIDS. When public health agencies saw women, their statewide public health initiatives put on them the onus of prevention both sexually and reproductively. Working to remove the burden of prevention, feminists created alternative public health publicity that educated women on how transmission occurred and how to protect the health of themselves and their partners. Aiding in the diagnosis of greater numbers of HIV-positive women and widening women's access to Medicaid, as well as disability and other social service benefits through the SSA, the revision of the CDC's AIDS definition in January 1993 signaled a major victory for HIV-positive women.

The outcomes of these fights call into question the conditions necessary for activist success. The ACT UP member Kimberley Christensen identified several factors that helped activists achieve their goals in the 1980s and early 1990s. Drawing inspiration from past civil disobedience

struggles for social justice, AIDS activists educated themselves and harnessed the power of the media to raise awareness of issues and put pressure on the government to act. Activists also effectively exploited the
tactics, skills, and social status of different individuals, acknowledging
that protest is a privilege that not everyone can participate in evenly.[167]
The successful campaigns animating this chapter—from taking on
Cosmopolitan magazine to the CDC—attest to the effectiveness of these
strategies. Moreover, they prove Schulman's and Hubbard's assessment
of the power of coalitions to effect progressive political change throughout US history.[168]

Activists' ability to pressure the CDC, FDA, SSA, and NIH to include
women in clinical research, add their symptoms to the legal definition
of AIDS, and grant them access to benefits and services also underscores Beatrix Hoffman's argument that throughout the twentieth century, activists found securing specific, discrete improvements that
benefited certain groups of patients easier than implementing comprehensive health reform or regulatory changes.[169] Moreover, women's
success in gaining access to clinical research, and the nature of that
inclusion—namely, to prevent mother-to-child transmission—proved
that federal agencies responded more proactively to the demands of
women as a class when they involved fetuses and infants. The FDA's
failure to reform its regulations to take responsibility for the potential
risks that trial participation posed to women's pregnancies also
reflected the neoliberalism of the era that shifted the burden of prevention to private citizens, and underscored the difficulty women faced in
securing treatment from pharmaceutical companies and federal agencies in ways that acknowledged their reproductive capacity but did not
violate their reproductive rights, as the government continued to place
the burden of preventing AIDS in infants on women.

As the women highlighting the links between AIDS and reproductive justice in this chapter noted, the discovery of AIDS in women

brought political risk. Public health messaging and policy made women responsible for preventing the birth of HIV-positive infants. Demonstrating how state recognition quickly tipped to state coercion out of purported concern for fetal health, those who failed to prevent conception faced punitive government intervention.

2

TESTING WOMEN

||||||||||||||||||||||||||||||||||||||||||||||||||||||||||||||||||||||||||||||||||||||||||||||||||||||||||||||||||||||||||||||||||||||||||||||||||||||||||||||||||||||||||||||||||||||

"IF A PREGNANT WOMAN TESTED positive for the AIDS virus, would you recommend an abortion?" one reporter asked the US Surgeon General Charles Everett Koop as he stood among a crowd of journalists and twenty-two television cameras at the National Press Club on March 24, 1987. All present anticipated that the surgeon general's words—the answer from a self-proclaimed evangelical Christian, nominated by the avowed antiabortion President Ronald Reagan—would be headlined on the evening news and next day's papers.[1] "If you wanted to give her all the possibilities that were available to her, you would have to mention abortion," Koop replied.[2] While Koop later reassured reporters that his personal opposition to abortion had not changed, his conservative advocates viewed his pronouncement as an evidence of his "re-thinking" on the subject.[3] Although Koop's commitment to public health compelled him to confirm that abortion was legal and possible in 1987, he was never motivated by a duty to affirm women's reproductive rights. Instead, like many other government officials, he was driven by a desire to protect children from HIV.

"One of the things I think is most important about this," he continued, "is my great concern for the babies who are born to positive mothers. I think no woman should contemplate a pregnancy without voluntarily wanting to be tested for the AIDS virus."[4] Reports that infants became infected primarily through mother-to-child transmission, that rates of transmission varied from thirty to seventy percent, that infants born with HIV would likely become seriously ill and cripple the state financially in the process, and that rates of AIDS in women and children were rising—3,601 and 737, respectively, in 1987—drove political and public health figures like Koop to call for testing to identify HIV-positive women and advise those who tested positive to not have children in the 1980s.[5]

Deep-seated cultural anxieties over infant mortality and disability in children informed Koop's advice. In the early to mid-twentieth century, lawmakers seeking to limit births among those considered "unfit" in order to promote Anglo-American dominance and avoid the expense of caring for unwell and disabled children in a for-profit health system in which care is considered a privilege and not a right introduced policies that restricted women's reproductive freedoms in the name of public health. This eugenicist thinking also informed the political response to AIDS in the 1980s, as conservative lawmakers and political commentators who expressed concern about the financial and moral cost of caring for HIV-positive children worked to limit the reproductive freedoms of multiply marginalized women with HIV.

Government figures tended not to match their rhetorical concern for fetuses and newborn children with structural support to help HIV-positive women get tested and, if positive, navigate their illness, their reproductive wishes, or the illness of their child. In line with the gutting of social welfare programs and a move toward a neoliberal social agenda that dovetailed with the expansion of the carceral state in the 1980s, the official response to AIDS in women shifted the responsibility for prevention away from the government and onto people with the fewest resources. Reflecting the historical treatment of women as the vectors of disease in men and children, the state placed this burden on women. Ideology trumped public health, as lawmakers restricted women's access to abortion care and other family-planning services that enabled them to control their reproductive health. The government also relied on private organizations to support infants whose parents had died of AIDS, or who came to care through removal. Underscoring the notion that protesting state neglect always brought the risk of state interference out of a purported concern for fetal health, lawmakers also passed legislation criminalizing the pregnancies of women who failed to prevent conception. Political figures vilified multiply marginalized HIV-positive women to justify the use of criminal penalties, seeking to absolve the government of the responsibility of investing in what Steven W. Thrasher has termed the "conceptual prophylaxis" of housing, education, and freedom from incarceration that protects people from disease and supports them in caring for their children.[6] Koop's speech at the Press Club therefore illustrates how HIV testing became interwoven with structural inequalities beyond homophobia and racist xenophobia, including the underacknowledged struggle over reproductive justice.

AIDS historians like Jennifer Brier and Anthony Petro have debated Koop's complex role in addressing AIDS, crediting his public health advice for countering the most extreme proposals of the religious and political right while also noting its contribution to what Petro called a "moral politics of public health" that nevertheless emphasized the conservative tenets of abstinence, monogamy, and personal responsibility.[7] A focus on Koop's actions also reveals the underexamined impact of abortion politics on AIDS and the role of AIDS on the development of the fetal rights movement in and beyond the 1980s. Putting public health before partisan politics, Koop earned the ire of conservatives who expected the surgeon general to advance their political agenda. Instead, he endorsed condoms and sex education in public schools as HIV prevention and refused to legitimize the concept of post-abortion syndrome (PAS) invented by the evangelical Crisis Pregnancy Center and other conservative activists to undermine abortion.[8] Koop not only upset his conservative former allies and surprised his critics through his endorsement of condoms and sex education, as Petro and others have argued,[9] but he also betrayed the hopes of those who expected him to use the institution of his office to deliver a practical blow against *Roe v. Wade*. Nonetheless, although Koop refused to hand the antiabortion movement a report with which to attack legal abortion, he equally refused to affirm its safety for women. Moreover, his conviction that life begins at conception furthered the discourse of fetal rights. These two views—that abortion is harmful to women and that the fetus is an unborn child whom the state needs to "protect" from "irresponsible" women and society from the moral and social cost of their care—have underpinned criminal penalties and abortion restrictions in the decades since. These measures have not helped infants or women. Rather, they have advanced the family values agenda of promoting sex and pregnancy in marriage, relying on the nuclear family to provide support for vulnerable groups in the absence of a social safety net, and punishing those who suffered from a lack of state support. As women with HIV fought for the right to make informed decisions about their bodies, including the right to have children on their own terms, the official response to AIDS eroded women's reproductive rights.

MATERNAL CONCERNS

On November 14, 1988, thirty-eight-year-old Carol Doe, a five-month-pregnant Haitian woman living in New York, visited Jamaica Hospital in New York City for a routine prenatal check-up. During the visit, Doe received a test for HIV as part of her prenatal care, and it came back positive. Three days later, Doe met Dr. Maurice Abitbol, the hospital's chief of obstetrics and gynecology. Since learning her test result, Doe decided she wanted to continue her pregnancy. A nurse recommended that she have an abortion, claiming that Doe was likely to transmit HIV to her baby. Dr. Abitbol agreed that Doe should terminate the pregnancy, adding that HIV-positive children placed a heavy financial strain on society. Doe was already a mother to a daughter born with spina bifida, and Abitbol claimed that giving birth to a HIV-positive child was worse. After pleading with Abitbol and other practitioners to allow her to continue her prenatal care with Jamaica Hospital's high-risk program, she was referred to King County Hospital, which Abitbol claimed provided superior care for HIV-positive women. Three weeks later, Doe received a second-trimester abortion at King County Hospital. The following year, the Center for Constitutional Rights—a New York–based legal advocacy organization that was founded in 1966 to advance civil rights legislation and in the 1980s offered help to people with HIV/AIDS facing discrimination in areas of employment, housing, and reproductive rights—filed a suit on Doe's behalf against Jamaica Hospital, Kings County Hospital, and the staff at both institutions, alleging that they breached their duties to provide appropriate care and get her informed consent.[10] Moreover, Doe claimed that her caretakers' conduct violated her rights as a person with a disability as protected by Section 504 of the Federal Rehabilitation Act.[11] Although Justice Scholnick of the New York Supreme Court found that the requirements of Section 504 did not apply, he ruled that Doe provided sufficient evidence to create an issue of fact as to whether Dr. Abitbol negligently offered inaccurate advice upon which she acted in deciding to have an abortion.[12]

Doe's experience was not unique. On May 14, 1987, the CCR organized a conference in Washington, DC, that brought together women from across the country to address the relationship between AIDS and reproductive rights. Rhonda Copelon, a law professor at the City University of New York who volunteered on reproductive rights cases at the CCR, and whose advocacy affirms what Margot Canaday has described as the leading role women lawyers played in addressing HIV/AIDS, shared stories that not only highlighted the reproductive restrictions HIV-positive women such as Doe faced but all multiply marginalized women navigating health policies that favored sterilization over abortion. Copelon told of how a doctor urged two pregnant Latina women from Arizona to take an HIV test. When they tested positive, he counseled them to abort their pregnancies, explaining that they could either pay for the procedure themselves or undergo sterilization at the state's expense. These women represented the many who early in the epidemic saw the desire on the part of medical professionals and federal agencies to control their reproductive decisions as undermining their right to become pregnant or to carry a pregnancy to term.[13]

Throughout the twentieth century, the outbreak of diseases that caused congenital disorders raised questions over who had the authority to determine whether a woman could plan for, terminate, or continue a pregnancy. The political responses to these diseases had different implications for women's rights along the lines of race, class, health, sexuality, and ability. During the Progressive era, as reformers feared that increased immigration threatened Anglo-American dominance in US society and physicians warned that venereal disease increased sterility and harmed developing fetuses, several states—illustrative of their role in intermingling with reproductive rights—passed laws mandating premarital testing for venereal diseases, hoping to increase birth rates among white, married, "respectable," and "healthy" couples.[14] Driven by the same desire to decrease birth rates among the seemingly "unfit," namely, recent immigrants, Black Americans, poor people, people with physical and intellectual disabilities, and "promiscuous" women, numerous states also legalized sterilization and banned interracial marriage.[15] The eugenicist thinking that informed these policies also shaped the state response to other genetic disease outbreaks, including Huntington's chorea in the early twentieth century.[16] In the 1960s, following the outbreak of rubella, a movement of doctors, religious leaders, and lawmakers presented abortion as a necessary procedure that protected both women from giving birth to children with physical and intellectual disabilities and society from having to pay for their care. The fact that society perceived rubella as mostly afflicting white, heterosexual, middle-class women deemed responsible and respectable helped to liberalize attitudes to abortion.[17] In the presence of fetal defects, abortions for family and eugenicist reasons are perceived as acceptable by many. In its response to AIDS, the government told all "at risk" women—a designation that implied HIV impacted only certain women to the detriment of public health—to get tested and advised those who tested positive not to have children. As the obstetricians Howard L. Minkoff and Richard H. Schwarz noted, "The majority of births in Brooklyn are to women not in high-risk groups and most women in high-risk groups do not have antibody [sic]."[18] The government's response to HIV drew on the same tactics used to tackle congenital diseases in the past.

Whether or not doctors like Abitbol provided substandard care, their view that HIV-positive women should end their pregnancies aligned with prevailing medical opinion. Physicians and public health professionals published articles in prominent medical journals such as JAMA, and key professional bodies, including the American College of Obstetricians and Gynecologists, released statements supporting the position that HIV-positive women should postpone pregnancy or end their pregnancies if already pregnant, citing the possibility of them transmitting HIV to their infants and the chance that pregnancy might accelerate their own illnesses.[19] These recommendations followed CDC guidelines, published in 1985, urging women considering pregnancy to get tested for HIV and advising those who tested positive to "delay" or postpone pregnancy "until more is known about perinatal transmission of the virus."[20] All states bar New Jersey followed the CDC in advising HIV-positive women to avoid pregnancy.[21] The advice mirrored that given to women in the context of Huntington's chorea and rubella, whom physicians and social workers told to delay or end pregnancy either through abortion, abstinence, or sterilization.[22] Although the CDC did not offer suggestions for how a woman might delay becoming pregnant, women's health advocates such as the physicians Carola Marte and Kathryn Anastos argued that without the prospect of a vaccine or cure coming soon, and in light of the increasing limits placed on abortion access in the form of public funding restrictions and physical harassment, the government could only achieve its goal of preventing the birth of HIV-positive infants if HIV-positive women did not have children.[23] Without access to legal and affordable abortion, they and other feminist health workers feared that doctors might encourage women to undergo sterilization against their will. As Jennifer Nelson noted, the threat of involuntary sterilization increased in the absence of legal abortion.[24]

Physicians spoke more candidly beyond the pages of academic journals. At a 1988 conference on AIDS in the workplace, the director of the CDC's AIDS program, James Curran, described undetected cases of AIDS in pregnancy as "a national tragedy" and asserted that the imperative to test pregnant women for HIV exceeded that of rubella or syphilis because AIDS "is much, much, much, much worse. With AIDS, the baby will die and the mother will die." Curran raised alarm not only about AIDS mortality but, dovetailing with federal efforts to reduce health-care spending under Reagan, he also raised concern about the cost HIV-positive children posed to the state. Through the 1981 Omnibus Budget Reconciliation Act, Reagan introduced block grants that gave states less money for health and welfare programs but greater discretion over how to spend it, enabling them to reduce the number of people eligible for support. He also refused to commit more federal resources to address AIDS.[25] Vilifying people reliant on state aid, Reagan in his policy agenda shaped a political discourse hostile to welfare, which crystalized a decade later in the major welfare reform of President Bill Clinton.[26] As Congress worked to shrink the federal contribution to Medicaid, Curran also argued that HIV-positive women should avoid pregnancy to reduce health-care costs. The "small state" rhetoric of the Reagan administration, which exploited deep-seated racist and gendered stereotypes about who is deserving of state support, informed Curran. Arguing that as the expense of pediatric AIDS exceeded that of adults, and that "Babies with AIDS have no parents"—a sweeping statement that lacked qualification—Curran protested that the burden of care would fall to the state. Although Curran's concerns over AIDS mortality were not unfounded—in 1988, HIV/AIDS was listed as the underlying cause of death for 249 children aged younger than fifteen and 1,430 for women aged 15 to 44—calling HIV-positive women who wanted to become pregnant illogical betrayed his disregard for the multifaceted reasons behind a woman's wish to have a child.[27] Such inflammatory comments, reprinted in mainstream media outlets like the *Washington Post*, contributed to the presentation of HIV-positive women who became pregnant or continued a pregnancy as selfish and created a perception of "crisis" in which coercive testing policies and advice appeared more acceptable.[28] Some male journalists agreed on the necessity of abortion in the presence of diseases, callously noting, "any pregnant woman who has the lethal AIDS virus" or whose newborn "will have a non-fatal affliction such as spina bifida or Down's syndrome . . . won't find me barring the door to the abortion clinic."[29] These comments reveal assumptions about who should decide whether and when pregnancies continue or end and when it should be appropriate. Here, male journalists echoed the view of leading male physicians that the moral and social cost of caring for sick infants outweighed the rights of HIV-positive women and their prospective children—a view which reflected the anti-welfare politics of the period in which they operated as well as the deep cultural anxiety about infant mortality and disability in children as seen throughout the twentieth century.[30]

The historical association between genetic testing, the eugenics movement, and racist, classist, and ableist reproductive control informed women's health advocates and activists' concerns over federal and state efforts to test HIV-positive pregnant women and infants.[31] Since the discovery of AIDS in the early 1980s, male and female AIDS activists called for voluntary, anonymous, or confidential —as opposed to mass, mandatory —HIV testing to protect against discrimination in employment, insurance, housing, medical services, and reproductive rights.[32]

States approached HIV testing differently and lacked uniformity in the application of this public health measure. Authorities required doctors to test all pregnant women in Florida and Michigan, and in Rhode Island, doctors did not need maternal consent to test newborns. Oregon directed medics to reveal the names of infants who tested positive at anonymous testing sites. In 1987, New York mandated that doctors offer counseling and voluntary testing to all pregnant women.[33] Testing infants for antibodies only revealed the HIV status of the mother, as infants receive antibodies against infections from women while in the womb that they keep for a period after birth. An infant that tested "positive" may not have become infected with the virus. Instead, many women first learned of their positive status when doctors found HIV antibodies in the blood of their newborn child.[34] Women's health advocates criticized the strategy of using an infant's test results as a "proxy" for a woman's status, instead of offering voluntary testing, counseling, and follow-up treatment to all women considering pregnancy and all pregnant women giving birth. Moreover, widespread cuts to prenatal care and family -planning services, and abortion restrictions that limited women's ability to translate knowledge of their status into action, raised concerns that health authorities might use the test results against women.[35]

During the 1980s, the CDC and state health departments also carried out large-scale, anonymous testing on newborn infants to track rates of HIV in women. Doctors did not obtain the consent of patients because the results were intended to direct education and services and not identify individuals with HIV.[36] In 1989, calls to "unblind" the results of the New York State Department of Health's anonymous study on newborns raised alarm that, under the guise of "fetal rights," health authorities might reveal the status of HIV-positive women without their consent and use the results against them.[37] In 1993, the New York State Assemblywoman Nettie Mayersohn (D-Flushing, Queens) introduced legislation requiring doctors to inform parents of the HIV status of their child without their consent "for the purpose of saving the infant's life," which "must be our first concern."[38] Mayersohn dismissed the fact that women could voluntarily learn their status and that of their child, and that identifying an infant with HIV also revealed the status of its mother who never consented to the test.[39] Other commentators noted that her "Baby AIDS" bill did not connect women to health or social care, undermining the claim that revealing the results would help women.[40] In 1989, doctors at New York's Harlem Hospital anonymously tested all newborns to track rates of maternal drug use. Doctors reported 364 women in the study to Children's Services for using drugs during pregnancy, of whom 245 had their infants removed at birth and placed directly into foster care. Thirty-nine of the children had HIV.[41] The debate around "unblinding" test results drew on the language of fetal rights to reinforce the perception that the state needed to intervene in the reproductive lives of women on behalf of infants.

The passage of HIV criminalization laws in the 1980s raised the stakes of testing initiatives. Driven by what the sociologist Trevor Hoppe described as the combined impetus to control disease through coercion and punishment and regulate sex and gender norms in the postwar period, eight states—Florida, Georgia, Idaho, Michigan, Missouri, Oklahoma, South Carolina, and Washington—enacted HIV exposure or nondisclosure laws before 1989. Implemented in mostly Republican states, these laws reflected the reach of the political agenda to "criminalize sickness." Lawmakers initially used the media panic over sex workers "carrying" AIDS to the "general" population to pass laws making HIV-specific offences felonies. These laws targeted sex workers but then were applied to all people living with HIV.[42] In 1990, the government reinforced these efforts through federal law, passing the Ryan White CARE Act, which provided states with funding for AIDS services. The act also made receipt of federal funding dependent on a state's willingness to use criminal laws to prosecute any HIV-positive person who knowingly exposed a non-consenting adult to HIV.[43] Forty-five states enacted measures that made possible the criminalization of HIV exposure and transmission, and this legislation continues in thirty-five of them. The Ryan White CARE Act not only criminalized sexual activity but also made possible the criminalization of HIV-positive women's pregnancies. The broad wording of these laws enabled the prosecution of HIV-positive women in relation to their pregnancies in most states.[44] While little data exists on the numbers of women prosecuted for transmitting or exposing their child to HIV, the reported cases confirm that state authorities have used positive test results to detain women because of their pregnancies and assume custody of HIV-positive children.[45]

The notion that the state should protect "innocent" citizens from the supposedly "immoral" behavior of people with HIV overlapped with efforts to punish women for using substances that allegedly harmed their fetuses during pregnancy. In 1985, the publication of a dubious medical study claiming that crack cocaine use during pregnancy harmed fetuses dovetailed with a moral panic about rising rates of drug use in Black communities and the supposed decline of Black families, both of which lawmakers, in political backlash against women's and civil rights, blamed on Black single mothers.[46] The report sparked public outcry that empowered law enforcement to target drug users as well as drug dealers, including pregnant women.[47] The focus on crack cocaine revealed the racism underlying these initiatives, just as the disproportionate targeting of women in public hospitals exposed class biases. Although white women used cocaine at a similar level to Black women, Black communities tended to smoke it in crack form.[48] Moreover, medical professionals also tested the urine of Black pregnant patients without their consent more regularly, reporting those who tested positive to the police and child welfare services.[49] Judges also tended to prosecute the Black women whose cases came before them at higher rates than white women.[50] The media representation of crack babies as Black solidified the association between the new so-called underclass of infants supposedly destined to grow into "troublesome" children, just as the media discussion of fetal alcohol syndrome framed it as an "Indian problem" for which judges sent Native women to prison and removed children from their care.[51] That doctors who tested women for drugs also tested them for HIV underscores how the war on crack cocaine overlapped with the AIDS epidemic to put multiply marginalized women who wanted to have children at risk of punitive state intervention.[52]

As Carol Mason argued, abortion opponents' calls for "fetal protection" took on a new meaning in the context of state efforts to regulate women of color's pregnancies. While antiabortion advocates pushed for restrictions like the partial-birth abortion ban to stop white women from ending their pregnancies, the threat of punishment disproportionately leveled against Black and Native American women encouraged them to end their pregnancies, suggesting that a racist desire to not only protect fetuses from the actions of women but society from the social and financial cost of supporting children described as "undesirable" and "degenerate" drove these measures.[53] State and federal legislation that criminalized HIV transmission and exposure, coupled with the vilification of women wanting to continue their pregnancies, surely encouraged abortion in general. As Koop noted, "In major obstetrical clinics on the East Coast, where the population has a high incidence of AIDS virus . . . women who are pregnant under 13 weeks are being advised to have abortions and about 50 percent of those, I understand, are indeed having abortions."[54] Criminal legislation encouraged abortion without lawmakers endorsing the procedure out loud.[55]

Two days after the National Press Club incident, Gary L. Bauer, assistant to the president, told Marlin Fitzwater, assistant to the president for press relations, that if anyone asked, "Did Surgeon General Koop advocate abortion for women whose unborn children test positive for AIDS?" to reply: "Dr. Koop answered a hypothetical question about the availability of information on abortion in our society. As you know, this Administration is opposed to abortion on demand. Dr. Koop has a distinguished record as an advocate for the right to life of all unborn children. We simply do not believe that the way to fight this disease is by killing the patient."[56]

Bauer's comments exemplified the political discourse that framed the ongoing debates over abortion, reproductive justice, and AIDS by 1987. The 1976 Hyde Amendment prohibited using Medicaid funding for an abortion unless the pregnancy threatened a woman's life. The Supreme Court upheld the decision to refuse federal funding for "nontherapeutic" abortion one year later in *Beal v. Doe* and *Maher v. Roe*.[57] Following the federal government, many states stopped funding "medically unnecessary" abortions, framed by opponents as "abortion on demand."[58] Moreover, in remarking on "the right to life of all unborn children" and identifying a fetus as a "child" separate from a woman, Bauer drew on the rhetoric of the advancing fetal rights movement that worked to elevate the status of a fetus to that of a child in the post-*Roe* years.[59] During this time, antiabortion activists also appropriated the language of the women's health-care movement in arguing that women suffered permanent psychological damage after undergoing an abortion in a phenomenon known as PAS.[60] Historians such as Sara Dubow have adeptly shown how the political culture of the 1980s and 1990s increasingly presented the interests and rights of pregnant women as distinct from those of the fetus.[61] Nonetheless, histories of abortion in the late twentieth century have underacknowledged how the emergence of the AIDS epidemic contributed to this development, addressing how in this case the "patient" became the "unborn" instead of the woman who carried it. The actions of Surgeon General Koop reveal how AIDS shaped the debates over fetal rights in the 1980s, and the importance of adding the history of AIDS to the battle over reproductive justice.

DR. KOOP AND THE AIDS QUESTION

The remit of the US surgeon general is to deal with the cause, control, and prevention of disease. In April 1989, the journalist Margaret Carlson published a profile on Koop in *Time* magazine, explaining how "Koop was expected to be a figurehead like most Surgeon Generals, with little authority and few staff or duties."[62] Nominated by the sitting president, the position of surgeon general is a partisan role. During his heated confirmation battles, National Organization for Women (NOW), the American Public Health Association (APHA), and several other progressive organizations, lawmakers, and medical professionals argued that Koop's personal beliefs, in particular his rigid opposition to abortion, made him unsuitable to serve as the nation's chief public health official.[63] According to the regulations, Koop was also too old for the job. Nonetheless, Republican congressmen worked hard and even bent the rules to get Koop into office, convinced he would advance the religious right's health agenda. Congress voted to lift the age restriction and confirmed Koop as the thirteenth surgeon general by a vote of 68 to 24 in November 1981.[64] Despite his commitment to take the responsibilities of his office seriously, his boss, Assistant Secretary for Health Edward Brandt, marginalized him during his first term in office.[65] Koop took a more active role after James O. Mason replaced Brandt in 1984 and, in the words of Carlson, he "quickly shook things up."[66] He wrote reports denouncing smoking while advocating for the rights of disabled children. He applied the same public health pragmatism that drove his approach to smoking and other public health issues to tackling one of the greatest health crises in US history.[67]

Koop described AIDS as a disease "made for a Surgeon General." But his first major opportunity to speak publicly about the disease did not come until February 1986 when, midway through his second term in office and five years after the CDC first reported on cases of AIDS-related diseases, Reagan instructed Koop to "prepare a report on AIDS for the people of the United States."[68] Koop's exclusion from the initial government AIDS response allowed him to develop an understanding of the disease grounded not in politics but in science.[69] As a result, Koop denounced the most extreme proposals of the political and religious right to control HIV as medically inappropriate. In so doing, he broke with social conservatives in the administration and pursued an agenda rooted in pragmatic public health.

Koop sought the input of organizations leading the early AIDS response. Over the next several months, after receiving reassurance from Secretary of Health and Human Services Dr. Otis Bowen of his sole authority over the report, he invited twenty-seven groups representing AIDS advocacy, business, politics, education, health, labor, and religion to his office at the NIH and conducted meetings that shaped his perspective on AIDS. In addition to consulting government experts like the immunologist Dr. Anthony Fauci from the NIH, Koop and his team met with groups ranging from the National Hemophilia Foundation, the Christian Life Council of the Southern Baptist Convention, the National Education Association, the National Coalition of Black Lesbians and Gays, and the National Minority AIDS Council. The information these diverse organizations shared informed Koop's understanding of methods of transmission and prevention. They confirmed that HIV did not spread through nonsexual, casual contact, disproving the need to quarantine people with HIV/AIDS or deny them housing, employment, or public education. The meetings also informed the report's frankness, which emphasized that HIV is spread through blood and semen as opposed to "bodily fluids." In October 1986, after seventeen drafts, Koop was ready to reveal his report.[70]

AIDS organizations, advocacy groups, politicians, and the press waited anxiously for Koop to release the first major government health report on AIDS. Koop began by confronting the "rumors and misinformation" about transmission, namely, that HIV was spread through casual, nonsexual contact. Moreover, he argued that the reticence in dealing with the subjects of "sex, sexual practices, and homosexuality" undermined education efforts, especially among youth and racial and ethnic minority communities. Imploring that "this silence must end," Koop proposed three solutions. First, he called for candid discussions about sexual practices, both homosexual and heterosexual, and suggested that sex education in school begin as early as possible "so that children can grow up knowing the behaviors to avoid to protect themselves from exposure to the AIDS virus." Second, he stated that the use of a condom, aside from abstinence, provided the best protection against infection during sex. Third, he denounced the quarantining of people with HIV/AIDS and mandatory blood testing, as HIV did not spread through casual contact and, as with syphilis, mass blood testing was "unnecessary, unfeasible, and cost prohibitive." The PHS distributed twenty-two million copies of the report through newspapers, members of Congress, public health organizations, and parent-teacher associations, breaking the almost total silence that had characterized the White House response to the epidemic thus far.[71]

Koop's endorsement of condom use, sex education, and his frank description of HIV transmission offended conservative advisers to the president, in particular White House aides Robert "Bob" Sweet, Carl Anderson, Becky Dunlap, and Gary Bauer, as well as Secretary of

Education William Bennett, whom Koop admonished for failing to see the necessity of school-based sex education. For Koop, the "death threat posed by AIDS mandated school-based education," and he recommended that sex education begin as early as possible.[72] Members of Reagan's Domestic Policy Council (DPC), such as Bennett and HHS staff, including Koop, also disagreed on the tone of HHS-led AIDS education initiatives, including whether schools should address "the moral context of sex education about AIDS" or treat it "purely as a public health matter."[73] The DPC and HHS eventually agreed that the federal government should consult educators, providing them with accurate health information, but not mandate a specific curriculum, leaving the delivery of AIDS education to local schools.[74] The right-wing activist Phyllis Schlafly nonetheless commented that Koop's report "looks and reads like it was edited by the Gay Task Force," accusing him of teaching "safe sodomy" to third-graders.[75] Koop betrayed the hopes of such prominent figures on the political right who saw him as failing to promote the conservative tenets of abstinence, fidelity, and heterosexual marriage as HIV prevention.

In contrast, the groups with whom he originally met to prepare the report received it positively. Gil Gerald, executive director of the National Coalition of Black Lesbians and Gays, praised Koop for exceeding his expectations in addressing "the issue of AIDS in Black and Brown communities."[76] Gary B. MacDonald, executive director of the AIDS Action Council, similarly wrote to "congratulate and commend" Koop "on the excellent report to the nation on AIDS that you released today [which] will do much to combat fear and hysteria, and, we hope, to encourage rational, scientifically-based responses to this crisis."[77] Koop received numerous letters echoing these sentiments from members of the medical community as well as the public, who thanked him for his "forthright leadership on AIDS."[78] Journalists similarly praised the report for urging "Americans to put aside prejudices they may have against homosexuals and intravenous drug users, to help victims of this epidemic and to stop talking nonsense about quarantines, universal blood tests and tattoos for those who test positive," and for setting a "standard for other government officials—federal, state and local—in dealing with AIDS and its victims."[79] Many praised what they saw as an "honest" report, absent the biases that informed the political right's response to the epidemic.[80]

When Reagan first nominated Koop to the position of surgeon general in early 1981, many activists, politicians, and medical professionals saw the appointment in terms of the larger threat the Reagan administration posed to legal abortion. Their concerns arose from Koop's involvement in the provocative antiabortion film *Whatever Happened to the Human Race?*, which he narrated and produced with evangelical theologian Dr. Francis Schaeffer.[81] Nonetheless, after six years in the job, Koop surprised his supporters as well as his critics. Democrats and organizations originally opposed to Koop's confirmation now backed him, while Republicans who had formerly offered support now denounced him. Koop's call for a larger government role in fighting AIDS, coupled with his endorsement of condoms, sex education, and clean needles, infuriated his conservative former allies and pleased his new supporters.[82] In the year following the publication of his AIDS report, conservatives in the administration felt betrayed again after Koop refused to condemn abortion as psychologically harmful to women. In this context, Koop's new detractors criticized his AIDS response for not only morally offending most Americans but also for taking resources away from what they deemed the more pressing issue of PAS. The same sense of duty to uphold medical standards that shaped Koop's AIDS response now shaped his response to PAS. In refusing to lie against the scientific evidence, he counterbalanced antiabortion advocates who invented nonmedically recognized, political concepts such as PAS and "partial-birth abortions" to attack women's reproductive rights.[83] Seeing abortion as a medically viable, if morally undesirable, HIV-prevention option, Koop argued that abortion opponents should challenge the procedure on moral grounds over the sanctity of life, not women's health.[84] While his duty to uphold public health drove him to offer legal, available, and nonpermanent ways for HIV-positive women to prevent conception, his stated aim to "protect" fetuses from the women of whose bodies they were a part advanced the view of women's bodies as harmful hosts. The absence of a surgeon general's report affirming the safety of abortion for women equally left room to question it. Moreover, Koop's promotion of the idea that life begins at conception and a fetus is an unborn child informed abortion restrictions that similarly drew on and furthered the discourse of fetal rights.

THE ANTIABORTIONIST SURGEON GENERAL AND THE BUREAUCRAT

The emergence of the AIDS epidemic in the early 1980s converged with the fraught battles over abortion and reproductive rights, which did not always fall neatly along party lines. Several Republican women supported Planned Parenthood and abortion. Others in the Republican party, such as Sweet, a senior member of the Office of Policy Development in Reagan's DPC and a former chemistry teacher from Maine, represented the larger push toward a more coercive approach to reproductive health care that accompanied the rise of the fetal rights movement. Whereas pro-life conservatives like Sweet felt that Koop owed the administration a report damning abortion as harmful to women as payment for his AIDS report, women's health advocates such as Faye Wattleton of Planned Parenthood worried about the implications of a government report claiming that abortion caused mental trauma in women.[85] Beginning her career as a nurse at the Miami Valley Hospital School of Nursing in Dayton, Ohio, and serving as president of the local Planned Parenthood chapter, Wattleton represented reproductive justice activists fighting to resist the political, legal, deceitful, and violent strategies of those seeking to obliterate women's access to abortion in the late 1970s and early 1980s.[86] Similar to Wattleton, whom Planned Parenthood elected in 1978 as its youngest and first Black president, Black women often spearheaded these efforts.[87] An abortion opponent committed to fulfilling the duties of his office, Koop straddled this broader divide within the Republican party over abortion. As with AIDS, none of the stakeholders knew how the surgeon general would approach writing a public health report on the subject.

In January 1987, three months after Koop published *The Surgeon General's Report on Acquired Immune Deficiency Syndrome*, Reagan invited a group of antiabortion leaders to the White House and informed them of his plan to direct "the Surgeon General to issue a comprehensive medical report on the health effects, physical and emotional, of abortion on women." Reagan promised to produce a "thorough and solid body of public health information on the effects of abortion on women," because "growing numbers of women who've had abortions now say that they have been misled by inaccurate information. Making accurate data on maternal morbidity available to women before an abortion is performed is an essential element of informed consent."[88] Koop's efforts frustrated antiabortionists who viewed his actions, in particular his completion of Reagan's instruction to prepare a "report to the American people on AIDS" in 1986 and his refusal to complete Reagan's instruction one year later to publish a medical report on the health effects of abortion on women, as a missed opportunity to strike a practical blow against *Roe v. Wade.*

Koop retraced the initial steps he took to prepare his AIDS report in planning his report on abortion, seeking to balance what he described as his private principles with public service.[89] Koop approached AIDS as a public health rather than a moral issue, while treating abortion as an issue of morality that therefore lay beyond the scope of his office. However, since *Roe*, the antiabortion movement had worked to prove the negative psychological impact of abortion on women. Reagan's call for an abortion report tapped into these same "woman-centered" antiabortion arguments that appropriated the language and tactics of the women's health movement, claiming that abortions often caused long-term psychological damage.[90] In making calls for "informed consent," Reagan also lifted the language of women's health activists who wanted to ensure that pregnant women and women considering pregnancy understood the possible risks and benefits of HIV testing. Evidence of the disconnect between rhetoric and action, as feminist health advocates fought for free or affordable quality health care for all women, the Reagan administration cut funding to the social programs that provided women with nutrition, maternal, and reproductive health care.[91]

Reagan's actions earned him the ire of some Republican women who supported Wattleton's efforts to protect a woman's right to abortion. Margaret J. Atwood, a "life-long Republican" from Connecticut, wrote to tell the "pig-headed" president that she would "never vote again for any person who is against abortion" as "no man should legislate against Women's rights."[92] In May 1987, Pandora M. Cooke from Alabama signed a petition from Wattleton to the White House concurring that Reagan's "efforts to make medically safe abortions illegal will cause untold suffering for millions of women." In an accompanying letter, Cooke told the president, "As a thirty-five-year-old mother of one, wife, career woman, and Christian, the moral rights and responsibilities of each of us must be upheld. . . . *The disservice that would be done in deleting the freedom of choice would be as criminal as unnecessary abortion.*" Asserting, "You cannot regulate how a woman feels about her body and an unwanted or unhealthy pregnancy, anymore [sic] than you can regulate free commerce and trade," she called on the president to "rethink" his "position" as "in this case, even fence-sitting would be better."[93] Opposition to abortion did not unite conservative women in this period.

The election in 1980 of Ronald Reagan as US president energized those in the antiabortion movement who had helped him win office.[94] From the outset, antiabortion advocates within government worked to separate "the Federal government from the performance of and referral for abortion."[95] Immediately after *Roe*, abortion opponents in Congress worked to recriminalize the procedure through the passage of a Human Life Amendment.[96] As efforts to pass a congressional amendment undoing *Roe* waned but calls to cut welfare grew, antiabortion activists shifted tactics, focusing on restricting access to legal services for low-income women.[97] In addition to the 1976 Hyde Amendment—the first major victory for antiabortion activists—this strategy also involved proposals to amend Title X of the Public Health Service Act, the federal program funding reproductive health services for low-income women. The amendment prohibited health-care workers in Title X family -planning clinics from providing patients with abortion referrals or information and required clinics to physically and financially separate its abortion-related activities funded through other sources from its Title X activities. The Supreme Court affirmed the constitutionality of the policy, known as the "domestic gag-rule," in the 1991 case *Rust v. Sullivan*, but Bill Clinton rescinded it when he came to office one year later.[98] The proposal to amend Title X proved additionally controversial when, in January 1987, Robert E. Windom, assistant secretary for health, reprimanded abortion opponent Jo Ann Gasper, the deputy assistant secretary for population affairs, for sending letters to ten regional health directors informing them that Planned Parenthood's "support" for abortion put it in violation of the PHS Act without authorization.[99]

The incident with Gasper upset antiabortion members of the administration as well as Congressmen like Jesse Helms (R-NC), who demanded her reinstatement.[100] Koop suspected that Reagan called for the abortion report to placate their concerns. He also speculated that the report represented an attempt on the part of the president to "distract me from my blunt and realistic approach to AIDS."[101] Despite its efforts to thwart abortion access, the Reagan administration, over two terms, failed to end legal abortion.[102] Whatever Reagan's motive, Koop accepted the assignment with the assurance of his sole control over the report. Although he believed that the question of abortion and its health effects on women could not draw on the same kind of "unassailable" and "correct" scientific data and interpretation as the AIDS report, Koop got to work.[103]

Koop and his team met with national organizations on both sides of the abortion debate. As he had with the AIDS report, he planned to synthesize several different perspectives in his recommendations. Although seemingly neutral, the bipartisan consultations that began with meetings with Planned Parenthood and other women's health activists testified to the connections Koop established with these groups through his work on AIDS.[104] A delegation from Planned Parenthood and other pro-abortion groups gave presentations that provided extensive information on the alleged connection between abortion and mental and physical health issues. The meeting concluded with Wattleton drawing on her personal experiences to communicate the different factors informing a woman's wish to end a pregnancy.[105] Working as a nurse in Harlem in the mid-1960s, Wattleton had witnessed hundreds of women who, like others across the country, visited the hospital suffering from the complications of an incomplete abortion.[106]

As with many of his other former critics, Wattleton's opinion of Koop changed because of his AIDS work. Wattleton assumed a role in educating the public about HIV/AIDS in the 1980s and credited Koop for refusing to back down on his position that people use condoms to prevent transmission of the virus. For Wattleton, Koop's AIDS interventions earned him the "guarded support" of those originally worried that he might forsake public health advice to pursue an ideological agenda.[107] Commenting on the unexpected alliance that developed between Koop and Planned Parenthood, a journalist writing for the *Washington Post* observed, "It isn't often that Planned Parenthood and the Reagan administration see eye to eye, but a national crisis has brought them together on at least one subject: AIDS. A report issued earlier this week by Surgeon General C. Everett Koop drew praise from the family-planning group specifically because it urges sex education in schools at the earliest possible grade."[108] Planned Parenthood credited Koop for pursuing a public health response to AIDS.

Just over one year into the planning of the surgeon general's report on abortion, the growing pressure the administration exerted on Koop matched his growing conviction of the infeasibility of the task. Most of the evidence he and his team had gathered from their interviews consisted of anecdotes of women who regretted their abortion and others who said it saved their marriage. But anecdotes, argued Koop, did not make statistics.[109] While stories long served as a powerful tool for women to assert credible knowledge about their bodies and lives, in this case, statistics worked more in women's favor.[110]

Members of Reagan's DPC, such as Sweet, grew increasingly frustrated as Koop explained that he could not reach a defensible conclusion on the question of whether abortion harmed women based on the existing evidence. Moreover, he noted that a thorough study of the issue would cost between $10 and $100 million. Koop suggested that he could either meet with the president to explain the problem or put it in a letter. Bauer advised Koop to continue with his report, and a White House staffer echoed that the president never changed his mind.[111]

As Koop expressed his misgivings about the abortion report, antiabortion members of the administration continued to protest the seemingly misplaced nature of the surgeon general's priorities. Sweet told Nancy Risque, deputy assistant to the president and cabinet secretary, "After listening to Dr. Koop last Wednesday I had the clear impression that he was not interested in doing research on post abortion syndrome, felt it couldn't be done or would cost $1 billion . . . . Abortion is the most frequent surgical procedure used in medicine today. Yet we spend virtually nothing to research the impact of this traumatic event on women, physicians and nurses to say nothing of the baby." He complained, "AIDS on the other hand is a recent phenomenon with a total estimated infected US population of less than four tenths of one percent and we are spending nearly $1.5 billion on AIDS in 1988 alone." He implored, "In God's name what is wrong with us? Where are our priorities? Have we lost our moral compass? The blood of our children crys [sic] out to us from the ground. Will no one listen?"[112] Conservatives like Sweet appropriated the language of fetal rights to oppose a compassionate and humane public health response to AIDS.

Koop appeared to confirm Sweet's concern that he cared more about AIDS than PAS as, in May 1988, in one of his last acts as surgeon general, he, along with the CDC, sent an eight-page, condensed version of his AIDS report to all 107 million households in the US. Costing approximately $20 million and unprecedented in its size and sexual content, the brochure explained, "You can become infected by having sex—oral, anal or vaginal—with someone who is infected with the AIDS virus."[113] Someone in Reagan's administration circled the words "vagina," "penis," "rectum," and "anal intercourse" on their copy, with an annotation that asked, "Is this appropriate for children? Won't parents be offended?"[114]

In addition to taking offense over the brochure's content, antiabortionists like Sweet also argued that the "unsolicited" amount of money spent on AIDS took resources away from the more pressing issue of recriminalizing abortion. Sweet called for the government to put as many resources into publicizing the surgeon general's report on abortion as it had on promoting the AIDS brochure. The government should send a mass mailing, argued Sweet, "with a great deal of publicity along the lines of the Surgeon General's report on AIDS." Moreover, drawing on the fetal right movement's use of audio and visual materials to promote the concept of fetal personhood in this period, Sweet called on the government to circulate "a high-quality, colorful booklet that is simply and clearly written describing fetal development at different stages, including the baby's capacity for pain; a description of the different abortion procedures and their effect on the baby; their possible effects on the mother; and, services for women seeking alternatives to abortion."[115] For Sweet, the proactive steps Koop took to respond to AIDS revealed how little institutional weight he put behind affirming the medical credibility of PAS.

On January 9, 1989, two years after Reagan ordered Koop to prepare a report on the health effects of abortion on women, Koop wrote to the president explaining that the lack of scientific research on the effects of abortion on women's health prohibited him from writing one.[116] In refusing to tow the antiabortion line, Koop was condemned by Sweet for missing his opportunity to "educate the American people and put our priorities back in order."[117] The administration continued to fight to secure the abortion report for the president before he left office. Risque sent Reagan a memo recommending that he direct the HHS to proceed immediately with the design of a survey to produce "reliable raw data" upon which to base a study on the health effects of abortion on women. Although the recommendation had a tick next to it, the opportunity passed with George H. W. Bush's incoming administration.[118] Whereas the *Washington Post* journalist Michael Specter remarked, "Many conservatives assumed the abortion report would present Koop with an opportunity to even the score," after alienating them over AIDS, abortion opponents and religious leaders accused Koop of betraying the antiabortion movement.[119] But the absence of a surgeon general's report affirming the safety of abortion for women also left room to question it.

In the early 1990s, articles published in medical journals affirmed that PAS, as a medical syndrome, did not exist.[120] Although Koop refused to lie against the scientific evidence, the idea that abortion harmed women, and that the procedure constituted the "slaughter of the unborn," informed legislation restricting abortion access from the late 1980s onward. Koop left office in October 1989, a few months after the Supreme Court, in *Webster v. Reproductive Health Services*, upheld the right of states to deny women access to abortion counseling and procedures in all publicly funded facilities and to require testing for viability if a woman was twenty or more weeks pregnant. The preamble to *Webster* drew on Koop's language of fetal rights, stating "the life of each human being begins at conception" and "unborn children have protectable interests in life, health, and wellbeing."[121] *Webster* set a precedent for further restrictions.[122] In the 1992 case *Planned Parenthood v. Casey*, the Supreme Court allowed states to restrict abortions during the first trimester of pregnancy—something which *Roe* prohibited—as well as require a twenty-four-hour waiting period before abortion and parental consent for minors.[123] Other states introduced restrictions, including mandated counseling before an abortion, wait times, and warnings about the procedure's psychological risks.[124] These restrictions made abortion more expensive and less accessible for all women, and especially low-income and young women, and women of color with restricted access to health care, in the following decades.[125] Although victories for the antiabortion movement, these rulings were framed as defeats by those seeking to overturn *Roe*, an interpretation that galvanized the more extreme branch of the Republican party to push for further restrictions in the 1990s and 2000s.[126]

The Reagan era ended with a stalemate at multiple levels for multiple people. The antiabortion movement did not secure their abortion report and the *Webster* decision stymied Planned Parenthood and Faye Wattleton, as well as doctors, other abortion providers, and those seeking abortion. The period also ended with the development of new factions that emerged to address the perceived "crisis" of infants neither prevented nor aborted but born to women living with HIV. This constructed "crisis" furthered the argument that HIV-positive women should not have children, which underwrote interventions into their reproductive freedoms.

BOARDER BABIES WITH AIDS

Whether women with HIV continued their pregnancies through choice or a lack of alternative options, for an approximately ten-year period between discovering perinatal transmission in 1985 and the approval of AZT for pregnant women in 1994, political figures and public health practitioners debated how to best address the needs of infants in the epidemic. While the historical literature on young people with AIDS tends to focus on school-aged children like Ryan White, an Indiana teenager who contracted HIV through a blood transfusion in the early 1980s, and whose name is attached to the largest federally funded program for HIV, a focus on infants demonstrates how efforts to address perinatal AIDS dovetailed with the monitoring of women of color's pregnancies as part of the war on crack cocaine and the strengthening fetal rights movement.[127] Many of these children lost parents or guardians to AIDS mortality or to child welfare services that removed them from their care.[128]

In a photograph taken in the summer of 1987, five women join hands and form a closed circle as they crouch down on the floor, all their faces bar one obscured by the angle of the camera above them. Four of the five women hide their faces, wishing to remain anonymous. "If you show my face, I will lose my kids," one woman says.[129] The documentary photographer Ann P. Meredith took the picture at a women's support group for HIV/AIDS in San Francisco. In March 1987, Meredith had attended the first workshop on AIDS at the Eye Photography Gallery in the city. A participant at the workshop stood up and recounted the story of Meredith Miller, who had her two children removed from her care. She felt isolated as one of the few women known to have HIV, but she was not alone. Other women Meredith met spoke of losing custody of their children or worrying about who would care for their children if they died, or making the painful decision to put their children up for adoption.[130] Rhoda, a single mother of three, who previously felt relieved when she found an experimental drug trial that accepted women, tried not to worry that researchers had belatedly discovered that the drug caused vaginal cancer in mice. She did worry about what might happen to her children in the future.[131]

The public discussion of HIV-positive women tended not to reflect the deep pain, anxiety, and grief they expressed about their illness and its effect on their children, or the structural inequalities that may have hampered their ability to provide for their care.[132] Instead, reporters often associated HIV-positive women's pregnancies with drug use and risky sex that took place outside of marriage. Describing HIV-positive infants, frequently depicted as poor and Black, "languishing" in pediatric wards, "abandoned by their mothers," this coverage perpetuated the historic devaluation of Black women's caregiving and underwrote government interventions into their reproductive lives.[133] Moreover, focusing on the social cost of such children reflected the anti-welfare politics of the period and underscored the perception that they posed a financial burden to society. Evidence of the gap between rhetoric and reality, new private charities, and not the government, took the initiative to establish foster homes to house affected children. Cuts to welfare services, which deepened family poverty and the likelihood of a child entering foster care, undermined the government message, shared through images of white, establishment women like First Lady Barbara Bush cradling Black children at AIDS houses, of its concern for children.[134] The need for privately run AIDS houses served as an example of the Reagan administration's reliance on private solutions to social problems.[135]

Throughout the decade, reproductive justice activists articulated the need to protect the rights of HIV-positive women to decide whether and when to have children. At the same time, a diverse coalition of organizations mobilized to protect a woman's right to abortion. New and existing organizations, such as the Committee for Abortion Rights and Against Sterilization Abuse, Reproductive Rights National Network, National Black Women's Health Project (NBWHP), Planned Parenthood, NOW, and the American Civil Liberties Union (ACLU) deployed a range of tactics in the fight to keep abortion legal and, critically, to make it accessible to all.[136] The Hyde Amendment already denied women who received Medicaid access to federal funds for abortion services. Since the passage of *Roe v. Wade* in 1973, the antiabortion movement had worked to decrease abortion access with the goal of recriminalization. Through decreases in federal and state funding, new restrictions, such as viability testing, parental consent laws, and mandatory waiting periods, and the pervasive harassment leveled against those seeking and those providing abortions, women increasingly found abortion, in the words of Marlene Gerber Fried, "legal but inaccessible."[137] By the 1990s, Medicaid plans covered abortion in only twelve states.[138] Gutting public funding for abortion forced women who could not afford to pay for one to continue their pregnancy.[139] Some abortion clinics also refused to perform abortions on HIV-positive women, further limiting their options to "delay" pregnancy.[140]

While abortion remained a prevention option for some, religious organizations, medical professionals, and other nongovernment actors began establishing structures for children and infants whose parents had died of AIDS or who came to foster care voluntarily or involuntarily through removal.[141] Mirroring politicians who promoted adoption as an alternative to abortion for young, poor, and unmarried pregnant women through policies such as the Adolescent Family Life Act in this period, conservative policymakers endorsed private foster homes as an expedient way to seem proactive in supporting children in the epidemic without contradicting their antiabortion stance, and to promote the conservative principles of volunteerism, individualism, and nonstate action.[142] In his 1985 State of the Union address, Reagan praised Clara Hale, a philanthropist who in 1970 established Hale House in New York to support infants and their mothers navigating substance use and related issues.[143] At the close of the decade, Barbara Bush offered children another symbolic gesture when she visited AIDS houses for HIV-positive children.

Those who established AIDS houses set out to respond to the needs of what journalists termed "boarder babies with AIDS."[144] "Boarder babies" referred to HIV-positive infants who, like infants apparently born addicted to crack cocaine and other substances, were deemed healthy enough by doctors to leave hospitals but, without parents or legal guardians, lacked a permanent home.[145] Journalists relayed that such infants often remained in hospital longer than medically required while waiting for placement in a foster home—financially crippling the medical system in the process.[146] Pediatricians at Harlem Hospital estimated that infants who lacked alternative means of accommodation stayed an average of 339 days at the hospital, four times the length of those with accommodation, with an average lifetime cost of hospital care at $90,347 per child, more than three times that of adults.[147] Medical professionals explained that a fear of contagion surrounding HIV-positive children inhibited foster-care placement.[148] The steps states such as New York took to remove children from hospitals mirrored the "dumping" of severely ill people from emergency rooms as a result of Medicaid cuts in the 1980s.[149]

In April 1987, Koop organized a workshop for "Children with HIV and Their Families" at the Children's Hospital of Philadelphia to field recommendations on how to reduce the "tremendous burden of this devastating condition especially among children."[150] Dr. Elaine Abrams and Dr. Stephen Nicholas, pediatricians at the Harlem Hospital, drew on racial stereotypes that linked Blackness with criminality when they presented institutionalized AIDS houses as a solution to address the "crisis" of boarder babies who, like "crack babies"—coded as Black in political and popular discourse—grew up to display aggressive behavior that arose partly from a "familial predisposition."[151] Abrams and Nicholas' proposal to establish AIDS houses to support these "abandoned" children drew upon similar rhetoric of the foundling hospitals created to care for so-called forgotten children in the early nineteenth century. The founders established both types of institutions to not only support children but to ease the financial strain they placed on city services. Describing the children who entered these institutions as "forgotten," "unwanted," or "abandoned," these discussions flattened the complex factors rooted in structural inequities that informed why a child came into care.

The legislation passed to support infants in the epidemic similarly stigmatized HIV-positive women. The 1988 Abandoned Infants Assistance (AIA) Act allocated funding to public and private organizations to carry out residential care programs for infants "abandoned" by mothers who used substances, as well as those with HIV. The act defined such infants and children as those who were "particularly difficult to place in foster homes" and aid they were "being abandoned in hospitals in increasing numbers by mothers dying of AIDS, or by parents incapable of providing adequate care."[152] Describing children who had lost parents to death, severe illness, or other factors as "abandoned" was especially cruel considering that child services involuntarily removed some children from the custody of HIV-positive women at birth.[153] The bipartisan support for this legislation reflected the power of the symbol of the child to move lawmakers to act.

That same year, Dr. Nicholas, in partnership with the Catholic Archdiocese of New York and other organizations, converted a four-story, red brick, former convent in Washington Heights into a residence for twenty-four HIV-positive children.[154] Named New York's Incarnation Children's Center, its opening coincided with that of Grandma's House, a residence for HIV-positive children located near Logan Circle in Washington, DC, which was funded through the DC Commission on Social Services and run by the sisters Debbie Tate and Joan McCarley for infants born with HIV.[155]

In March 1989, Barbara Bush visited Grandma's House and embodied the maternal role women have often assumed in their support of orphanages and unwed mother's homes. Dressed in a smart red suit with her signature pearls and gray permed hair that signaled respectability, photographers captured images of her embracing a baby, kissing a toddler, and playing with three young girls.[156] Through this coverage,

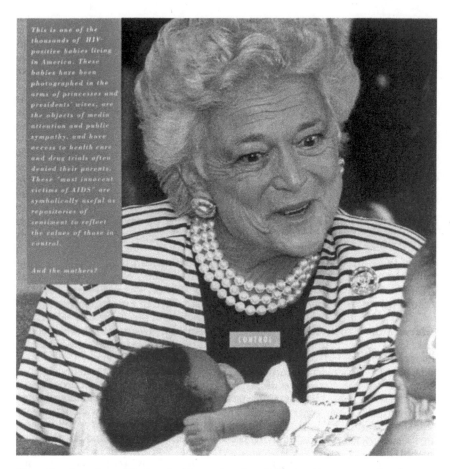

This is one of the thousands of HIV-positive babies living in America. These babies have been photographed in the arms of princesses and presidents' wives, are the objects of media attention and public sympathy, and have access to health care and drug trials often denied their parents. These "most innocent victims of AIDS" are symbolically useful as repositories of sentiment to reflect the values of those in control.

And the mothers?

CONTROL

Fig. 3. Gran Fury, Control [Barbara Bush], 1989. Gran Fury Collection. Manuscripts and Archives Division. The New York Public Library. Astor, Lenox, and Tilden Foundations.

the media presented Bush as an altruistic alternative to the women vilified as too "sick" or "disorganized" to care for their children.[157] In contrast to reports of "boarder babies" that erased the experiences and perspectives of HIV-positive mothers, the media depicted Bush as the respectable face of womanhood.

The images of Bush cradling and playing with HIV-positive children epitomized the "guilty-innocent" binary that shaped assumptions about who deserved sympathy for their illness, which often fell along racial, class, and gender lines and which, as the AIA Act underscored, also informed legislation.[158] As the art activist collective Gran Fury depicted in their 1989 poster "Control," Bush's visit played into the binary between "guilty" mother versus "innocent" child, as well as "guilty" mother versus "supportive" woman.

Noting, "With perinatal transmission of HIV on the increase, one would expect someone to be interested in the women bearing these children. Unfortunately, that has not been the case," the physician Janet Mitchell of the Harlem Hospital similarly highlighted the irony of the state marginalizing women's needs while expressing concern about their pregnancies.[159]

Critics of the antiabortion movement charged them with hypocrisy for expressing concern over the pregnancies of poor and non-white women, and claiming to care for Black fetuses, while doing nothing to support Black children, adolescents, and adults.[160] As the art historian, queer theory scholar, and AIDS activist Douglas Crimp noted, rhetoric about child welfare in the context of AIDS did not translate into funding for prenatal care, childcare, education, or other programs that helped children.[161] The government did not address AIDS by investing in services that would help women raise children with dignity but promoted messaging that blamed women for their illness and passed legislation that punished them for having children.

The deep investment of women in the health of their pregnancies, future children, and their newborns cast a very different light on the rhetoric that identified them as a health threat to their children. The emergence of AIDS houses in the late 1980s coincided with the results of the ACTG 076 trial, which proved the effectiveness of the antiretroviral drug AZT to block perinatal transmission of HIV. In 1994, the PHS recommended that pregnant women with HIV take AZT to reduce the risk of perinatal transmission of the virus.[162] The use of AZT during pregnancy led to a sharp drop-off in pediatric AIDS cases from the mid-1990s onward that eased much of the moral panic over mother-to-child transmission.[163] Nevertheless, the introduction of effective medicine also put women at increased risk of coerced HIV testing, as the CDC began recommending that states test women unless they specifically declined it (the opt-out approach), a measure that relies on physicians giving women clear information about the test to ensure informed consent. Several states, including North Carolina, Alabama, and Arkansas, ignored this recommendation, either requiring or allowing physicians to test pregnant women without their consent.[164] New testing guidelines went hand in hand with increased prosecution, as the introduction of AZT also empowered courts and social services to intervene in women's medical care on behalf of their fetus or child.[165] Nonetheless, whereas health advocates Marte and Anastos raised concern that "eliminating congenital HIV infection can be achieved only if HIV-infected women never have children," the FDA's approval of AZT during pregnancy in 1994 at least gave women who could access the drugs the possibility of reducing perinatal transmission without undermining their right to choose to have a child.[166]

CONCLUSION

Reflecting on his time as surgeon general, Koop said he felt misunderstood. He regretted that "people of faith never understood what I was trying to do as the Surgeon General to prevent the spread of AIDS," despite his "whole program in reference to AIDS" being "thoroughly pro-life . . . especially . . . pro-life concerning children." He followed that he "was certainly misunderstood when President Reagan asked me to write a report on the effects of abortion on women—a misguided effort to focus on women instead of the fetus."[167] Although Koop's commitment to his office compelled him not to lie against scientific evidence and to offer legal, available, and nonpermanent ways for HIV-positive women to prevent conception, his focus on preventing the birth of sick and disabled children and what to do with children neither prevented nor aborted but born to women living with HIV effectively erased HIV-positive women from the story. Framing the needs and interests of fetuses as separate from those of women, and the pregnancies of multiply marginalized women as undesirable, the official response to AIDS as reflected in Koop contributed to the false notion that fetuses are autonomous beings, that women's bodies are harmful to children, and that the state should intervene to protect society from the moral and social cost of marginalized children's care.

The notion that women pose a threat to their pregnancies contributed to the erosion of women's reproductive rights in the following decades. Since the 1980s, medical professionals and law enforcement officials have tested, arrested, and detained several hundreds of mostly low-income and non-white women for actions taken during their pregnancies that allegedly harm their fetuses. Law enforcers have also punished women, mostly those believed to have used illegal drugs, on account of their HIV-positive status. Moreover, the testing of newborns and infants for HIV set a precedent for testing newborns and pregnant women without their consent, resulting in charges for drug delivery, manslaughter, homicide, and other crimes.[168] The notions that life begins at conception and that a fetus is an "unborn child" requiring protection have also informed a plethora of abortion restrictions at the state level since the 1980s.[169] The criminalization of pregnancy does nothing to help women or their children. Rather, the specter of punishment, and the fear, stigma, and shame that it engenders, deters women from seeking HIV testing, treatment, and prenatal care, putting their health, which includes their pregnancies, at risk.[170] As Jennifer Brier and Celeste Watkins-Hayes noted, the specter of mistreatment has driven some women to withhold knowledge of their HIV status, disrupting the popular AIDS activist refrain that silence equals death.[171] Instead of supporting women, these measures punish them for having sex outside of heteronormative marriage.

As politicians shifted their focus away from debates over AIDS, abortion, and motherhood by the mid-1990s, lesbian women became central figures in the ensuing battles over what sex education looked like. Chapter three explores how the debate over women and AIDS shifted to lesbian women in the 1990s, as Republican lawmakers who believed that Reagan had not gone far enough to restore "family values" pushed national politics further to the right, and as the sharp drop-off in cases of perinatal HIV following the approval of the use of the AZT drug in pregnancy in 1994 eased much of the moral panic over perinatal transmission. As lesbian women organized to provide lifesaving sex education, conservative politicians intervened to censor articulations of their nonreproductive, nonnormative sex acts in the public sphere.

3

WOMEN'S FIGHT FOR
SAFER SEX

⁣⁣||||||||||||||||||||||||||||||||||||||||||||||||||||||||||||||||||||||||||||||||||||||||||||||||||||||||||||||||||||||||||||||||||||||||||||||||||||||||||||||||||||||||

AT 3 A.M. ON SUNDAY September 27, 1992, four young, white supremacist men threw a Molotov cocktail into the basement apartment of Hattie Mae Cohens, a twenty-nine-year-old lesbian woman, and her forty-five-year-old gay friend, Brian H. Mock, in Salem, Oregon, killing them both.[1] Several weeks later, on November 3, Oregon citizens turned out to vote on Ballot Measure 9, a referendum that the conservative group Oregon Citizens Alliance proposed on amending its state's constitution to classify "homosexuality" as "unnatural and perverse" and in need of being "discouraged and avoided." Arguing that gay men and lesbians deserved "no special rights," the initiative sought to prohibit governments from promoting, encouraging, or facilitating homosexuality.[2] Journalists viewed the referendum campaign as the backdrop for the attacks in Salem and elsewhere that were motivated by racial and homophobic hate.[3] As the murders of Cohens and Mock illustrate, the battles over sexuality and gender in the 1990s—refracted through a politics of race and involving not only gay and lesbian rights, but also abortion, censorship and pornography, sexual harassment, and welfare reform—played out not only in debate but also in violence and sometimes death.

That summer, on the other side of the country, six women involved in the New York gay and lesbian activist scene—Ana María Simo, Sarah Schulman, Maxine Wolfe, Anne-Christine D'Adesky, Marie Honan, and Anne Maguire—mobilized to form a direct-action group dedicated to raising lesbian women's visibility amid the current wave of statewide, homophobic initiatives. They called themselves the Lesbian Avengers.[4] The murders of Cohens and Mock inspired the group to choose fire eating as their trademark,[5] as homophobic attacks often came in the form of firebombing queer spaces.[6] The Lesbian Avengers' appropriation of arson took the Salem attack as a particular incident that crystalized anger and made it part of the symbolic response to homophobic violence on the side of queer people. In October 1992, the Avengers built a shrine for Cohens and Mock in the West Village and, during a memorial held on Halloween, they ate fire, chanting, "The fire will not consume us. We take that fire, and we make it our own."[7] The following April, these burgeoning lesbian networks that emerged from the earlier work of ACT UP, reproductive justice, and other progressive organizing in the 1970s and 1980s, demonstrated remarkable mobilizing capabilities when they organized the first "Dyke March" in Washington, DC, during which more than twenty thousand people joined the Avengers eating fire outside of the White House.[8] When Dee DeBerry, an HIV-positive lesbian woman, made plans to join the march, her neighbors threatened to firebomb her house. In defiance, DeBerry traveled to the nation's capital from her home in Tampa, Florida, only to return to find her house destroyed. In June, the New York Avengers traveled to Tampa and held a vigil at the site of her home.[9] The violence directed at DeBerry typified the hate and hostility aimed at sexual minorities in this period, just as the Avenger's actions typified the grassroots resistance to it.

The murders of Cohens and Mock, the Oregon referendum, and the founding of the Lesbian Avengers did not happen in isolation. They represented the conservative backlash to advances in gay, women's, and racial rights since the social justice movements of the 1960s and 1970s, as well as lesbian women's resistance to such hostility that built on decades of mobilization by diverse groups of women.[10] The tough-on-crime, anti-welfare, neoliberal agenda of a new conservative coalition that brought Reagan to power in the 1980s to restore conservative "family values," and which advanced in the 1990s under a Clinton administration that acquiesced to the far-right faction of the Republican Party, led by Newt Gingrich (R-GA), speaker of the US House of Representatives, rendered diverse gay women and men like Cohens and Mock hyper-visible and therefore vulnerable.[11] The emergence of the AIDS epidemic a decade earlier simultaneously raised the stakes of women's organizing, as securing education, social services, and treatment for lesbian women became a matter of life and death.

Since the epidemic's outset, lesbian women struggled for recognition as individuals living with and dying of HIV/AIDS, especially from public health agencies, as well as from some other lesbian women and gay men. In the mid-1990s, following a decade of organizing on the part of a diverse coalition of HIV-positive women and their allies to change the CDC's AIDS definition to include symptoms pertaining to women, some lesbian AIDS activists coined the phrase "the myth of lesbian immunity" to describe the belief that women could not transmit HIV sexually to each other or contract HIV through other behaviors that put them at risk of infection.[12] This myth arose in part from the sex and gender assumptions of CDC epidemiologists who, in the first decade of the AIDS crisis, failed to take seriously the possibility of women transmitting HIV sexually to other women, treating women as the transmitters of HIV perinatally to infants or heterosexually to men as sex workers.[13] The myth also resulted from the debates over what constituted lesbian identities that occupied lesbian feminists in the early 1970s and 1980s.[14] In the wake of AIDS, some lesbian feminists wanted to emphasize that a person's vulnerability to HIV derived not from how they identified but what they did. They argued for an expanded understanding of their identities that acknowledged that many women who had sex with other women, whether they identified as lesbian or not, engaged in other activities that might bring then into contact with the virus, including having unprotected sex with men, using drugs, receiving blood transfusions, and undergoing artificial insemination.[15] In 1992, building on years of AIDS work, the activist Amber Hollibaugh founded the Lesbian AIDS Project (LAP) at the Gay Men's Health Crisis (GMHC) in New York City to reach a diverse community of women. Shortly thereafter she commissioned the filmmaker and visual artist Cynthia Madansky and the performance artist Julie Tolentino Wood to design a safer sex handbook for lesbians.

The LAP produced their brochure against the backdrop of the prejudice toward those who rejected the racialized normative sex and gender roles that the "family values politics" of the 1990s prescribed and within the context of fear that such hostility evoked. Designed to overcome the lack of accurate and accessible medical information available to lesbians about HIV/AIDS, the handbook simultaneously intervened in ongoing debates within lesbian communities over the meaning of lesbian identity as it related to sexual practice. Moving away from rigid ideas about what it meant to be a lesbian woman to a focus on explicit sexual practice and behavior, the handbook contributed to the emerging queer politics of the 1990s that emphasized the fluidity of sexuality and identity.[16]

The political right's campaign to censor the handbook underscored the difficulties women faced in securing lifesaving access to education, research, and treatment as nonreproductive, sexual agents who used their bodies not for procreation but for pleasure. Unlike the medics, lawmakers, and conservative figures who called for interventions into the reproductive lives of HIV-positive women to "protect" fetuses from

HIV, and society from providing for the cost of caring for sick infants, the political right did not view lesbian women's bodies as a threat to HIV in infants. Rather, as much of the moral panic over mother-to-child transmission eased with the approval of AZT for use in pregnancy in 1994, they co-opted lesbian AIDS activists' safer sex information and framed it as dangerous homosexual propaganda in need of censorship for the sake of symbolically protecting America's children. In distorting and demeaning the brochure, the campaign silenced lesbian women's right to sexual self-determination in the public sphere and highlighted the historic difficulty women faced in securing their rights as citizens without making claims on the state as mothers.[17] It is not surprising that the LAP, like the Lesbian Avengers, encountered such backlash. Operating within a political context that rendered nonnormative sex taboo, both organizations subverted the sex and gender prescriptions of the 1990s while rejecting the tactics of gay and lesbian groups that "degayed" AIDS in an attempt to make it more politically palatable—a strategy that would have blunted the effectiveness of their safer sex interventions.[18] Moreover, coming from other progressive movements, these activists were already invested in critiquing state power in more systemic ways than that which some gay white men with greater privilege first brought to activism because of AIDS.[19]

The journey of the *Safer Sex Handbook for Lesbians* reveals how the AIDS epidemic shaped conceptions of lesbian identity at the end of the twentieth century and how such conceptions were tied to politics, medicine, and sexual practice. That members of the political right co-opted and distorted women's safer sex materials as dangerous homosexual propaganda underscores not only the long-standing centrality of the symbol of the child to civil rights battles over gender, sex, and race, but the centrality of lesbian women to a longer history of government surveillance, regulation, and punishment of nonnormative and non-procreative sexual acts.

CHALLENGING THE "MYTH OF IMMUNITY"

Early in 1988, Alice Terson decided to take an HIV test. She expected the result to come back positive because of the behaviors in which she had engaged: "I drank and used drugs for most of my adolescent and adult life. Repeatedly sharing needles and practicing unsafe sex, I was at risk many years before anyone in this country even knew that HIV existed." Writing for the inaugural LAP newsletter, *LAP Notes*, in April 1993, Terson stated that thirteen years into the epidemic, many still failed to take seriously the possibility of woman-to-woman transmission. Her biggest fear came from what she saw as the universal belief that lesbians could not contract HIV or develop AIDS. She argued that lesbians "often forget that our behaviors vary," and that many self-identified lesbians had unprotected sex with men, with other women, and with people who injected drugs, and engaged in other behaviors that might bring them into contact with the virus. Terson decided to take the risk of being "out" as an HIV-positive lesbian to challenge the denial among lesbians, the public health system, and society at large about the vulnerabilities of women who had sex with women. Lesbians were not immune simply because of their sexual identity, explained Terson.[20] Or, as Amber Hollibaugh later put it, "Lesbianism is not a condom."[21]

AIDS caused a reckoning within the lesbian community over what it meant to be a lesbian woman, especially as it related to sexual practice. Historians of sexuality have long examined the converging forces shaping the conceptions of lesbian identities throughout the twentieth century and the shifting terminology used to signify lesbian life. Changes in what society understood as female homosexuality ranged from the "romantic friendships" of women passionate for other women in the early twentieth century, to the butch/femme categories prominent at midcentury.[22] In the late 1960s and early 1970s, members of the women's movement looking to affirm women's rights to sexual pleasure with other women while rejecting the need for women to define themselves emotionally, economically, and erotically in relation to men began referring to themselves as "lesbian feminists."[23] Those involved in this movement debated the nature and meaning of lesbian life and its role in dismantling patriarchal society, questioning, for instance, the timeless or socially constructed nature of lesbian identities, whether lesbianism denoted an erotic or political experience, and how and whether lesbian women seeking to end male domination should live and organize "separately" from men.[24] Lesbian feminists never reached a consensus on these questions, with their different approaches revealing racial as well as class and sex divisions within the women's movement. Some lesbian feminists of color, such as the twin sisters Barbara and Beverly Smith, co-authors of the Black feminist Combahee River Collective Statement, critiqued the single-issue ideology and practice of lesbian separatism that failed to address women's intersectional oppressions.[25] At the same time, the lesbian feminists Deirdre English, Amber Hollibaugh, and Gayle Rubin questioned whether the inclusion of all women in the political project of lesbianism called for by such prominent writers as Adrienne Rich erased the erotic aspects of lesbian life.[26]

The debates occupying lesbian feminists also informed the "sex wars" of the 1970s and 1980s, in which feminists asked whether pornography and role-playing sex acts advanced or undermined the larger project of gender and sex equality. In the early 1970s, white, radical feminists such as Andrea Dworkin and Catharine MacKinnon, as well as some Black writers like Alice Walker and Audre Lorde, condemned certain sexual practices such as sadomasochism for objectifying women and perpetuating white male dominance, and presented pornography as a form of sex discrimination requiring regulation. Pro-sex feminists disagreed, maintaining women's right to engage in any consensual sex act from which they derived pleasure.[27] While members of the lesbian feminist movement sympathized with both positions, many supported the arguments of prominent sex and gender theorists such as Rubin that radical feminists' interpretation of the relationship among sex, gender, and oppression, including Dworkin's rejection of gender binaries, stigmatized sexual minorities who engaged in butch/femme relationships.[28] Radical feminists similarly challenged repressive sex and gender norms and sought to empower individuals, not the state, to seek legal remedies for pornography's harms.[29] Nonetheless, in working with the Reagan administration, testifying before Reagan's Attorney General Edwin Meese's Commission on Pornography in 1986, they appeared to legitimize the government censorship of women's bodies and desires.[30]

The lesbian feminist and sex wars debates shaped how some lesbian women responded to AIDS.[31] For the pro-sex, lesbian feminist activist Hollibaugh, AIDS made urgent the need to challenge assumptions about what it meant to be a "real" lesbian and to foreground the aspects of lesbian sexualities and other behaviors that she accused anti-pornography feminists of shaming, and of some lesbian women of rendering hidden or taboo. Hollibaugh maintained that the focus on prescriptive ideas about what it meant to be a "real" lesbian woman, as opposed to a focus on explicit sexual practice and behavior, lent a false sense of security to the white, middle-class, and monogamous women whose membership in the lesbian feminist community led them to believe that HIV posed little threat to them, regardless of their actions.[32] In the wake of AIDS, Hollibaugh wanted to interrogate and broaden the definition of the term "lesbian" to recognize not only women who self-identified as lesbian but also those who desired, and had sex with, both women and men. In so doing, she hoped to connect with women from diverse racial, ethnic, and class backgrounds in spaces like prisons, shelters, and drug recovery centers who might not have identified as lesbians but who needed specific information and support in ways that addressed their sexuality.[33]

The intimate relationships between women who identified as lesbians and men who identified as gay in ACT UP underscored Hollibaugh's argument that desire did not always align with notions of identity and community. The ACT UP members Maria Maggenti, Marion Banzhaf, and Zoe Leonard each described having sexual relationships with men in the organization, sometimes alongside intimate relationships with other women. As the former ACT UP/Chicago member Deborah Gould later recalled, ACT UP facilitated mixed-sex erotic as well as political relationships that challenged the typically segregated nature of lesbian and gay life in this period.[34] Their hesitancy to express these relationships openly, fearing that other ACT UP members might question their authority as lesbian women, suggests how women's efforts to silence aspects of their sexual lives to fit within a community hampered HIV-prevention efforts.[35] Moreover, while the ACT UP and Lesbian Avenger member Sarah Schulman felt that lesbian women should not spend time advocating for lesbian safer sex given the lack of official evidence proving woman-to-woman HIV transmission, others, such as Maxine Wolfe, argued that the imperative for safer sex was less about proving the existence of same-sex transmission than expanding the category of "lesbian" to reflect the diversity and range of lesbian lives. Besides, as Wolfe noted, epidemiologists did not know the actual risk of women transmitting HIV to each other because little data existed on the prevalence of HIV in fluids such as menstrual blood, which researchers treated as "a non-issue." Instead, much of the evidence about same-sex transmission came from women's testimonies, reflecting how official neglect drove women to become authorities on their own bodies.[36] The lesbian critic and AIDS scholar Cindy Patton similarly called for a transformation of dominant notions of lesbian identity to accommodate alternative lives and techniques. Patton argued that as the greatest risks for lesbian women came from actions not typically associated with the lesbian community—namely, drug use and sex with men—addressing AIDS involved interrogating the very notion of who was a lesbian, and who was included and excluded from the lesbian community.[37] Lesbian feminists who used ACT UP to experiment both sexually and politically contributed to this goal.

Speaking of the variety of lesbian self-identification, Hollibaugh wrote, "We call ourselves by many names or none at all, and our needs are complex and varied." Cynthia Madansky, an artist and assistant to the director at the LAP, similarly challenged the "false sense of security that 'it can't happen to us,'" arguing that "the perpetual myth in the lesbian community that we are not at risk contributes to the silence, invisibility, and isolation of those among us who are living with HIV/AIDS."[38] The safer sex educator Catherine Saalfield agreed, stating, "We tell ourselves that we don't have to worry since HIV-positive lesbians don't exist. It's a lame justification, based on our fantasies and enforced by our own silence."[39] Along with lesbian feminists in ACT UP, their expansive conception of lesbian life that focused on bodies and behaviors as opposed to prescriptive labels contributed to the emerging queer politics of the 1990s that similarly rejected rigid identity categories.[40]

A self-described "lesbian sex radical, ex-hooker, incest survivor, Gypsy child, poor-white trash, high femme dyke" from Bakersfield, California, Hollibaugh cited "numerous, varied, and passionate" reasons for participating in AIDS work that combined her queer, feminist, class, and racial politics.[41] Similar to other lesbians, her involvement in the lesbian and gay movement compelled her to support those in the community affected by AIDS and resist the political right's use of the epidemic to advance their homophobic agenda.[42] Moreover, her desire to do explicit sex work that addressed the diversity of women's sexualities, and to represent the women who had relationships with, or desire for, other women but whose class or racial background placed them outside the boundaries of the mainstream lesbian and AIDS movement, drove her activism.[43] Similar to the mostly white lesbian activists who founded the women's caucus of ACT UP/NY, as well as the New York Lesbian Avengers, and whose involvement in other progressive organizing informed their intersectional approach to AIDS activism, Hollibaugh understood that AIDS affected diverse groups of women marginalized because of their race, gender, and class.[44] Specifically, she wanted to provide resources to low-income women of color who had sex with women that addressed the same-sex aspect of their lives, as existing information tended to focus on topics of drug use or sex with men.[45] Hollibaugh therefore worked to support an often-invisible community of women who had sex with women.

Hollibaugh began her paid AIDS work as an HIV test counselor and hotline worker in New York before joining the AIDS Discrimination Unit of the New York City Commission on Human Rights.[46] In 1992, she launched and became director of the LAP, the first organization dedicated exclusively to addressing lesbian issues related to HIV/AIDS. In the 1980s, the lesbian documentary photographer Ann P. Meredith described women as the "hidden population" in the AIDS epidemic.[47] Echoing Meredith, Hollibaugh described lesbians with HIV as "the disappeared" population in lesbian communities. She launched the LAP for the sake of reaching them.[48]

For Hollibaugh, challenging the "myth of lesbian immunity" involved centering the lives of a diverse constituency of women who had sex with other women and who, for reasons of economic necessity, desire, or both, also injected drugs, had sex with men, and found love and intimacy in other women. Hollibaugh used her past experiences to clarify the confusion between visibility, identity, and behavior, claiming to have engaged in all the behaviors that might bring women into contact with HIV while also identifying as a lesbian woman. In so doing, she rejected the prescriptive ideas about what it meant to be a "real" lesbian that other activists, such as members of the Daughters of Bilitis, a lesbian homophile organization, had advanced to win credibility in the mid-twentieth century, and which were often tied to ideals of whiteness, middle-classness, and monogamy, and emphasize that behavior, and not identity, determined a woman's vulnerability to HIV.[49]

Lesbian activists' efforts to center multiply marginalized women in the response to AIDS signified their efforts to reframe AIDS as an intersectional women's health issue. Lesbians with HIV challenged the notion that lesbian women primarily acted as the caregivers of men in the epidemic as opposed to people navigating their own illness, and to show that AIDS, like breast cancer, rape, alcoholism, and poverty, was also a woman's health issue.[50] In addressing AIDS as a disease that compounded other health inequities, lesbians were often more alert than their white, gay counterparts to tackling AIDS as a political and health crisis related to both sexuality and gender. Their efforts challenged the perspectives of diverse women in the lesbian community who saw AIDS as a predominantly gay male issue. For example, the lesbian separatist Naja Sorella, the lesbian feminist and founder of the Women's Cancer Resource Center in Berkeley, California, Jackie Winnow, and the poet June Jordan expressed frustration at suffering from other diseases, such as breast cancer and chronic fatigue, "while Lesbians put their physical, emotional and financial energy into AIDS."[51] With experience navigating the dual burdens of sexism and homophobia, often alongside racism and classism, in health care, lesbian women intervened in the epidemic not only in solidarity with gay men but also on behalf of themselves and other women.

As evidence of the changing understanding of AIDS as a disease of behaviors and not identities, lesbian activists pointed to several studies showing that due to the prevalence of violence against lesbian women, their engagement in unprotected sex with both men and women, and use of intravenous drugs, women who had a sexual history with other women had a greater risk of contracting HIV than women who did not. Studies conducted at the Bronx-Lebanon Hospital and Montefiore Hospital found that more than thirty percent of HIV-positive women had had a same-sex partner. A Seattle study similarly found a five-fold increase in the infection rate for women who engaged in same-sex behaviors compared to women who only had sex with men. Studies carried out in California showed that one-fifth of a sample of female intravenous drug users identified as either bisexual or lesbian.[52] In October 1993, the San Francisco Department of Public Health published a "Women's Survey" based on 498 women in the San Francisco area showing that while the prevalence of HIV infection among lesbian women did not vary much according to age or race, lesbian and bisexual women had an HIV-infection rate three times higher than that of heterosexual women.[53] The report also pointed to the direct connection between violence and HIV, whereby 32.1 percent of lesbian and bisexual women surveyed reported nonconsensual sex with men, and 5.8 percent reported nonconsensual sex with women, thereby underscoring the importance of emphasizing how gendered violence increased women's vulnerability to HIV.[54] The studies confirmed the need for HIV interventions that addressed the particular realities of women who had sex with women.

These studies angered activists already outraged at the CDC's failure to track HIV risk among lesbian women. The early death of twenty-six-year-old Joan Baker from AIDS-related complications on September 3, 1993, became a further rallying cry for members of the San Francisco Lesbian Avengers. Thirteen years since the emergence of the AIDS epidemic in the US, Baker's death symbolized the overdue need to recognize the vulnerability of lesbians, bisexual women, transgender lesbians, and all women who had a sexual history with other women regardless of how they identified. Baker tested positive for HIV in 1986 at the age of eighteen. She left her home in Riverside, California, to move to the Bay Area, seeking a surrogate community, and she spent the next several years campaigning alongside groups like the Lesbian Avengers for education and services for women living with HIV.[55] "It doesn't matter how I got it," Baker explained. "It's the fact that I have been diagnosed and I am coming out as a woman with AIDS, because a lot of lesbians still think that they can't get AIDS, and I am here to say that it can happen." One month after her death, on October 23, members of the Lesbian Avengers, ACT UP/San Francisco and ACT UP/Golden Gate, the San Francisco WAC, and the Lyon-Martin's Health Services held a political funeral for Baker that saw hundreds of women

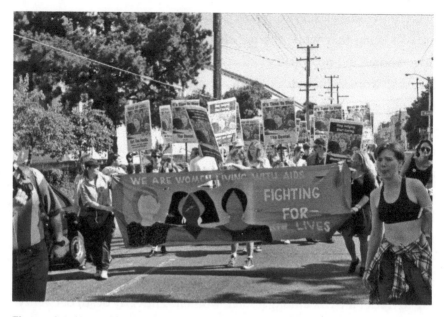

Fig. 4. Political Funeral for Joan Baker, October 23, 1993, Lesbian Avengers collection 96-10. Courtesy of Gay, Lesbian, Bisexual, Transgender Historical Society.

and men march from Dolores Park into the Castro playing drums and holding signs that featured images of Baker, reading: "We Are Women Living with AIDS," "It's Time to Stop the Denial," and "Wake up Call. Get the Facts: Women Who Fuck Women Can Contract HIV/AIDS."[56] The response to Baker's death underscored the integral role lesbian women with HIV played in their communities.

The concurrent publication of the San Francisco Health Department's "Women's Survey" and the death of their friend Joan Baker led the San Francisco Lesbian Avengers to create leaflets and posters protesting the CDC's failure to collect statistics on HIV among lesbian women, including "Lesbians Get AIDS Just Like Joan Baker," "Dykes Get AIDS. How? The Center for Disease Control doesn't have a clue," and "We Demand a Definitive Study of Woman-to-Woman Transmission of HIV!"[57] The chapter organized a demonstration targeting the CDC's policies as part of a larger campaign that criticized the federal government for "its complete failure to address the issues surrounding dykes and AIDS." The San Francisco Avengers made three demands: first, that the CDC study the possibility of woman-to-woman transmission; second, that it fund outreach efforts directed at lesbian and bisexual women; and, third, that the agency revise its definition of "lesbian" as a woman who had only ever had sex with other women, which erased the diversity of women's sexual lives. On August 13, 1994, twenty-one Lesbian Avengers took these demands to the CDC's Bay Area office, covertly located at the San Francisco International Airport. As some women wrapped their peer's pelvises in saran wrap, others unfurled a 20-foot-long banner which read, "Dykes demand the CDC study woman-to-woman AIDS transmission." The women planned to target the CDC with faxes to its headquarters and phone calls to its AIDS information hotline in the following months.[58]

Lesbian AIDS activists therefore worked not only to make visible the varied behaviors that made lesbian women vulnerable to HIV but also for the CDC to properly monitor and research HIV among women who had sex with women. In the early 1990s, the CDC began using the term "men who have sex with men" (MSM) in its surveillance reports to separate men's sexual behaviors from their identities.[59] The CDC's creation of a medical classification that moved beyond identity categories reflected the need to address occurrences of HIV among men who may not have self-identified as gay but who had previously been in a same-sex relationship. The CDC did not develop an equivalent term for women who had sex with women but may not have identified as lesbian or bisexual. The CDC's failure to do so reflected the marginalization of women who had sex with women within the health-care system. Due to the intersection of sexism and homophobia, lesbians, on average, lacked adequate health insurance because of their struggle to access private insurance through their partner or work, or public insurance because of age and parenting status. Moreover, they often chose not to disclose their sexuality to health-care providers for fear of discrimination, further rendering themselves invisible to the medical and scientific research establishment.[60]

By the early 1990s, the percentage of women assigned "no identified risk" was consistently double that of men.[61] The CDC collected data on HIV/AIDS from the reports of physicians across the country and did not require them to ask HIV-positive women about their sexual orientation or same-sex practices.[62] Instead, CDC epidemiologists counted women who reported having had sex with a man at any time since 1978 as a heterosexual contact.[63] If physicians did report cases in which women cited woman-to-woman contact as their only risk behavior, the CDC classified these as "unknown," "other/undetermined," or "no identified risk."[64] CDC epidemiologists did not list woman-to-woman transmission as a possible exposure category in its surveillance data, despite repeated cases of women reporting this as their only risk for HIV since the early 1980s.[65] Many lesbian women with HIV had no recorded risk factor. Instead, researchers placed women like Lynette "Cookie" Hubbard, who identified as a lesbian all her life, received a HIV-positive diagnosis in 1989, and died in June 1993, in the opaque "other" category.[66] CDC researchers thereby erased or heterosexualized lesbian-identified women and collected no data on the numbers of women diagnosed with HIV/AIDS who identified as a lesbian or had a same-sexual history. Moreover, CDC staff members, such as Ann Duerr, admitted not knowing how the viral load in cervical and vaginal secretions changed during sexual arousal and climax.[67] Duerr's comments underscored the lack of priority epidemiologists placed on understanding how HIV acted in women's bodies during sex after studies from the 1980s suggesting the low prevalence of HIV among sex workers assailed the initial panic over women infecting men.[68] The CDC's failure to collect data on woman-to-woman transmission or investigate how HIV acted in women's bodies during sex reflected the US public health services' historic treatment of women as either— depending on their race and class—the passive recipients or active spreaders of STDs, but heterosexually, as mothers, sex workers, or wives.[69] The normative assumptions about sex and gender that shaped CDC epidemiologists' conditional understanding of AIDS also reflected the conservative political climate committed to maintaining prescriptive sex and gender roles in which they operated.

The CDC also used a hierarchy of exposure categories to assign one HIV transmission category for each reported case of AIDS and categorized a woman as the highest risk only if they reported more than one possible exposure. The hierarchy for infection in women was: 1) intravenous drug use; 2) receipt of blood products; 3) heterosexual contact with an HIV-positive man; and 4) no identified risk.[70] In contrast, from 1986 onward, the CDC grouped men with both a history of sexual contact with other men and intravenous drug use in a separate exposure category that acknowledged the dual sources of exposure, identified on the 1986 report as Homosexual Male and IV Drug Abuser. Researchers did not layer categories of risk for women who had sex with women and erased women from the multiple modes of exposure categories—obscuring understanding of the disease's reach in women as well as the ways in which different behaviors that brought women into contact with the virus overlapped.[71] The data collection methods that failed to track or categorize the same-sexual sources of transmission for women and the lack of official medical studies on the possibility of woman-to-woman transmission sustained the notion that women who had sex with women constituted a "low-risk" group. This assumption rendered infected women vulnerable to misdiagnosis from doctors who assumed their illness was not AIDS-related and left unaddressed the vulnerabilities associated with women's same-sexual relationships.

As major areas regarding HIV in all women remained underresearched, and an unknown number of lesbians and women who had sex with other women continued to contract HIV and die without recognition of a diagnosis, lesbian health activists and advocates argued for official studies on lesbian practices and more information about

HIV in menstrual blood, vaginal and cervical secretions, and other discharges. The artist Zoe Leonard who, alert to the overlap between safe-sex negotiation and drug use in lesbian communities, also worked with men to advocate for clean needles in the 1980s and 1990s, argued, "In order to get the information the scientists needed and we needed . . . we just had to stop worrying and arguing about identities and identification. We just had to talk about what are doing [sic]? What are the fluids involved? Where are the fluids going? What is coming into contact with what?"[72] Leonard's sexual relationships with men and women shaped her perspective on the need to move away from opaque identity categories to focus on behavior. Throughout the twentieth century, white, middle-class lesbian activists often de-emphasized the nonnormative and sexual aspects of their relationships as a political strategy to win credibility from heteronormative society.[73] The hidden aspects of women's same-sex relationships culminated in the sentiment, as articulated by Dr. Charles Schable, who conducted HIV transmission studies for the CDC, that it wasn't necessary to address the risks for lesbian women because "lesbians don't have much sex."[74] Studies showing that lesbian-identifying women reported having sex more often and with a larger number of partners than straight-identifying women contradicted Schable's depiction of lesbian women as asexual and highlighted the need to challenge the misconceptions about lesbian sexuality and identity driving the lack of medical focus on lesbian vulnerability.[75]

In the absence of full institutional recognition and support, and mirroring the educational initiatives of activists such as Dázon Dixon Diallo, who provided sex education to low-income, women of color in Atlanta, the LAP filled the gap in knowledge about HIV and lesbian women.[76] The LAP ran a series of sexual and empowerment workshops based on the sex-positive politics of Hollibaugh and others with titles such as "Feeling Good All Over" and "Living Examples: Lesbians and HIV in Three Acts," to teach lesbian, bisexual, and women who had sex with women, as well as service providers, ways to negotiate safer sex, address drug use, and connect with low-income women and women in sites like prison who wanted to learn more about HIV.[77] These initiatives, culminating in the publication of their *Safer Sex Handbook for Lesbians* in 1993, contributed to a larger movement to increase public awareness of the relationship between lesbian sexual practices and vulnerability with the aim to save lives in the wake of AIDS.

The political right did not view lesbian women's bodies as a threat of HIV in children. Instead, they judged their safer sex publicity as obscene homosexual propaganda in need of censorship for the sake of symbolically protecting America's children. During the 1980s, many public health agencies and condom manufacturers directed their safer sex campaigns at heterosexual women to prevent mother-to-child transmission of HIV. A decade later, lesbian activists published their own safer sex materials that centered sexual acts between women seeking to raise awareness of the reality of lesbian women's vulnerability to HIV and challenge the "myth of lesbian immunity" within lesbian communities and public health agencies. Male and female activists shared the goal of creating explicit pamphlets to educate communities about sexually transmitted diseases and address HIV through a discussion of pleasure.[78] As women worked to break the silences around lesbian sexuality to save lives in ways similar to queer writers such as Douglas Crimp and queer organizations like the San Francisco drag group Sisters of Perpetual Indulgence, their efforts opened them up to political attack.[79] The political backlash to the frank tone and imagery of the safer sex handbook revealed women's struggle to assert their rights as nonnormative, nonreproductive sexual agents in and beyond the AIDS epidemic at the end of the twentieth century.

THE *SAFER SEX HANDBOOK FOR LESBIANS*

The LAP did not write the *Safer Sex Handbook* for children. The women for whom the LAP produced the booklet already engaged in sex and wanted to know how to do it more safely. Like other prevention materials, the handbook explained how to do this and sought to save lives. Unlike sex education projects designed for family use, such as Koop's *Understanding AIDS* booklet published five years earlier, the authors took an uncensored approach. Coming from the pro-sex faction of the women's movement that rejected what they saw as the sexual moralism of anti-pornography feminism, Hollibaugh, Madansky, and Tolentino Wood wanted to offer an alternative to clinical, sterile, and condescending sex education and explore a safe and shame-free lesbian sexuality.[80] They adopted a purposefully explicit tone and visuals—emphasizing the fun and raunchy aspects of safer sex. It emerged from a specific desire to promote pro-sex lesbian erotics that differed even from the sexual education offered in feminist anthologies like *Our Bodies, Ourselves*. Feminist politics not only informed the LAP's decision to use explicit language and imagery, but the authors also recognized the medical necessity of sex education that featured sex organs and acts. Its success shocked people, highlighting that the need for sex education not only for school-age children but also women exploring what a pro-sex, lesbian future free from sexual violence on the part of men might look like.

The publication of the *Safer Sex Handbook* brought debates over what constituted lesbian identities and life from lesbian communities to the mainstream political arena. Lesbian AIDS activists' efforts to reach the broadest number of women attracted the attention of a political right working to narrow the parameters of sexuality and gender threatened by the emergence of a sex-positive, non-patriarchal sex education. As was the case for women seeking recognition as people affected by HIV/AIDS to secure benefits, services, and treatment in the 1980s, lesbian women's safer sex activism a decade later came with prescriptiveness and political risk.

AIDS brought political focus to the sexual aspects of lesbian life. Throughout much of the twentieth century, the police and a hostile public frequently threatened and persecuted women, and especially women of color already vulnerable to racist harassment, judged to have transgressed the gender norms associated with sexuality.[81] Nonetheless, the federal government generally focused less on regulating same-sex relationships between women in comparison to their efforts to regulate those between men. As Margot Canaday outlined, the burgeoning federal bureaucracy of the early twentieth century paid closer attention to male homosexuality, deciding that homosexuality among women was a problem that deserved federal attention only later, when women became fully integrated into the masculinized military in the 1940s. According to Canaday, sexism drove this differential treatment. "Male perverts mattered so much to the state" in the early twentieth century "because male citizens did." Moreover, as state agents found sex between women harder to define, they also found it more difficult to police.[82] In making visible some of the specific sexual behaviors that women engaged in for the sake of public health, the *Safer Sex Handbook* opened lesbian women up to political backlash, demonstrating how vulnerability assisted visibility in the fight for the rights of sexual and gender minorities in US history.

In 1993, Hollibaugh commissioned the pro-sex filmmaker Cynthia Madansky and performer and activist Julie Tolentino Wood to write a safer sex handbook for the lesbian community. Designed to counter the widespread lack of accurate information on HIV, the LAP set out to produce a sex positive, explicit, and "informative yet erotic" guide. Like contemporaneous, lesbian-directed safer sex guides, the resulting twenty-sided-brochure, entitled *The Safer Sex Handbook for Lesbians*, promoted women's sexual agency.[83] The handbook contained explicit guidance on learning "erotic and comfortable techniques for practicing safer sex," offering strategies for integrating gloves, plastic wrap, latex barriers, clean sex toys, and implements into sex. Acknowledging that these practices also rendered women vulnerable, the handbook contained information on intravenous drug use and a short paragraph at the end on sex with men.[84]

Madansky and Tolentino Wood wanted to equip lesbian women with the vocabulary and confidence to share their sexual desires to protect themselves in the epidemic. For the authors, women who slept with other women, no matter how they identified, needed basic medical information about the transmission of HIV and other STDs during sex. They sought to provide this information openly and without prejudice.[85]

GMHC printed 61,000 copies of the *Safer Sex Handbook*, created in 1993, within a year, most of which they distributed for free through word of mouth to people and organizations who wanted to learn about safe sex for women who had sex with women. The LAP also distributed the brochure internationally to AIDS organizations, as well as to prisons; physicians; at New York's Gay Pride celebration in 1993; Tolentino Wood's New York City bar, the Clit Club; the Community Health project; the Lesbian and Gay Community Center; and through the mail. By the end of 1994, the LAP and GMHC had printed 67,000 leaflets.[86]

That year, the evaluation research department at GMHC held four focus groups composed of thirty-two Black, Latina, Caucasian, and Asian women to evaluate the effectiveness of the handbook among the diverse lesbian communities for whom it was designed. Topics covered in the focus groups ranged from the handbook's distribution, layout and design, language, and content. The participants generally responded positively, appreciating the brochure's realistic and nonjudgmental tone and its inclusion of sexual activities typically unaddressed in safer sex literature. One woman highlighted the section on less common sexual activities that presented a diverse view of lesbian lifestyles. Others agreed that the brochure made safe sex seem appealing: "All other things I've read says to do this [practice safer sex] 'cause there's an epidemic . . . [but this brochure] . . . makes lesbian [safer] sex sound good." Many also praised the explicit nature of the photography, especially the cover, which, featuring a Black woman cupping her breasts and vagina with her hand in a latex glove, conveyed the brochure's message of

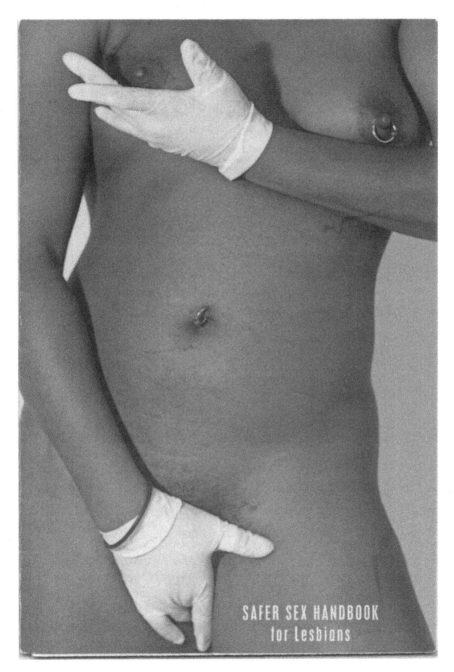

SAFER SEX HANDBOOK
for Lesbians

Fig. 5. *Safer Sex Handbook for Lesbians*, by Cynthia Madansky and Julie Tolentino Wood, Lesbian AIDS Project–Gay Men's Health Crisis, Inc., 1993, 1999, 2000. Courtesy of Gay Men's Health Crisis (GMHC) and the Lesbian Herstory Archives.

promoting erotic safe sex for women from diverse racial and ethnic backgrounds. The group suggested that the images helped create a positive feeling about lesbian sex.

The women who participated in the focus groups also expressed relief over the availability of a pamphlet that addressed their desire to practice safe sex. While their praise was not unanimous—some viewed the language and visuals as too explicit and critiqued aspects of its scope and content—the response the handbook received outside the lesbian community proved the most divisive.[87] The political right's vitriolic anti-gay and anti-woman agenda as seen throughout the HIV epidemic's first decade coalesced to impede lesbian activists' efforts to curb the spread and effects of the disease. The political debates over women and AIDS during the early 1990s departed from those of the previous decade in that they centered the performance of specific sexual acts between women, including HIV-positive lesbians, as the government intervened not to prevent women from transmitting HIV to infants but from showcasing a deviant lifestyle to children.

DO YOU KNOW WHERE YOUR DAUGHTERS ARE?

Conservatives acted quickly. Within a year of its publication, political and religious activists co-opted the handbook and weaponized it as evidence of the need to symbolically protect America's children from the alleged threat of gay recruitment. The strategy of evoking the symbol of the child to shore up white, male, heterosexual power dated back to nineteenth-century debates over race. Conservatives in the twentieth century similarly used the image of the child and the language of child protection to warn against the dangers of racial integration, as well as communism, abortion, and homosexuality seen as threatening the status quo. In the 1970s, white parents seeking to preserve the racial, class, generational, gender, and sexual hierarchies following the social justice movements of the 1960s worked to deny gay and lesbians, Black

Americans, and women of all races the full benefits of citizenship under the banner of child protection. In 1977, one of the most notable proponents of this strategy, the actress Anita Bryant, became the spokesperson of a campaign led on behalf of the organization Save Our Children (SOC) to repeal a gay civil rights ordinance in Dade County, Florida. SOC borrowed from the tactics, arguments, and people leading the contemporaneous fight to block school integration, as well as the Equal Rights Amendment (ERA), that they viewed as similarly undermining public order, warning of the potential for openly gay teachers to recruit children if granted access to them in school.[88] The success of the SOC campaign inspired other discriminatory campaigns. In 1978, the California State Senator John Briggs sponsored Proposition 6, a statewide initiative that sought to prohibit gay individuals from working in public schools in California.[89]

The LAP created the safer sex handbook within the context of the moral panic over gay recruitment that the political right weaponized to attack gay and lesbian rights at the end of the twentieth century.[90] In 1993, evidence of his search for a politically expedient "third way" between an increasingly far-right Republican party and Democrats, Clinton reneged on his campaign promise to end the ban on lesbians and gay men openly serving in the military through his policy of "Don't Ask, Don't Tell."[91] Three years later, he doubled down on the exclusion of gay men and lesbian women from traditional family structures when he signed the Defense of Marriage Act, which allowed states to not recognize same-sex marriages performed elsewhere, and defined marriage for federal purposes as the union of one man and one woman.[92] In 1996, Clinton also signed a major piece of welfare legislation ending single mothers' and children's entitlement to cash aid through the Aid to Families with Dependent Children program, which had been in existence since the 1960s. The program which replaced it, Temporary Assistance for Needy Families, marked the culmination of Republican efforts to shift support for the perceived, racialized "nonworking poor" from state agencies to private families and organizations since the Reagan era.[93] As the political right withdrew its support from communities rendered "undeserving" of state help and worked to restrict the participation of openly gay men and lesbians in public life, they used the *Safer Sex Handbook* as evidence of the need to remove any references to gay men and women from public schools in the name of child protection.

In 1989, a group of teachers in New York City began designing a multicultural curriculum for first-grade students to celebrate the city's racial and ethnic diversity. The authors dedicated three pages of the 443-page "Children of the Rainbow" curriculum to encouraging teachers to discuss lesbian and gay lives at school. They also listed Michael Willhoite's children's book *Daddy's Roommate* and Lesléa Newman's *Heather Has Two Mommies* and *Gloria Goes to Gay Pride* on a recommended reading list. These references to gay families proved the most controversial aspect of the curriculum, sparking citywide protests that involved the Roman Catholic Bishop of Brooklyn and Queens, Thomas V. Daily.[94]

Mary A. Cummins, a white grandmother and president of the school board in District 24 in Queens, led the campaign against what she described as "dangerously misleading lesbian/homosexual propaganda."[95] On the heels of Cummins's protest, a socially, racially, and ethnically diverse set of parents from Manhattan to Queens began challenging the curriculum based on its gay and lesbian content.[96]

The Board of Education did not mandate that schools teach the curriculum, but Cummins's refusal to adopt any syllabus that acknowledged gay men and lesbians riled the chancellor of New York City Schools, Joseph A. Fernandez, enough to suspend the entire school board in District 24 in the fall of 1992. Already facing opposition for his endorsement of AIDS education and condom distribution in high schools, Fernandez asserted, "There will be no changing the requirement that, at some time in the elementary grades, diverse family structures be recognized and acknowledged as loving, caring households."[97]

Fernandez's commitment to promoting both racial and sexual diversity failed to convince many parents of the need to bring discussions of gay and lesbian lives into the classroom. In February 1993, following months of heated political debate over the future of the city's public school system, the New York City Board of Education forced Fernandez to reinstate District 24's school board and terminated his contract as chancellor.[98]

The inaugural New York Lesbian Avenger action took place on September 9, 1992, the first day of school, in support of the Rainbow Curriculum. Wearing outfits that imitated Catholic school uniforms with tops that read "I was a lesbian child," sixty women played bass drums, handed out lavender balloons, and carried banners that read "Ask About Lesbian Lives" and "Teach About Lesbian Lives" as they marched down Metropolitan Avenue to P.S. 87, an elementary school at the center of District 24 in Queens. Like the public service announcement that asked, "Do you know where your children are?," they asked, "Do you know where your daughters are? (At the Lesbian Avengers' back-to-school-party!)"[99] With slogans "We recruit" and "I was a lesbian child," the group appropriated the scare tactics of the political right over gay recruitment and took the conservative message that society should promote heterosexuality in all children and replaced it with one that affirmed their stake in promoting sexual diversity in the classroom. Centering themselves as part of the national family, the Avengers demonstrated how gay rights organizations conformed to, navigated, and subverted the "family values politics" of the late twentieth century.[100]

The protests over the Rainbow Curriculum fed into a larger national debate about the types of sex education schools should offer young people in the wake of AIDS. In New York City, Cardinal John O'Connor, a member of Reagan's 1987 HIV/AIDS commission and a friend of Mary Cummins, used his platform to denounce condoms, clean needles, abortion, and gay rights while promoting abstinence-only sex education in the city's public schools. In December 1989, his outspoken position led to ACT UP and WHAM!'s notorious 4,500-strong "Stop the Church" protest at St. Patrick's cathedral.[101] In October 1986, Koop made the controversial call for sexual education to begin at home and in school "at the lowest grade possible" so that children can grow up "knowing the behaviors to avoid to protect themselves from exposure to the AIDS virus."[102] In December 1994, President Clinton fired his surgeon general, Joycelyn Elders, for her recommendation to incorporate masturbation into school-age sex education. Throughout the 1980s and 1990s, AIDS made urgent the divisive question of what sex education should look like.[103]

On February 12, 1994, New York University hosted a Conference of Peer Education for HIV educators between the ages of fourteen and twenty-four. Nineteen organizations sponsored the event, including GMHC and the New York City Board of Education's High School HIV/AIDS Resource Center.[104] The organizers only allowed young people, and a small number of adult speakers, to attend the event. John Hartigan, an attorney from the organization Hands Off Our Kids, which opposed sex education, two members of the HIV advisory council from the Board of Education, and affiliates of Parents for the Restoration of Values in Education tried unsuccessfully to register for the conference. When this attempt failed, they recruited and sent a fourteen-year-old boy on their behalf to collect materials, attend the workshops, and write up a report.[105]

GMHC volunteers set up a table at the conference and put out copies of some of their leaflets and brochures. These included Listen Up!, a pamphlet aimed at educating Black and Latino teenagers about condoms, as well as the Safer Sex Handbook that someone accidently displayed.[106] Stating his age as seventeen, the fourteen-year-old boy collected both pamphlets and brought them back to the adults.

A few days later, armed with his new evidence, Hartigan sent letters of complaint to Ramon C. Cortines, the new chancellor of the New York City schools, demanding that he abolish the Board of Education's

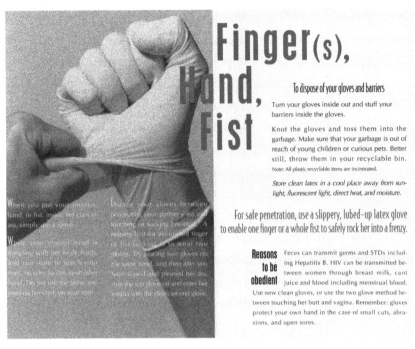

Fig. 6. *Safer Sex Handbook for Lesbians*, by Cynthia Madansky and Julie Tolentino Wood, Lesbian AIDS Project–Gay Men's Health Crisis, Inc., 1993, 1999, 2000. Courtesy of Gay Men's Health Crisis (GMHC) and the Lesbian Herstory Archives.

HIV/AIDS Resource Center and ban GMHC from public schools. Cortines decided to move the HIV/AIDS Resource Center to a Board of Education building in Brooklyn to bring it more closely under his control. He also suspended GHMC from entering schools for a year.[107]

The New York press picked up and sensationalized the story. Mona Charen of the *New York Post* accused GMHC of using "the occasion to engage in homosexual propaganda."[108] Lynda Richardson of the *New York Times* shared details of the handbook, including "Vulgar words and phrases many considered shocking and unsuitable for children," which Cortines argued "possessed no educational value."[109] According to Madansky, to justify the handbook's censorship, opponents focused most on the two pages on "fisting," which they framed as a fatal and sadistic act.[110] The focus on death revealed the extent of the political right's distortion of the handbook's aim, which sought to provide women with frank safer sex information to save lives.

This reporting bolstered the political right's campaign to discredit the *Safer Sex Handbook*, which the New York Board of Education censured in 1994.[111] The censorship campaign coincided with congressional Republicans' use of the handbook to advance their own misogynistic and homophobic agenda to erase women's bodies from the public sphere and silence their articulations of nonnormative sex.

The Reverend Louis P. Sheldon, a Presbyterian minister from Washington, DC, cut his teeth campaigning to bar openly gay and lesbian teachers from California schools in the 1970s.[112] In the early 1980s, he founded the Traditional Values Coalition, a network of churches based in the conservative area of Orange County, California, to oppose gay rights. This work earned him the ear of prominent Republican lawmakers, such as House Speaker Gingrich.[113] A decade later, he used the controversy around the conference and the safer sex handbook as evidence of homosexual recruitment in schools.[114] Mary Cummins sent Sheldon the handbook, and on March 28, 1994, he joined Duffy, the talk-show host of the radio program "Live in LA" to discuss it. Duffy began describing the handbook for the audience: "a book that's about three inches by five inches." Using titillating language, the conversation that unfolded belittled it, with Duffy telling listeners, "What you can see is a nude woman. I'm assuming this is a woman . . . this person has latex gloves on. There's no polite way to say this, friends, on her left breast there is a ring that has been pierced through the nipple. There is in her belly button a pierced ring that goes through her belly button." Evoking a common conservative refrain, both men agreed that they were "not homophobic" but equally refused to "affirm a lifestyle of vaginal fisting." Sheldon explained:

> The bottom line to this, uh, Duffy, is that they're telling these young children how they can counsel lesbians not to get HIV virus infection. . . .

And they say this about themselves: that lesbians are now into vaginal fist-ing. I've heard of homosexuals, gays, into rectal fisting, but this is vaginal fisting. And I want to tell you that a woman can die—the vaginal, the vagina is not made to have a fist placed in it for such purposes as this book-let is trying to say. And what their purpose in this booklet is to say to young children, you must wear a latex glove. As you do vaginal fisting, wear a latex glove. Then it goes on to tell you all these other things.

And as we showed this on the floor of the Congress, as men and women were coming into the floor of the Congress, we went there with fear and timidity and I tell you we prayed before we went, 'cause I've never given out pornography. I don't participate in any kind of pornography. But when these were sent to me by dear Mary Cummins, a 74-year-old grandmother, president of School District 24 in Queens, New York, she said "Lou, you've got to tell the Congressman." I gave it to Congressman Mel Hancock; Mel Hancock said, "I will instruct the sergeant-at-arms not to touch you. You may give this out on the street, at the foot of the steps of the House side of the U.S. Capitol as they come in to vote." And we did that.[115]

Sheldon took the brochure to Representative Mel Hancock (R-MO) on Capitol Hill. In March 1994, as the House of Representatives began debating Clinton's reauthorization of the Elementary and Secondary School Act, which provided $12.5 billion to the nation's public schools, Hancock introduced an amendment barring federal funding to any school district that "affirms a homosexual lifestyle" in its programs. The House passed a less severe version of Hancock's amendment.[116]

Undeterred, Sheldon took his cause to the Senate. On August 1, 1994, seven years after Senator Jesse Helms (R-NC) proposed an amendment that blocked federal funding for safer sex materials produced by and for gay men, Senator Bob Smith (R-NH), with the help of Helms, intro-duced a new amendment designed to stop any school system that received federal funding from running "a program or activity that has either the purpose or effect of encouraging or supporting homosexual-ity as a positive lifestyle alternative."[117] He told his colleagues, "There are some materials here that are so obscene that I cannot show them to the public. I cannot display them here and I cannot hold them up. I cannot quote from them, because to put them on the airwaves in any way, shape, or form would be considered obscene." Instead, he invited colleagues to study the materials at his desk, which included the *Safer Sex Handbook, Talk About Sex, Listen Up!, Heather Has Two Mommies,* and *Daddy's Roommate.* Smith convinced most of his colleagues, and the amendment passed 63 to 36. Seeking to blunt the amendment's homophobic angle, Senator Edward Kennedy (D-MA), one of the few advocates for progressive AIDS policies in Congress, proposed a successful amendment that blocked federal money to schools that encouraged any sexual activity, homosexual or heterosexual.[118] Seven years after the 1987 Helms Amendment, lesbian safer sex, created to provide women with the lifesaving information on HIV transmission that the government failed to give, became the vehicle for homophobic AIDS legislation. The shift in focus toward lesbian sexuality highlights the success of women AIDS activists in making visible the sexual practices of women who have sex with women for public health purposes and, equally, the risk that such visibility engendered.

In the wake of political backlash, the LAP continued to push for medical recognition and services. A breakthrough came in 1994, when the CDC created an internal working group, chaired by Dr. Mary Guinan, on woman-to-woman HIV transmission to review the literature on the topic.[119] On April 21–22, 1995, the CDC held a meeting on Lesbian HIV Issues, the first convened to discuss at a policy level HIV risk among women who have sex with women.[120] The CDC hosted the two-day meeting in Decatur, Georgia, which brought together CDC staff, including its AIDS director, James Curran, and eighteen community-based activists focused on lesbian and women's health issues, including Hollibaugh from the LAP, Eileen Hansen of WAN, Marj Plumb of the Office of Gay and Lesbian Health Concerns, and Lisa Silverberg of the National Gay and Lesbian Health Association.[121] Participants offered perspectives on the risk of HIV transmission among women who have sex with women, the factors and conditions affecting lesbian women in the epidemic, and their HIV-prevention needs. They highlighted the dearth of information available to people who planned prevention programs for such women, as well as the need for health-care professionals to better understand the behavioral risk factors, such as substance use, sex with men, artificial insemination, as well as heterosexist biases around sexuality that made self-identified lesbians and bisexuals, as well as all women who had sex with women, vulnerable.[122]

The meeting informed CDC epidemiologists' outputs, culminating in the publication of a CDC-funded, special issue of the *Journal of the American Medical Women's Association* on HIV in women. In 1990, the CDC epidemiologist Dr. Susan Y. Chu co-authored a paper that classified lesbians as "women who had sexual relations only with female partners."[123] In 1995, she contributed to an article in the special issue that acknowledged that identity did not predict behavior and which used the term "women who have sex with women" (WSW) to mark women's sexual subjectivities. The article also called for prevention interventions that "address behaviors that put WSW at risk for HIV infection, including injection drug use and unprotected penile sex," and asserted that the "possibility of sexual transmission of HIV via female-to-female sex should not be discounted."[124] That four women authored the paper suggests the greater responsiveness of women scientists' to women's non-childbearing demands.

The historic 1995 meeting represented women AIDS activists' indefatigable efforts to press the CDC to recognize lesbian and bisexual women and take seriously their specific health needs in the epidemic. This gesture, albeit significant in signaling the institutional acknowledgment of the range and diversity of women's sexual lives, came too late for an unknown number of women who died of an illness that many doubted they could contract. The CDC also did not introduce the transmission category WSW in its subsequent surveillance reports, as the percentage of women placed in the "other" exposure category consistently surpassed that of men.[125] Moreover, activists also noted that education alone could not end the epidemic. As Dázon Dixon explained, "giving out condoms and safety squares (dental dams) and ideas on erotic safe sex" could not overcome the economic, social, and power barriers tied to "racism, sexism, classism, ableism, ageism, and homophobia" that were also "directly and indirectly killing people."[126] Deborah Bybee, author of a health survey of lesbian women in Michigan, agreed on the imperative to make health care "a right rather than a privilege for lesbians and for all individuals."[127] The Clinton administration's failure to implement universal health care in the 1990s ensured that it would remain a privilege only for some into the next century.[128]

One year after the Decatur meeting, in 1996, scientists at the international AIDS conference in Vancouver reported that the combination of three, recently FDA-approved antiretroviral drugs, including a protease inhibitor, dramatically improved the health of people living with HIV.[129] The medicines only worked if people regularly took them. Lesbian AIDS activists turned their attention toward supporting women with limited access to the new medicines to fight for health care.

CONCLUSION

In the early 1990s, the LAP sought to reach as many women as possible to overcome the "myth" that lesbian women were not vulnerable to HIV. Public health agencies' slowness to recognize or track lesbian behaviors during the epidemic, treating all women as heterosexual or erasing them as "other," perpetuated this myth, but it also arose from the debates over what constituted lesbian identity that occupied lesbian feminists in the late 1960s and 1970s. For Amber Hollibaugh, involved in the wider battles over sexual expression and regulation, AIDS made urgent the need to emphasize that vulnerability to HIV infection was not about how people identified but about what they did, and so argued for an expanded understanding of their sexual identities that acknowledged that many women who had sex with women also engaged in other activities that might bring them into contact with the virus. Lesbian feminist AIDS activists like Hollibaugh and others at the LAP, as well as the women, and men, who used ACT UP to experiment both politically and sexually, exploded rigid identity categories in ways that contributed to the development of queer politics in the 1990s.

The popular, pro-sex, anti-patriarchal sex education of the LAP attracted backlash from members of the political right. For Madansky and Hollibaugh, the political campaign waged on behalf of individuals such as Mary Cummins and Mel Hancock to censor the *Safer Sex Handbook* prohibited a frank discussion of lesbian sexuality. In 1996, Madansky reflected that she "read this move toward censoring the handbook as symptomatic of a desire to silence the articulation of lesbian sexuality."[130] In her article published the same year, "Seducing Women into a 'Lifestyle of Vaginal Fisting,'" Hollibaugh explained that the lesbian community remained divided about lesbian risk of HIV infection when the political right attacked. Conservative politicians whose debates around HIV and safer sex largely obscured lesbian women during the first decade of the epidemic now silenced lesbian women in their attempts to provide lifesaving information to women who had intimate relationships with other women.[131] Their campaign, waged in the name of child protection, illustrates how the strategy of evoking the symbol of the child, the nuclear family, and the nation shaped gay and lesbian rights organizing at the end of the twentieth century.[132] The evocation of parental rights, family values, and child protection set the terms of other rights battles in the 1990s, for instance in the 1992 Supreme Court *Planned Parenthood v. Casey* ruling that young women lacked the maturity, experience, and judgment to consent to an abortion without their parents' knowledge.[133] The strategy of rhetorically and visually censoring women's bodies also informed the subsequent battles over the partial-birth abortion ban in the late 1990s and early

2000s.[134] The history of the *Safer Sex Handbook* underscores the challenges women, as well as others who engaged in nonreproductive, nonnormative, and anti-normative sex, faced in living free from prescriptions about their bodies and lives, and with full institutional support, against the backdrop of political efforts to restore a conservative vision of society at the end of the twentieth century.

Conservatives evoking family values politics not only silenced women's expressions of nonreproductive and nonnormative sexuality in the public sphere, but they also removed from it altogether the women who they believed forfeited their right to make claims on the state when they broke the law. Lesbians in organizations such as the San Francisco Lesbian Avengers and ACT UP supported women in their fight for decent medical care in prison. In July 1995, the San Francisco Avengers traveled 150 miles southeast of the Bay Area to join demonstrations that the California Coalition for Women Prisoners (CCWP), a prison advocacy group, organized on behalf of women prisoners living with HIV/AIDS and other reproductive and chronic health complications at the Central California Women's Facility (CCWF) in Chowchilla, California.[135] Lesbian women in progressive organizations helped sick women in prison take on the state in what marked the next chapter in women's fight against AIDS.

4

MURDER BY PROXY

IN 1992, JOANN WALKER, a forty-one-year-old, HIV-positive woman from Sacramento, California, received a four-year, four-month prison sentence for the theft of a $200 jacket. The judge sent Walker to the CCWF in Chowchilla—one of twenty-four prisons built in rural, conservative areas between 1982 and 1994 as part of the state's turn toward "tough on crime" politics.[1] Other women were incarcerated in this period of vast prison expansion under similar circumstances to Walker: as mothers, suffering from a host of mental and physical health complications, sent to prison for nonviolent property, public disturbance, or drug offenses.[2] Upon arrival at the facility, women like Walker encountered staff who not only neglected their specific health-care needs but actively obstructed their efforts to address them, keeping women locked up and sick based on the assumption that society needed "protecting" from them. The abuse that Walker and other women at CCWF experienced was not unique. Prison staff across the country frequently stigmatized and overlooked the needs of people in prison believed to have forfeited their constitutional right to health care by virtue of their incarceration.[3] Walker's response to mistreatment was not unique either. Like other women, the shock and horror of inhumane prison conditions led her to protest in prison and beyond. As "the paper pusher, the information getter, the HIV/AIDS advocate," Walker "raise(d) pure hell" at CCWF because "there is no other way to get things done."[4] Her efforts to educate other women about HIV/AIDS reflected the leading role Black women played in addressing the epidemic since its onset. Women's activism against AIDS in prison demonstrates how their fight against the co-occurring neglect of their health-care needs and interference in their efforts to secure proper treatment shaped the wider battle over prison health care in the late twentieth century. With the high stakes of life and death, women met abuse with powerful activism.

As the shared experiences of Walker and many other women illustrate, cases of HIV existed in women's prisons from the 1980s onward, but the political and public health response to HIV/AIDS inside prison largely mirrored the public response to the epidemic in society at large. It focused predominantly on male incarcerated persons, many of whom also experienced discrimination at the nexus of racism and classism and suffered crippling mistreatment and neglect.[5] As in other arenas of the US epidemic, prison officials and public health agencies often neglected women's specific health-care needs, leaving women to fill the gap left by a lack of institutional recognition and support. The dearth of focus on HIV in women's prisons is particularly noteworthy as from the mid-1980s onward, studies repeatedly found that—owing to the convergence of trauma, poverty, racism, physical and psychological abuse, drug use, and sex exchange—rates of infection among women in prison often matched and sometimes surpassed those among men.[6]

Women who organized in response to these conditions did not physically rebel in the manner more commonly associated with prison protest.[7] Many may have struggled to do so given their health complications. Instead, they started small prison support groups with the aim of providing critical education about HIV/AIDS. These support groups, similar to other AIDS initiatives led by women of color, continued the feminist practice of women listening to, educating, and supporting one another, as in earlier decades of the women's movements.[8] Moreover, women also continued the long tradition of people in women's prisons agitating—as scholars such as Victoria Law and Emily Thuma have shown—sometimes violently, for change.[9] In 1987, women at Bedford Hills Correctional Facility in Westchester County, New York, established ACE (AIDS Counseling and Education), one of the earliest HIV/AIDS peer support groups in the country. Other institutions replicated the Bedford Hills program, often marking the beginning of women's collective action against HIV/AIDS inside.

About 2,500 miles west of Bedford Hills, the efforts of a small group of women aiming to educate one another about HIV/AIDS at CCWF culminated in a class-action lawsuit against the state of California. Prison authorities frequently denied women at CCWF adequate medical treatment, but locking up women far away from home in institutions, cut off from networks of support, did not stop them from seeking outside help to improve the provision of health care at the facility. Prison guards routinely worked to suppress the women's efforts by blocking their communication with outside organizations; confiscating their educational materials; placing those deemed to have broken prison rules in the special housing unit, also known as solitary confinement; and threatening to remove their parole.[10] The women persevered despite these restrictions, successfully initiating contact with external activists, lawyers, and advocates. The action the women took to improve the conditions of their confinement culminated in a lawsuit against the State of California in 1995. The case, *Shumate v. Wilson*, did not focus exclusively on HIV/AIDS. Rather, as people with HIV/AIDS sued several state departments of corrections across the country,

Shumate continued the feminist practice of beginning with one health issue and expanding it to address a range of other problems, tackling HIV/AIDS alongside a multiplicity of health crises afflicting multiply marginalized women, thereby broadening our understanding of what constitutes AIDS activism.[11] Unlike other cases that typically focused on the discriminatory treatment inside male prisons, *Shumate* used the denial of women's multiple health needs to expose the inhumanity of California's prisons at the end of the twentieth and turn of the twenty-first century. Although the State of California agreed to improve the health care in its prisons in a settlement reached with the plaintiffs in 1997, women's fight for state treatment as a group deserving of care persists today.

As the field of carceral studies and histories of the AIDS epidemic expand, there is a danger that the contemporary focus on men is recapitulated in the historiography.[12] The field-defining work of scholars such as Michelle Alexander, Elizabeth Hinton, and Julilly Kohler-Hausmann has outlined how the ideological commitment to "tough on crime" politics since the 1960s—in which politicians rely on punishment to address social issues—resulted in the US incarcerating a greater proportion of its citizens than any other country in the world. Criminal justice scholars have also highlighted the racial disparities of the law-enforcement strategies that constituted the federal "war on drugs," as well as the intersections among systemic violence against women and the expansion of what the sociologist Beth E. Richie has termed "America's prison nation."[13] The work of feminist criminal justice scholars such as Richie, as well as Angela Davis, Victoria Law, and others, has in turn shifted attention toward women's incarceration.[14] Despite this shift, accounts of women protesting AIDS in prison often received less public attention than how male prisoners, prison authorities, and policymakers responded to the epidemic in men's prisons. Tracing the battle between women prisoners seeking access to treatment and care and the correctional systems of New York and California brings the history of the AIDS epidemic into conversation with the gendered and sexual dynamics of the carceral state.

Women's fight for treatment in prison reveals how the misogyny of an already gendered criminal justice system intensified with late twentieth-century prison expansion.[15] The combined misogynistic, racialized, and privatized parameters of the modern carceral state disproportionately harms women living at the intersection of multiple forms of discrimination, especially along the lines of race, class, gender, sexuality, health, and disability. In failing to adequately prepare to deal with the reproductive and chronic illnesses that are common in women, the carceral state provided an example of what Kate Manne argued happens when "institutions and other social environments" are "differentially forbidding . . . or hostile toward women."[16] Moreover, the poor health care inside women's prisons serves as an example of what Moya Bailey termed "misogynoir" in practice—the anti-black misogyny that renders Black women uniquely vulnerable to medical abuse.[17] Women living with HIV/AIDS and other illnesses in prison had a distinct set of needs, for which the expanding criminal justice system was not only ill-prepared but unwilling to address. Prison officials assumed a healthy young male, not a woman with reproductive and chronic illnesses, as its model prisoner, and implemented health-delivery systems in which inmates received care only when they requested it.[18] Making women's ability to access regular care dependent on the responsiveness of mostly male prison guards continued the history of those in positions of authority denying women's pain, especially for women of color.[19] Moreover, demonstrating, with the rise of neoliberal politics, how far a commitment to punish replaced a duty to care, lawmakers in California who committed billions of dollars toward building new prisons allowed prisons to make people in their custody pay for their care.[20] Women whom the state deemed undeserving of support—and who, due to social and economic inequality linked to racism and other vectors of discrimination already experienced disproportionately high rates of diseases such as HIV/AIDS—suffered from the increasingly privatized and politicized nature of public health at century's end.

The experience of living within a racist, misogynistic, and privatized prison system shaped the women's organizing on the inside, inspiring forms of mutual aid between prisoners and compelling the formation of inside-outside alliances. Their organizing well illustrates Juanita Diaz-Cotto's assessment of the variety and power of women prisoners' political resistance.[21] As people in women's prisons across the country experienced abhorrent medical conditions akin to those at Bedford Hills and CCWF, the HIV/AIDS activism of women at those facilities is notable for combining less obviously disruptive acts, such as peer education, with traditional examples of political activism, such as filing lawsuits. Their actions open avenues to explore the ways in which different activist strategies work and why. Brought together in confinement, the women built supportive alliances with others in prison across lines of racial, class, sexual, and health difference, and, as in the case of CCWF, with external advocates with greater traditional means to take up their cause. Living at the intersection of multiple forms of discrimination, they were well placed to confront the systemic oppressions that threatened their lives. Equally, the inability of the women at CCWF to fundamentally improve the delivery of care at women's facilities spoke to the challenge of taking on California's prison system amid the bipartisan commitment to using prison expansion to "fix" social, political, and economic problems in the late twentieth century.[22]

INSIDE PRISON WALLS

The outbreak of AIDS in the early 1980s made urgent the question of how to contain HIV within prisons. The steps taken to address the issue of AIDS in prison in the 1980s and 1990s varied according to state and facility. Some prisons took the advice of the public health community and made available condoms, drugs, and cleansing solution to sanitize hypodermic needles. Others refused, believing that such measures condoned homosexual activity and drug use. Instead, they tested and segregated HIV-positive prisoners, arguing that isolation protected not only uninfected incarcerated persons in and out of prison, but HIV-positive prisoners themselves.[23]

Following the FDA's approval of AZT in 1987, the introduction in 1996 of combinations of three antiretroviral agents (also known as antiretroviral therapy or ART) to suppress a person's viral load and recover immune function shifted the meaning of HIV from a lethal virus to a chronic, manageable condition.[24] As effective treatment options became available, the increased cost of distributing more effective medication directed the response of correctional authorities to HIV/AIDS in prison.

Prison authorities varied in their approach to dealing with AIDS because of the costly treatment. Jan Diamond, a physician at the California Medical Facility at Vacaville State Prison, explained how the introduction of AZT changed prison authorities' priorities over testing. The California legislature initially pushed to introduce mandatory testing of prisoners and quarantine those who tested positive in an effort to curb transmission, but when "AZT became accepted therapy for treating asymptomatics, they quickly figured out how much it would cost to really know who had the virus and they dropped their push."[25] According to Matthew Purdy, as the annual cost of treating an HIV-positive incarcerated person rose from approximately $2,000 in the 1980s to $13,000 in the 1990s, "drugs are not being widely prescribed in some prisons even though doctors acknowledge that it is unethical not to."[26] States willing to spend more money to address AIDS did not necessarily take a more progressive approach. Instead, as the former incarcerated person John Zeh noted, less funding often resulted in fairer treatment in terms of "reduced mass testing, less segregation, and . . . the early release for" people with AIDS "needing costly long-term care."[27] The high cost of treating HIV drove other, more progressive prison officials, such as William Hall, the correctional assistant director for health services in Washington, DC, to distribute condoms and clean needles.[28] The lack of access to effective medicines in prison reflected the situation in society at large. In a hybrid public-private, for-profit health-care system, only the insured, and those living in a city or state that covered the medication, benefited from the medical advances.[29]

While Hall recognized the financial and medical efficacy of providing condoms as HIV prevention in male prisons, few acknowledged the need to take comparable steps to prevent transmission in women's prisons, either through education or supplying prophylactics, such as condoms for voluntary or coerced sex during conjugal visits or with guards, dildos, or dental dams. While the onset of HIV/AIDS led some prison authorities to more closely police women's physical contact, the lack of concern about the sexual transmission of HIV among women perpetuated the "myth of lesbian immunity" that assumed women could not contract or transmit HIV to each other and reflected the broader denial of sex in all prisons.[30] Aware of the prevalence of same-sex activity in women's prison and the possibility of woman-to-woman transmission through blood or vaginal fluids, Felicia Davidson, a program coordinator at the Women's Project in Little Rock, Arkansas, advised women to use bread sacks, cookie wrap paper, "any kind of barrier to keep from sharing fluids," as "some protection is better than none."[31] In November 1992, a lesbian woman incarcerated at the New York Albion Correctional Facility wrote to the LAP explaining that prison officials dismissed the possibility of woman-to-woman HIV transmission. The woman asked LAP to "please send me everything you have for gay women and HIV" due to the inadequate resources on the disease available to women at the facility.[32]

The scaling up of the carceral state from the mid-twentieth century onward failed to prepare for women's needs. The slowness on the part of prison authorities to respond to women's reproductive and chronic illnesses resulted in part from the fact that the medical treatment offered in most prisons catered to healthy, young men. Dr. Corey Weinstein, former chair of the Jail and Prison Health Committee and member of the governing council of the American Public Health Association, explained in a 1997 interview with the reporter Nina Siegal of the *San Francisco Bay Guardian* that the military developed the "sick call" system, in which prisoners only received care when they requested it, because in the military, "most of the people are healthier than the norm."[33] A system designed for healthy young men failed women, as well as men, living with multiple health complications requiring regular care.[34] The lack of maternity and gynecological care available to women in prison posed a particular danger for women living with HIV/AIDS at high risk of cervical cancer and other reproductive health complications.[35]

The military-inspired model that Weinstein described required women with health problems to visit sick call and persuade a prison guard with minimal medical training, whom the California Department of Corrections and Rehabilitation (CDCR) renamed Medical Technician Assistants (MTAs), that the problem justified seeing a qualified medic.[36] The MTAs, to whose authority women were expected to be subordinate, also served as the gatekeepers to receiving proper care. Making women's ability to secure regular treatment dependent on the whim of nonspecialist prison guards, who were also responsible for discipline and who repeatedly failed to take their health complaints seriously, continued the practice of heteronormative, male-led, and male-dominated medical institutions denying women proper treatment.[37] An inmate with sickle cell anemia reported that the prison staff at CCWF frequently denied her the regular medical treatment needed for her condition, so every month "like clockwork" she went into crisis, forcing staff to rush her to the closest medical community center for emergency treatment. She explained that the center "more or less stated that they don't do preventative care."[38] Thus, women who arrived at prison with multiple health complications—including chronic physical and mental health problems that arose from past experiences of trauma and abuse, drug use, involvement in sex work, or a lack of access to community health care, as well as reproductive health needs—were failed by the system because they were unable to access regular care.[39] Due to these factors, women in prison, on average, suffered health complications at higher rates and requested health services more frequently than men.[40] That such chronic illnesses are expensive to treat likely accounts for the prison's preference for using the sick call system to provide sporadic, rather than consistent, care.[41] But state actors were not only motivated by a desire to cut costs. Employing MTAs cost the CDCR more than hiring nurses to do the job. Releasing older incarcerated persons and those with severe and life-threatening illnesses would have also saved the prison money. Driven by an ideological commitment to incapacitate, the CDCR's policies of the late twentieth century lacked efficiency as well as humanity.[42]

Sick and fatigued, prison staff forced women at CCWF to queue outside once a week in either the baking California sun, the rain, or freezing cold to request sick call with no guarantee of being seen.[43] Women experiencing severe sickness probably questioned whether joining the sick call queue was worth it. Prison officials in states with similarly large prison populations and high incarceration rates, such as Florida, Texas, and Alabama, also required incarcerated persons to queue up daily or weekly to receive their medicines, which the prisons sometimes ran out of, demonstrating their disregard for inmate health.[44] The so-called pill line or med line removed confidentiality, and those too sick to line up did not receive their drugs. Moreover, medicine collected in the pill line did not always come with clear instructions on when and how to take them or guidance on their potential side effects, making drug regimens difficult to maintain.[45] Failing to take medicines correctly puts people at risk of developing drug resistance, which can be fatal. The largest prison systems across the US forced sick women to navigate health-delivery systems designed for healthy young men.[46]

In frustration and fury, women protested. The outbreak of HIV/ AIDS in the 1980s made explicit the inadequacy of medical care in prison. Women at Bedford Hills began educating and counseling other women and fostering a community of support.[47] Kathy Boudin and Judith Clark, two white, former members of the Weather Underground, a radical left-wing organization, whose role in the 1981 Brink's robbery brought them to Bedford Hills, contributed to the early efforts to address HIV/AIDS.[48] The grassroots experience that Clark and Boudin brought to the prison influenced their role in the organizing efforts among its women prisoners. The mistreatment the women with HIV/ AIDS and other illnesses experienced at the facility moved other inmates. Katrina Haslip, for example, a Black Muslim HIV-positive activist, advocated on behalf of other women with HIV in prison and established the ACE-OUT program to support women leaving prison. She continued her work after she left Bedford Hills in 1990, joining the campaign to change the CDC's AIDS definition. She died in December 1992 of bacterial pneumonia, a condition she petitioned the CDC to recognize as a symptom of AIDS. She died one month before the agency added the condition to their AIDS definition, and was therefore not officially registered as having died of AIDS.[49] With diverse racial, class, religious, sexual, and health backgrounds, Haslip, Boudin, Clark, as well as Doris Moices, Ada Rivera, Gloria Boyd, Awilda Gonzales, and others mobilized around the shared goal of securing proper medical attention for themselves and their peers.[50]

Haslip, Clark, Boudin, Moices, Rivera, and Boyd vowed to educate themselves, staff, and other inmates about HIV to combat the fear and prejudice that typified the prison community's attitudes toward AIDS at Bedford Hills. Prison guards isolated women known to have HIV in the in-patient care unit (IPC), where the medical staff often knew little about the disease and avoided physical contact with their patients.[51]

Officers interacting with HIV-positive women often wore gloves and masks, an unnecessary measure, as people knew that HIV does not spread through casual contact. This stoked fears among the prisoners, who sometimes acted violently toward women with HIV or those with HIV-positive relatives. The women visited those housed in the IPC to provide support.[52]

Building on the consciousness-raising tradition of the intersectional feminist health movements of the 1960s and 1970s, the women at Bedford Hills set up prison support groups that took women's stories and perspectives seriously. They also educated women about HIV and its causes, the experimental drugs they were denied access to following a ban on testing drugs on people in prison, available treatments, and its transmissions to empower women and combat stigma. In 1988, the women secured permission from the prison administration to create the ACE program at Bedford Hills, one of the first and most comprehensive prison support groups for women prisoners in the country.[53]

The fact that they did not physically resist oppression in ways similar to women prisoners during the strikes at the Massachusetts Correctional Institution in Framingham, Massachusetts, in 1972, and the California Institution for Women (CIW) in 1973, or during the 1974 August Rebellion at Bedford Hills, did not make them passive.[54] Like women prisoners who empowered themselves through education, they set up prison support groups with the aim of educating one another and petitioning for proper treatment and a better quality of life.[55] Other women prisoners across the country based their support groups on ACE, such as the Pleasanton AIDS Education and Counseling Program that the political prisoners Linda Evans and Laura Whitehorn established at California's Federal Correctional Institution at Pleasanton.[56] At the York Correctional Institution in Connecticut, Felicia Crowe, an HIV-positive prisoner, wrote letters to the warden, the medical unit, and the mental health unit until they approved her HIV support group.[57]

Prison officials rarely responded to the women's respectful requests in kind. Instead, they interpreted women's efforts to protect their health as a challenge to prison authority. Following the historic punishment of women deemed "dangerous" and "unruly" for demanding improved prison conditions, prison staff committed to maintaining the prison order frequently detained women who agitated for change in solitary confinement.[58] In California, the CDCR expressly prohibits "acts of disobedience or disrespect" that might result in "violence or mass disruptive behavior," as well as "participation in a strike or work stoppage." The power of these rules lies in their vagueness. Women isolated for acts deemed to have threatened prison security also risked losing their parole.[59] Despite the potential penalties and regardless of administrative approval, women prisoners continued to challenge the conditions of their confinement in facilities across the country, eventually connecting with outside support.

THROUGH PRISON WALLS

The medical disaster inside California women's prisons turned many sick women into activists. One of the first preventable deaths that mobilized women at CCWF involved Dianna Reyes, a forty-three-year-old Latina woman with diabetes. On June 18, 1991, Reyes joined the sick-call line to get her insulin. The negligence of the medical staff irritated Reyes, and she and another woman became involved in a physical altercation. Officials sent them both to administrative segregation for a ten-day disciplinary isolation, where staff refused to give Reyes medical attention. Her health severely deteriorated until officers eventually realized they needed to act and transferred her to the hospital. A short time later, doctors pronounced her dead. According to prisoner Linda Eagerton, prison officials said that Reyes died of natural causes and added a total of ten years to the sentences of the women who refused to work that day.[60] Reyes's death underlined the medical negligence commonplace in California's women's prisons in the 1990s.

The gutting of social welfare services and advance of a neoliberal social agenda that championed individualism, volunteerism, and non-state action during the 1980s and 1990s exacerbated inequities in health care along race, sexuality, gender, and class lines, and converged with prison expansion.[61] That President Clinton won bipartisan support for expansive, punitive prison legislation while his plans for implementing universal health reform failed underscores how a political commitment to punish rather than provide care dominated the late twentieth century. In 1994, the same year that Clinton lost his fight for national health care, and two years before he introduced sweeping welfare reform, he signed the Violent Crime Control and Law Enforcement Act that increased budgets for law enforcement and prisons, and made grants available for states that implemented Truth in Sentencing programs designed to prevent the early release of incarcerated persons from prison.[62] Across the country, other states introduced punitive sentencing measures.[63] Promising new jobs in a faltering economy and the restoration of public order, many Californians mandated the use of prisons to "fix" a series of perceived "crises" in the last decades of the twentieth century. In November 1994, California voters approved Proposition 184, also known as "three strikes-and-you're-out" sentencing, which imposed automatic life sentences for repeat offenders without the possibility of parole. Legislators also passed new laws that expanded the criminalization of drugs and gangs.[64] Together, these laws swelled the state's prison population.[65] Coupled with lengthened sentences, California's prison population not only grew, but aged.[66] The increasing incarceration, homelessness, and precarity that resulted fueled the spread of disease. Steven W. Thrasher attributed the growth of HIV/AIDS in Black communities following the introduction of effective medicines to Clinton's domestic reforms.[67]

Harsher enforcement and sentencing practices drove women's prison growth in and beyond California. The prosecution of drug use that followed the moral panic over a "crack cocaine epidemic" in Black communities, combined with the increased targeting of quality-of-life and low-level, nonviolent offenses, such as petty theft, brought greater numbers of women—more likely than men to engage in these acts— into contact with the criminal justice system.[68] During the 1990s, female inmates came to prison mostly after convictions for nonviolent property, drug, and public order offenses and, to a lesser extent, acts of violence often carried out in self-defense.[69] With the introduction of "three-strikes" legislation, the broadening of offenses with mandatory sentence length, and stricter drug enforcement practices, the number of women in California's jails and prisons skyrocketed, increasing five-fold from 4,432 to 23,597 between 1980 and 2000.[70] In October 1990, CCWF, the largest women's prison in the state, opened.[71] Five years later, the Valley State Prison for Women (VSPW) opened across the road. Located approximately 150 miles southeast of San Francisco in the predominantly Republican-run Madera County, and covering 640 acres of land, the two compounds on either side of Road 24 constituted the two largest women's prisons in the world in the 1990s.[72] The offenses that brought women, with a median age of thirty-six, to CCWF—such as low-level embezzlement, petty theft, and violence carried out in self-defense—brought women to prisons across the country.[73]

Women faced several obstacles to accessing medical care in California's prisons. CCWF did not have a licensed infirmary. Management refused to hire an HIV/AIDS medical specialist and rarely let women see a gynecologist. Women with serious illnesses reported having to wait weeks to see a medically trained doctor, and the retired physician who treated HIV-positive women on C yard specialized not in women's health but pediatrics, flattening the differences between women's health and that of infants and children. In the absence of medical professionals, MTAs regularly examined and diagnosed the women.[74] Due to their limited or nonexistent medical training, MTAs frequently misdiagnosed women and prescribed the wrong drugs, which led to further illness and sometimes death. One woman with HIV-related thrush in her mouth reported that an MTA gave her vaginal suppositories to eat when they failed to acquire the lozenges she needed.[75] As the CDC based the initial diagnosis of AIDS on how HIV manifested in men, women experienced enough difficulty obtaining a HIV diagnosis without having to rely on guards with minimal medical training to recognize symptoms. The suffering women experienced at the hands of MTAs highlights the harmful, sometimes fatal, consequences of using systems designed to punish to provide care.

Prison officials not only placed on women the burden of convincing MTAs of their health needs but also the financial responsibility of requesting care. In 1994, the California legislature passed a law allowing the CDCR to charge a $5 co-pay to request a medical visit through sick call.[76] Although the law required prisons to provide care if an inmate could not afford to pay, women testified to having to choose between medical care visits or sanitary products because they could not afford both.[77] Moreover, the co-pay system only allowed the treatment of one health problem per visit, thereby failing to meet the multiple health needs common among women in California's prisons.[78] In December 1994, CCWF reduced sick call to once a week. As prison officials did not provide routine medical exams and all medical procedures went through sick call, this policy further impeded women's ability to access regular care.[79] Costing more to administer than the income it generated, the co-pay system, designed to raise money and reduce medical requests, proves how an ideological commitment to punish trumped efficiency in late twentieth-century prison systems.[80]

For Joann Walker, the medical neglect, segregation, lack of confidentiality, and the high stress that women prisoners with HIV experienced constituted "murder by proxy."[81] According to Walker, while CCWF officials offered voluntary testing to all inmates in theory, in practice they frequently denied HIV tests to women who requested one, informing them that they could only receive a test if they showed visible signs of sickness. This requirement proved particularly onerous for women given that the physical manifestations of HIV virus in women are often not visible, with death frequently coming from opportunistic infections such as cervical cancer and other non-visible diseases. Prison officials also denied women with HIV the ability to participate in the family visitation program and did not allow them to work in the kitchen or infirmary. Because of the housing segregation and loss of job opportunities and visitation privileges, many women hid their HIV-positive status or did not seek testing. As a result, although the CDCR reported that fifty women at CCWF had HIV in the early 1990s, Walker argued that the agency had no real idea of the actual number of HIV-positive women at the prison.[82]

Other discriminatory treatment that deterred inmates from seeking testing and treatment included guards segregating HIV-positive women in C Yard alongside signs reading, "Beware! There are HIV infected inmate persons housed in this facility!"[83] Women's confinement in a segregated yard automatically revealed their HIV status.[84]

These persistent health-care violations moved women like Charisse Shumate to act. In 1989, while in her thirties, Shumate received a life sentence for killing her abusive partner in self-defense.[85] As a Black woman with sickle cell anemia, a disease that significantly impacts Black communities, and around which Black activists had organized to protest government inaction, she represented the women whose mistreatment lay at the intersection of racial and gender marginalization.[86] CCWF did not hire a hematologist for women's sickle cell anemia, lupus, and other blood diseases, and Shumate received a blood transfusion for her illness only once every three months instead of the more regular transfusions necessary for severe and persistent anemia.[87] Shumate began educating women about the complications of sickle cell and HIV in women and the necessary treatment. At the same time, she fought to receive proper care for her illness and advocated for the right to compassionate release for terminally ill prisoners, a policy to allow those within six months of death to return home but which is notoriously difficult to secure.[88]

Instead of supporting women, prison officials hampered their efforts to learn more about HIV/AIDS, censoring the educational materials sent to them from outside organizations such as ACT UP/San Francisco, the ACLU National Prison Project, and the San Francisco AIDS Foundation.[89] In June 1993, a thirty-three-year-old HIV-positive woman named Brenda Lee Ivy wrote to the AIDS advocate Paul Collins requesting HIV information. He replied one month later to inform her that "on July 26, 1993, as per your request, I mailed to you a package containing literature on HIV/AIDS. Unfortunately, that package was returned to me today, stamped by your correctional facility as unauthorized correspondence."[90] Gina Marie Caruso wrote, "All of our mail is read and censored before it goes out of this institution . . . . You must understand the length and chance I'm taking to be heard. . . . I'm not the only one that has something to say there are several hundred women that are willing to speak out if only someone would listen." To stop prison officials from censoring her letter, Caruso sent it out with her cellmate on her release date.[91]

Joann Walker, Gina Marie Caruso, and their peers understood that bringing the inhumane situation inside CCWF to the attention of outside lawyers, activists, and politicians with more resources and greater political leverage increased their chances of improving health care at the facility. The number of organizations they contacted is a testament to the vibrant, progressive organizing that took place in response to HIV/AIDS and related issues in and around Oakland and San Francisco in this period. Oakland-based advocacy groups such as Legal Services for Prisoners with Children (LSPC) began receiving letters from women at CCWF almost as soon as the facility opened in 1990.[92] Twillah Wallace wrote to California State Assemblywoman Barbara Lee, acknowledging that "there are many important issues that needs the attention of someone from the outside and someone of power, as yourself."[93] Women contacted other politicians, attorneys, legal services, and people in positions of authority in California and beyond trying to get news out and make contact with outside organizations.[94] According to Nancy Stoller, people in California's women's prisons filed 1,269 complaints to attorneys between 1996 and 1999, 555 of which came from women at CCWF.[95]

News of inmate complaints brought the Fresno attorney Catherine Campbell and Dr. Corey Weinstein to CCWF in 1992. Together, they launched an independent investigation into the health care at CCWF after they toured the facility and heard accounts of MTAs denying women with sickle cell anemia, HIV/AIDS, epilepsy, and other health complications adequate care, including access to their regular medication. Campbell and Weinstein began conducting independent interviews with women prisoners and collecting data.[96]

In May 1993, Walker wrote to the Prison Issues Committee of ACT UP/San Francisco asking for support for women with HIV/AIDS at the prison.[97] ACT UP connected Walker to the prisoner rights advocate Judy Greenspan, a white activist who worked with ACT UP/San Francisco's Prison Issues Committee. Greenspan also worked as the AIDS information director for the ACLU's National Project and director of the Catholic Charities' HIV/AIDS in Prison Project in the Bay Area.[98] Her ongoing work with HIV-positive prisoners and connections with the women's, lesbian and gay, prisoner advocacy, AIDS activist, and criminal justice communities enabled her to become the bridge between the women in prison and outside organizations.[99] In 1993, after women at CCWF initiated contact, she helped launch the Coalition to Support Women Prisoners at Chowchilla (CSWPC), which offered grassroots support to women inside.[100] A formidable advocate, Greenspan went beyond the call of duty in corresponding with, working on behalf of, and supporting the women in CCWF. Her standing within various progressive communities enabled her to bring the health-care struggles of women prisoners to the attention of groups already involved in rights organizing around HIV/AIDS and prisons. In relaying the women's stories of medical neglect and the difficulty of obtaining information about HIV/AIDS in prison, Greenspan motivated activists to approach prison organizing from the vantage point of race, sexuality, and gender in the 1990s and early 2000s.[101]

Walker sent Greenspan a copy of the proposal for a peer education program that she and several other Black women living with HIV at the facility—including Deborah Paul—drafted in March 1993 "to provide support for CCWF inmates who are living with HIV and AIDS; to join the CCWF staff in educating the general population about HIV and AIDS; and to work effectively within the CCWF system and the larger community to promote awareness of our special care needs."[102] Because CCWF offered no formal HIV/AIDS education program, the women endeavored to start an informal prison support group focusing on HIV/AIDS, tuberculosis, and hepatitis C. They submitted the proposal for the prison administration's approval, but the warden initially ignored it. Greenspan sent copies to groups on the outside and asked them to send letters of support. With the help of outside pressure, administrators eventually approved the program on the condition that the four women did not question the prison's rules, policies, and staff's conduct, threatening to write them up if they did.[103] Despite approval, prison officials took no steps to implement the program and, in the meantime, Walker, Paul, and others visited the prison yards giving presentations on the disease to their peers.[104] Not long afterward, staff told Walker to stop her peer education efforts, citing her "negative" influence on other women.[105]

In July 1993, Walker sent Greenspan a copy of a petition she had initiated demanding that prison officials fire David Archer, an MTA accused of abusing women.[106] More than 450 women signed the petition that got Archer removed from C Yard. While the petition impressed Greenspan, who noted that "petitioning inside under the eyes of the prison guards is quite a feat," it also alarmed her because the "fact that so many women signed a petition was a strong signal that medical care was reaching a crisis point at CCWF."[107] One month later, in August 1993, Greenspan wrote to inform James Gomez, the director of corrections, of the deep concern arising from the multiple complaints she received from HIV-positive women at CCWF, including over the lack of medical care and the censorship of HIV/AIDS educational material. Greenspan, who copied journalists from leading local and national newspapers into the letter, argued that these actions aided the spread of HIV and created a life-threatening situation at the prison, and that she, writing on behalf of ACT UP/San Francisco, demanded an immediate investigation of medical services at the facility.[108]

Owing to the absence of institutional services for women with terminal illnesses at CCWF, prisoners also pushed for the compassionate release of dying inmates. In October 1993, Walker called Greenspan to tell her about her roommate, Betty Jo Ross, a thirty-five-year-old HIV-positive woman with deteriorating health.[109] Ross suffered from a series of serious AIDS-related ailments, including dementia, Mycobacterium avium complex, Cytomegalovirus retinitis, and a T-cell count of one. The doctor informed her that she had fewer than six months left to live, making her eligible for compassionate release.[110] Walker insisted that the warden grant Ross compassionate release, but Gomez denied this request twice on the grounds of Ross's "uncontrollable conduct and pattern of assaultive behavior."[111] Angry, Walker demanded that ACT UP/San Francisco and other groups act immediately. She began a petition for Ross's release that more than one thousand prisoners, all risking retribution, signed. She also made signs reading "Free Betty Jo" and "Don't let the system kill another PWA (Person with AIDS)," which the women pinned to their clothing.[112] Outside, ACT UP and the CSWPC began a "Send Betty Jo Ross Home for Christmas" fax and phone campaign, and organizations such as the Mobilization Against AIDS sent Gomez letters "strongly recommend[ing] that the inmate be granted an early release."[113] To the amazement of outside organizations who initially doubted Walker's ability to do anything for Ross, the CDCR released her on January 5, 1994.[114]

This remarkable victory helped attract further outside support for their cause. A few weeks after Ross's release, on January 29, the CSWPC held its first demonstration at the gates of the prison to demand quality medical care for the women inside. More than one hundred people from the Bay Area and California organizations, including ACT UP/San Francisco, the San Francisco AIDS Foundation, and LSPC picketed the prison to support the prisoners, demanding that it provide "quality health care for all women prisoners; hire an HIV/AIDS specialist; high nutritional diets and vitamin supplements for HIV+ prisoners; compassionate release for all terminally ill prisoners; support prisoner-initiated peer education efforts."[115] Greenspan sought the support of lesbian and gay groups, relaying that "many of the women inside Chowchilla . . . are lesbians of color who are fighting the worst forms of homophobia inside the prisons, compounded with the stigma of having HIV and AIDS."[116] Greenspan raised $800 to assist travel to the demonstration from the organization Resist.[117] Walker committed to writing to outside organizations and media "all day long if need be," putting a "call out around the world" to "help the HIV/AIDS incarcerated women at CCWF!"[118] The lesbian advocacy organization Out of Control published a letter in which Walker accused "The California Penal System" of treating "HIV/AIDS as if it is a crime!" and asked, "Does anyone out there care?"[119] She also secured radio interviews and a one-page profile on her three days before the protest in the *San Francisco Bay Guardian*, in which journalist Noelle Hanrahan observed, "Walker seems anything but weak."[120] Attorneys from Human Rights Watch also interviewed her.[121]

In the wake of the protest, CCWF officials assured the press of the adequacy of their medical services. Toby Wong, the public information officer, dismissed the women's claims as "biased" and denied the collective power of women's testimonies, claiming that information gathered "from just a few inmates" could not sustain a campaign.[122] Wong's discrediting of the women and their supporters resulted in editorials, such as one published in the *Merced Sun-Star* that dismissed women in CCWF's fight for humane care as "out of line."[123]

The dismissive response to the women's demands jarred with the deaths of several more women over a few weeks in early 1994. Sonja Staples and Jackie Jenkins both died of AIDS-related illnesses after MTAs failed to give them the appropriate medical attention long called for by their cellmates. Molly Reyes died one month later, on February 25.[124] The nonprofit advocacy group People with AIDS Coalition New York relayed news of these women's deaths in their monthly newsletter, *Newsline*.[125]

Walker became seriously ill with severe headaches in March. Every time she visited the sick call, the staff sent her away with the ibuprofen drug Motrin.[126] In April, she began coughing up blood and staff sent her to the outside medical center in Merced, where doctors diagnosed her with fungal meningitis that spread throughout her system. Following a three-week-long fax and phone campaign to both the warden and Gomez, a Fresno superior court judge granted Walker compassionate release. Two months later, on July 13, she died of AIDS-related complications in the care of her family in Sacramento.[127] After her death, Walker's friend Twillah Wallace wrote "the struggle will not end because you are gone" and continued Walker's fight for improved medical care at CCWF.[128] Through her prolific writing on the situation inside CCWF, Walker was a key spokesperson for women prisoners with HIV, and many of her articles captured outside media attention.[129] Walker's death—along with the deaths of Staples, Jenkins, and Reyes—prompted activists and lawyers to demand immediate, impartial legislative investigations.[130]

A few months before Walker's death, in the spring of 1994, Greenspan contacted Amnesty International and the US Department of Justice (DOJ) to provide details of the inadequate medical care and services available to women prisoners with HIV/AIDS and other medical problems at CCWF that she hoped might aid investigations into the conditions at the prison.[131] She also sent statements about the treatment of HIV-positive women to large media outlets such as the *San Francisco Chronicle* as "national coverage of this unique struggle, involving women prisoners organizing on the inside and the Coalition demonstrating on the outside, is essential to save lives and win better health care for the women at Chowchilla."[132] A few months later, the DOJ informed Greenspan of their intention to initiate an investigation of her allegations pursuant to Title II of the Americans with Disabilities Act of 1990 and Section 504 of the Rehabilitation Act of 1973, which prohibits discrimination against individuals with HIV/AIDS on the basis of their disability in public entities.[133]

DOJ investigators visited CCWF in August 1994 to interview women.[134] In September, after two years of independent investigations, Campbell and Weinstein decided to use the evidence gathered to launch a major class-action lawsuit against the CDCR. Within a year, Elizabeth Alexander of the ACLU National Prison Project, Ellen Barry of the LSPC, and Charles N. Freiberg of Heller Ehrman White & McAuliffe filed a suit in the US District Court for the Eastern District of California against California prison officials on behalf of state prisoners and parolees living under the custody and control of the CDCR. The DOJ investigation and subsequent class-action lawsuit compelled the district court to approach the medical mistreatment of people in prison from the vantage point of the chronic and reproductive health rights of people in women's prisons, including the disability rights of women with HIV/AIDS.[135]

FROM THE CELL TO THE COURT

The eleven attorneys' efforts to challenge the egregious health care in California's women's prisons built on the work of civil rights lawyers, who from the late 1960s onward began suing prison systems in the federal courts and arguing that prison conditions across the nation violated the Eighth Amendment's prohibition against cruel and unusual punishment.[136] In 1972, the ACLU established the National Prison Project to defend the civil and constitutional rights of prisoners.[137] In the 1976 case *Estelle v. Gamble*, the Supreme Court affirmed the constitutional obligation of jails and prisons to provide health care to those in custody, as the "deliberate indifference to serious medical needs of prisoners constitutes the 'unnecessary and wanton infliction of pain' . . . proscribed by the Eighth Amendment."[138]

The women's claims that the state's inadequate sick calls, use of MTAs, denial of medical care based on cost, and failure to provide proper chronic care endangered them appeared to put the California prison officials in violation of this ruling. But *Estelle* also placed a burden on the women to prove that the alleged negligence constituted a sufficient threat and that the officials acted with deliberate indifference to their health and safety.[139]

On April 4, 1995, twenty-six inmates at CCWF in Chowchilla, along with the CIW in Frontera, California, filed their class-action lawsuit, *Shumate v. Wilson*, in the US District Court for the Eastern District of California. Defendants included Pete Wilson, Republican governor of California; James Gomez, director of the CDCR; and Kyle S. McKinsey, deputy director for health care services for the CDCR.[140]

The plaintiffs sought reform of the prison's "knowing and deliberately indifferent failure to provide necessary care for serious medical needs," as well as relief to remedy alleged "policies, practices, acts, and omissions evidenc[ing] and constitut[ing] deliberate indifference to the rights of prisoners and violat[ing] the Cruel and Unusual Punishment Clause of the Eighth Amendment."[141] For her ability to lead and inspire, Charisse Shumate was chosen by the attorneys as the lead plaintiff.[142] The case alleged that defendants failed to supply numerous adequate health provisions, including sick calls, triage, emergency care, urgent care, follow-up care, chronic care, gynecological care, mental health care, medical equipment, specialty referrals, terminal care, dental care, medically necessary diets, health education, confidentiality, and complaints procedures. They also alleged that the delivery of medical care included unsafe delays and the disruption of prescription medications.[143] While the suit focused on two women's prisons—CCWF and CIW—Nina Siegal of the *San Francisco Bay Guardian* noted that "many of the problems alleged in the suit (and confirmed by various independent investigations) result from systemic problems built into the health care delivery system in women's prisons."[144]

During the 1980s, as HIV/AIDS spread throughout the national prison population, the ACLU and other legal advocacy organizations challenged the mistreatment of HIV-positive incarcerated persons, from the inadequate medical care they received to their isolation and exclusion from prison programs. Organizations filed several lawsuits on behalf of prisoners against various state departments of corrections, including those in Connecticut, Alabama, Pennsylvania, as well as California.[145] While some of these suits, such as *Doe v. Meachum* (1988) and *Harris v. Thigpen* (1990) also involved people in women's prisons, the settlements rarely addressed the distinct needs of women with HIV, including provisions for pregnancy-related and gynecological care and cervical cancer. The significance of *Shumate* lay not only in challenging the inadequate medical care in California's prisons but in foregrounding the multiple health-care needs of women prisoners with HIV/AIDS.

As *Shumate* progressed, the women involved in the lawsuit, Greenspan, and other advocates worried that "nothing will change unless we keep up a high level of public protest and scrutiny."[146] They organized regular protests outside CCWF and VSPW and the Sacramento Federal Courthouse.[147] At a demonstration held outside CCWF on July 8, 1995, which was endorsed by nearly thirty progressive organizations, activists reiterated their demand for "quality medical care for women prisoners," including the hiring of "an HIV/AIDS medical specialist" and prohibiting "payment" as a requirement for "care." It also called for

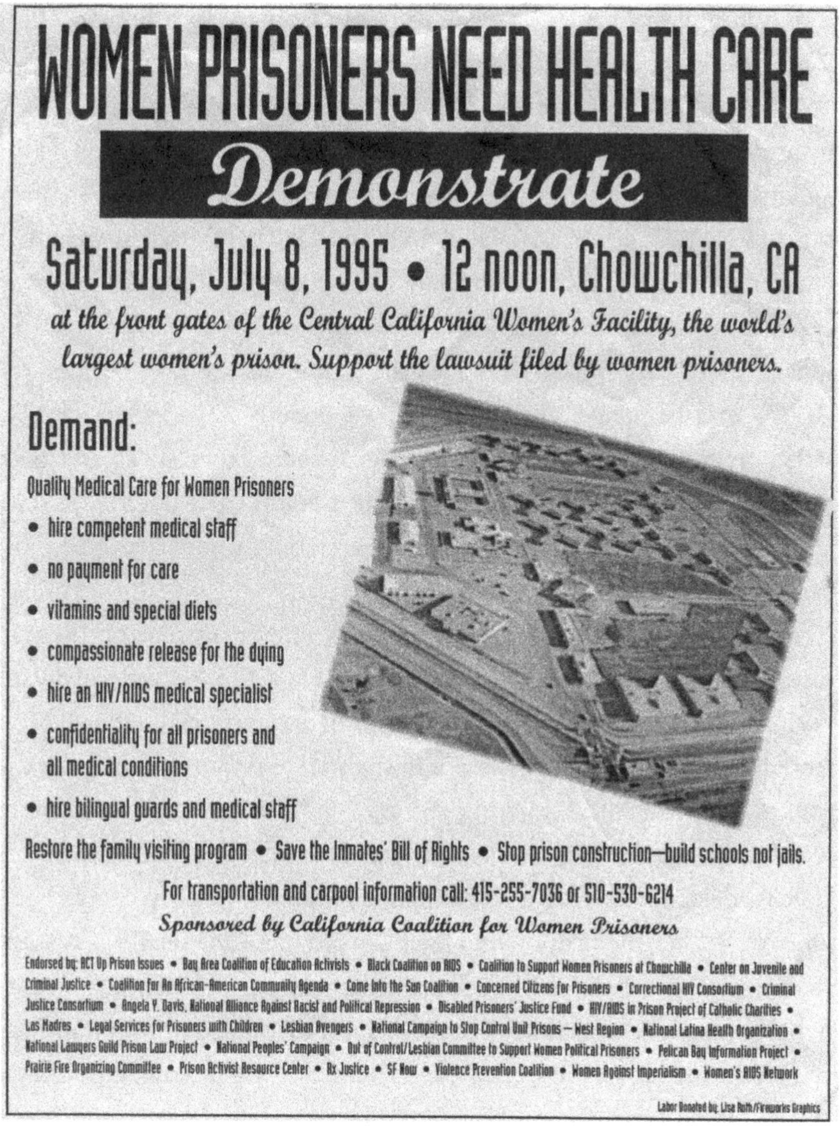

Fig. 7. Chowchilla Demonstration for Medical Care for Women Prisoners, July 8, 1995, Lesbian Avengers collection 96-10. Courtesy of Gay, Lesbian, Bisexual, Transgender Historical Society.

a shift in political priorities away from punishment to support, calling for the building of "schools not jails."

Judges do not make or decide laws in a vacuum. They are influenced by and respond to the historical context in which they operate and the actions of people in the streets. As Dorsey Nunn and Karen Shain of the LSPC, two other advocates who worked tirelessly on behalf of women in CCWF, told Greenspan, "lawsuits are not only fought in courtrooms, they are also fought in the public eye, through the media."[148] To this end, in May 1995 the women at CCWF founded the CCWP and launched *The Fire Inside*, a quarterly newsletter that provided women with a vehicle to publicize their experiences and raise public awareness of the ongoing institutionalized gendered, sexualized, racialized violence they and other women experienced in the carceral system.[149]

As activists continued to show up for women prisoners on the outside, CCWF officials on the inside threatened the *Shumate* plaintiffs with retaliatory treatment. Shumate claimed that officials labeled her a troublemaker for her involvement in the trial and that she accepted the role of lead plaintiff "knowing the risk could mean my life in more ways than one."[150] Her complaint, the first one brought against the CDCR, described how the "defendants have periodically delayed and interrupted her medication and have denied her a medically necessary special diet" for her "sickle cell anemia, heart problems, pulmonary hypertension and asthma." The complaint also alleged that Shumate received "inadequate medical care" because of the co-payment system.[151] Despite the threat of reprisal, Shumate stated she would "do it all over again. If I can save one life from the medical nightmare at CCWF Medical Department then it's well worth it."[152] A total of twenty-six complaints chronicled the systemic medical neglect and abuse at both women's prisons.

In August 1997, after two years of litigation and negotiation, and in what Shain of the LSPC described as a "win" for the women prisoners, the CDCR agreed to a court-approved settlement.[153] The CDCR pledged, among other things, to provide screening of contagious diseases and timely referrals for those in need of medical attention, stop untrained prison employees (the MTAs) from assessing prisoners' medical needs, and provide medications without delays.[154] Nevertheless, foreshadowing future struggles, the Shumate plaintiff Marcia Bunney expressed concern that prison officials "will never live up to this agreement, and I wonder how many women will have to die in here before they will really make a change."[155] On December 22, 1997, despite the women's concerns over certain provisions, Judge William B. Shubb approved the settlement and dismissed the case.[156]

The settlement required the CDCR to allow an independent, court-appointed team of five medical experts to monitor the prison's compliance over an eight-month period.[157] The first report showed that the facilities failed to adhere to state standards in several medical areas.[158] As the final report found them in compliance with 55 of the 56 terms of the agreement, the CDCR requested unconditional dismissal of the case in February 2000.[159]

The modestly improved medical situation did not last long. In early 2000, women reported delays in treatment and accused administrators of tampering with medical records. The women's attorneys submitted a motion to the court to reopen discovery in the case.[160] Judge Shubb denied the motion and dismissed Shumate with prejudice, meaning that the plaintiffs could never bring it again. Shubb's actions reflected the increased difficulty that incarcerated persons faced in pursuing lawsuits in federal courts in the expanded carceral system—a key means of petitioning for improved conditions—following passage of the 1996 Prison Litigation Reform Act. He closed the case in August 2000.[161]

As medical mistreatment persisted in California's women's prisons, the women and their advocates pursued further legal and political redress. Two months after the Shumate dismissal, on October 11 and 12, State Senator Richard Polanco (D-Los Angeles), chair of the Joint

Subcommittee on Prison Construction and Operations, led a two-day Joint Legislative Committee on Prison Construction and Operations hearing into prison conditions at two of California's women's prisons, CCWF and VSPW. During the hearing, fifteen women prisoners from CCWF and VSPW, as well as CIW, including Charisse Shumate and other *Shumate* plaintiffs, each spoke to the pervasive medical negligence at the prisons, including the failure to inform women who tested positive for hepatitis C.[162] As a prisoner co-infected with HIV and hepatitis C, Judy Ricci, who earned the nickname Dr. Juju for educating others at CCWF about both conditions, described the end-stage liver disease of another co-infected woman who had died the previous month:

> The first woman that died on September 6, 1999, I had seen this woman running around for months. She had pieces of Tampax and Kleenex stuffed up in her nose to stop the flow of blood. Her stomach (she was a little skinny woman) looked like a basketball. . . . Her eyes were literally the color of a pumpkin. I had never approached this woman, because while I knew what she had . . . I didn't want to break her confidentiality and I didn't want to offend her. But I couldn't help asking her, "Do you need some help?" . . . As a person who was informed, I could see and I knew what was happening to her, and it hurt that much worse, but anybody, even an untrained eye, could see that she was going to die. How did they release her from the hospital in this condition?[163]

Other women testified to the negative health impact of ongoing delays to testing and treatment.[164] They also spoke of the sexual abuse they experienced at the hands of prison staff.[165] What State Senator Cathie Wright (R-Simi Valley) heard over the course of those two days "curdled her stomach."[166] The hearing concluded with lawmakers agreeing to a follow-up study and recommendations.[167]

Women continued to die in California's prisons despite this political attention. The *Shumate* plaintiff Brenda Otto died of a heart attack on April 28, 1996. The heart attack followed two strokes for which staff denied her treatment in the infirmary.[168] Otto's death represented a larger pattern of fatal neglect at the prison, including the ongoing reliance on MTAs to treat women in violation of the *Shumate* settlement. Seven women, in their thirties and forties, died in November and December.[169] Three of the women were HIV-positive, while the cause of death for the other four remained undetermined.[170] Sixteen women died at CCWF in 2000, following nine in 1999 and ten in 1998.[171]

These women's deaths drew renewed public attention to the situation inside the prison.[172] Amnesty International highlighted the urgent need for an "independent investigation into deaths at California prison."[173] The seven deaths in December 2000 persuaded CDCR officials to allow another independent team of medical doctors to review the women's records, but their actions failed to prevent several more women from dying in 2001.[174] Charisse Shumate died at CCWF on August 4, 2001. Governor Gray Davis, a Democrat, refused to grant Shumate the clemency that the Board of Prison Terms recommended, and which needed his approval, a decision which reflected the bipartisan commitment to inhumane methods of punishment at this time.[175] Similar to many other women, Shumate died, away from her friends and family, in prison.[176] Twillah Wallace died on October 8, 2001, joining Walker, Shumate, Otto, and others as one of the original protestors and *Shumate* plaintiffs who did not survive their illness.

Like women of all races in CCWF and women of color beyond prison long denied adequate health care, Shumate suffered from mistreatment at the hands of often callous prison staff who refused to take her health complaints seriously. The medical mistreatment that Shumate and those living with HIV/AIDS and other health complications experienced in facilities such as Bedford Hills and CCWF since the 1980s underscores Thuma's argument that the modern carceral state functions as a source of further harm rather than safety and redress.[177] The efforts of Shumate and her peers to access treatment and care in a prison system that not only failed to prepare for but deliberately harmed them was striking given how much was against them. None-theless, the actions on the part of prison officials to destroy the women were matched by the efforts of women to get their stories out. As prison staff dismissed women's complaints and punished those who agitated for change, women believed that securing outside recognition and support offered the best chance to hold the prison system accountable for mistreatment. Their efforts culminated in a class-action lawsuit against one of the largest and most powerful prison systems in the US: a battle that the LSPC called a "modern day David v. Goliath."[178] After a remarkable five-year legal battle, their deaths highlighted the limited power of women in prison to effect institutional change. Nonetheless, women incarcerated inside CCWF and other California prisons have continued, with the CCWP, to protest the co-occurring neglect and abuse underpinning the carceral system.[179]

Activists' efforts can take years to bear fruit. At about the same time that the women filed *Shumate*, people in men's prisons filed two other cases, *Coleman v. Brown* (1990) and *Plata v. Brown* (2001), which similarly alleged that the CDCR's inadequate medical care violated the cruel and unusual punishment clause of the Eighth Amendment, as well as the Americans with Disabilities Act and Section 504 of the Rehabilitation Act.[180] *Coleman* and *Plata* laid the basis for the landmark 2011 decision in *Brown v. Plata*, in which the Supreme Court upheld a lower-court order for California to reduce its prison population, finding the state's overcrowded prisons in violation of the Eighth Amendment. But *Shumate v. Wilson* also set a precedent for change, raising public awareness of the inhumanity of the expanded prison system, especially toward women with HIV/AIDS and multiple other health conditions, at the turn of the twenty-first century. Women in prison and their allies have similarly fought for recent state-level policy wins in New York. For Laura McTighe, these fights for prison health care are part of the broader struggle for prison abolition.[181] Women's activism against AIDS in prison as reflected in the *Shumate* case shaped this battle. While the crisis health situation in California's women's prisons drove multiply marginalized women to fight primarily for adequate treatment, their activism opened ways to critique and challenge the ideology underpinning the warehousing of society's most sick and vulnerable in the era of mass incarceration.

CONCLUSION

Brought together in confinement, women at Bedford Hills and CCWF addressed HIV/AIDS alongside the multiple health crises afflicting them. They showed that women not only suffered because of the slowness of federal officials to acknowledge that HIV manifested differently in women's bodies, but also because prison officials ignored the multiplicity of health conditions that were also killing them. Experiencing, and witnessing, the impact of this daily neglect on themselves as well as their peers, women with HIV in prison did not confine their activism to HIV/AIDS but addressed the absence of all the health care that women in prison failed to receive. Although women risked abuse from prison staff, they braved further punishment to persistently push for care.

A key to the women's success in bringing the lawsuit came from their ability to articulate their needs and mobilize around their right to medical care and protection from cruel and unusual punishment as guaranteed by the US Constitution. As one advocate writing about *Shumate* in the May 1997 issue of *The Fire Inside* asserted, "women prisoners . . . believe that they have a constitutional right to medical care, that their punishment is being in prison and should not be compounded by being forced to live in constant pain and fear of death."[182] The state was responsible for providing health services to those in prison. The women also argued that prisons should not only protect their constitutional rights as citizens but also ensure their safety and dignity. The women's success centered on their ability to work across multiple identity categories around this shared goal. As Judi Ricci put it, "I believe that every person, Black, white, male or female, incarcerated or free, has a right to decent and responsible health care."[183]

In and out of prison, women with HIV and their advocates continued to challenge the co-occurring neglect and intervention obstructing their access to "decent and responsible health care" in the twenty-first century. Like the women in this chapter who sued the state of California to secure consistent, lifesaving care, their efforts have included developing a tool to prevent new cases of HIV, as the high cost of antiretroviral medicines limited their effectiveness in curbing the virus. Designed to empower women sexually, these tools which center women's sex acts and organs have struggled to win the political support required to bring them to market. At the same time, the political right intensified their campaign to gut abortion care, limiting women's access to the nonprofit spaces where they receive treatment for a host of health issues. In the twenty-first century, in a radically new treatment era, the state neglect of women's sexual health-care needs, combined with state interventions into their reproductive lives that represent the culmination of a forty-year political assault on women's health on the part of the political right, continues to perpetuate gender inequities and thwart efforts to end the HIV/AIDS epidemic.

5

THE FIGHT TO END AIDS

IN THE MID-1980s, teams of scientists from around the world began exploring the possibility that the spermicide nonoxynol-9 (N-9) could protect against HIV infection. As awareness of women's increased risk from HIV grew worldwide, scientists like Dr. Sharon Hillier, a professor of obstetrics and gynecology at the University of Pittsburgh, began looking to microbicides—substances containing compounds such as N-9 that come in gels, foams, creams, rings, and sponges—to empower women in the fight against HIV. Acknowledging that economic factors inform sexual behavior, scientists wanted microbicides to be available at the lowest possible cost. They hoped these short-acting products would cause few side effects and appeal to and reach the most diverse range of women.[1]

Their optimism about N-9 did not last long. At the 13th International AIDS Conference in Durban, South Africa, in 2000, scientists shared the disappointing results of an N-9 trial. N-9 did not protect women. In fact, the compound increased a woman's chance of infection, as it irritated the lining of the vagina, making it easier for HIV to infect cells. In addition, the lubricants on some condoms and other contraceptive products contained nonoxynol-9. Thus, contraceptives marketed at women as the best way to protect themselves sexually actually increased their risk of infection.[2]

The ongoing challenges scientists like Hillier faced in developing a woman-controlled and initiated microbicide product point to the gendered problems that have persisted in pharmaceutical research since the turn of the twenty-first century. Despite the medical community's initial enthusiasm for such a tool, none has not been brought to market in the US. Designed to cost as little as possible, the drugs were aimed at reaching economically marginalized women, including women in developing countries who are especially vulnerable in the epidemic. Drug manufacturers, however, questioned their profit potential and withheld the corporate investment needed to take the drugs forward until they could gauge the market for them.[3]

The prevention tools that are available are new treatments but with old problems. The research proving that a pill taken once a day can prevent HIV infection excluded cisgender women. The marketing of this treatment, called PrEP (pre-exposure prophylaxis), also gave the impression that researchers developed it for men. Compounding the research and advertising that associated this new tool with male sexuality and health, the Trump administration's political assault on women's nonprofit health spaces also put available prevention options further beyond the reach of women, resulting in real public health effects. The particularities of the US health market and regulation that gives private pharmaceutical companies freedom to pursue profit at the expense of public health, a freedom advanced by the global, neoliberal agenda of the Clinton administration in the 1990s, compounded the recent political attacks on women's health. Building on past efforts to make effective drugs available and affordable to vulnerable populations both in the US and globally since the 1980s, a coalition of activists challenged these particularities in court.[4] The impact of women's marginalization from the marketing and design of new prevention options underscores how privileging a male scientific and medical perspective over an intersectional feminist perspective disempowers women and undermines their health.

In the absence of free or inexpensive women-controlled products, women have struggled to afford drugs because of the deregulated pharmaceutical industry and struggled to control their sexual health because health-delivery systems are designed for men. Their efforts reveal how, since the 1980s, the campaign of those on the political right to censor women's non-childbearing bodies and neglect their nonreproductive, sexual health-care needs has blunted HIV-prevention efforts in the twenty-first century. By the mid-1990s, activists succeeded in getting the CDC to revise its definition of AIDS to include women's symptoms and moving the FDA to revise its guidelines to include women in clinical research. While federal agencies acted relatively quickly to include women in drug trials for the sake of preventing mother-to-child transmission in the early 1990s, they showed less urgency in approving a product to protect women sexually. Instead, pharmaceutical companies continued to marginalize women in the research and design of nonreproductive medicines that have come to market, just as the government failed to enforce its own guidelines requiring gender equity and inclusion for approval.[5] As a result, in a changed treatment environment, scientists, doctors, and women continue to know less about how the latest drugs work in women's bodies, mirroring the situation in the 1980s.

The story of microbicide research reveals the gender and racial dynamics underpinning not only the distribution but also the development of new HIV-prevention technologies.[6] As Celeste Watkins-Hayes noted, biomedical solutions alone cannot end AIDS.[7] Women's prevention activism in the twenty-first century underscores the need to not only tackle the uneven access to existing medicines along race, geography, gender, and class lines, driving the high rates of HIV/AIDS among multiply marginalized communities, but also to make available prevention methods that are designed with an intersectional awareness of the relationship between bodies and identities, power and inequality, and sex practices to tackle the gender and race inequities hampering efforts to "end" the epidemic. Free, women-controlled HIV-prevention tools seek to meet that need.

IN WOMEN'S HANDS

The mood at the 11th International AIDS Conference in Vancouver in 1996 felt hopeful for the first time in a long while. After years of searching for a cure or treatment for the virus, scientists shared the breakthrough news that combinations of antiviral drugs, including a new drug called protease inhibitors, drastically improved the health of people living with HIV.[8] With the advent of effective ART in the mid-1990s, the public health strategy for tackling HIV/AIDS shifted away from the prevention and management of a fatal disease to the treatment of a chronic illness.

The optimism of the Vancouver meeting did not last long. At the next conference in Geneva, two years later, scientists reported on the disappointing test results of a vaccine once thought promising.[9] To make matters worse, the high cost of protease inhibitors, which also caused severe side effects, limited their potential benefit.[10] The combination of therapies had an annual price tag of up to $20,000 in the US alone. As Dr. Toye H. Brewer of the University of Washington in Seattle explained, "just a minority of people around the world are going to benefit" from the new drugs.[11] Failures in vaccine research and the high cost of available treatments drove conference attendees to emphasize the importance of prevention in containing the epidemic as it entered its third decade.[12] As one journalist writing in 2006 put it, "If care and treatment were the buzzwords of the first 25 years of the pandemic, prevention is decidedly the key player of the next 25."[13] In 2000, the CDC reiterated the need to prevent new HIV infections, as the prevalence of AIDS in the country began rising again following the introduction of protease inhibitors in 1996.[14]

At the end of the twentieth century, amid the burgeoning international feminist movement that worked to address AIDS as part of a global women's health agenda, women scientists and advocates called for woman-controlled prevention tools to address the accelerating rates of HIV/AIDS among women and girls worldwide.[15] In 1990, Dr. Zena Stein, a South African epidemiologist based at Columbia University, published an article in the *American Journal of Public Health*, demanding feminist prevention methods be put on the public health agenda.[16] Participants at the first conference on women and HIV in the US, held in Washington, DC, in 1990, reiterated Stein's call for research into "methods women can use" to protect themselves during sex with men.[17] Feminist scientists, including Hillier and Dr. Zeda Fran Rosenberg, an epidemiologist for HIV prevention at the NIH, accepted Stein's call, turning their attention in the 1990s to developing HIV prevention methods that empowered women.[18] At the turn of the twenty-first century, journalists hoped that, within a few years, the availability of woman-controlled prevention tools could prevent millions of new infections worldwide.[19]

Advocates looked to microbicides as woman-initiated, cheap, easy to use, and undetectable prevention options. Microbicides contain drugs that are applied inside the vagina before or after sex to block STDs. They also come in both contraceptive and noncontraceptive forms. In 2000, the community educator and women's health advocate Megan Gottemoeller of the Center for Health and Gender Equality praised microbicides for taking "into account the contexts in which women are struggling to protect themselves."[20] As Watkins-Hayes had similarly argued, new biomedical interventions must address the context in which women use them to be effective. The ability to protect oneself without having to rely on the willingness of a sexual partner to use contraception is particularly important for women, given the gendered power imbalance in condom use. Male condoms are only effective in preventing HIV infection if a man agrees to wear one. Men can refuse to do so, including in acts of sexual violence, such as "stealthing." Due to its design, it is also difficult for women to hide use of the female condom—the only woman-initiated HIV-prevention method that the FDA approved in 1993—from sexual partners. That widespread sexual violence and poverty increases the risk of infection in women, coupled with the fact that women lack control over most available prevention methods, underscored the need for an affordable method available for women to use without relying on male consent.[21]

In 2009, Jane K. Stoever, a law professor at the University of California, Irvine, published a paper detailing how male supremacy in the bedroom undermines women's ability to protect themselves from HIV, other STDs, and pregnancy. One woman's husband accused her of cheating and threatened her life after she asked him to wear a condom. She found it "easier to engage in unprotected sex," despite knowing he used drugs and might have other sexual partners. A HIV-positive woman described how her boyfriend interfered with her treatment, flushing her medication down the toilet because she was "going to die anyway." These stories reiterated the necessity of woman-controlled prevention tools.[22]

Pharmaceutical companies did not share the scientists' enthusiasm for developing "efficient, widely available, and low-cost microbicides . . . to prevent sexually transmitted HIV infections."[23] The companies contribute to the development of drugs that are expected to generate profit. A 2002 report from the Rockefeller Foundation questioned the ability of the first generation of microbicides to make enough money to justify the investment in their development.[24] As Lori Heise, whose advocacy against gender-based violence brought her to microbicide work, explained, drug manufacturers assumed that the market for microbicides resided solely in countries with limited resources, where the product's effectiveness depended on its availability to users at low cost.[25] Moreover, unlike the contraceptive pill that women must take daily, microbicides are used on an as-needed basis, limiting the profit potential. Doubts over the product's ability to recoup the investment from its research and development dissuaded pharmaceutical companies, which already profited from birth control tools such as the oral contraceptive pill, which does not protect against viruses, from investing in a tool to protect women from HIV.

The responsibility for research and development therefore fell to nonprofit foundations, governments, and academic institutions without the resources to finance large-scale clinical trials, stalling the development of promising products. Advocates like Heise called on the federal government to spend more to meet this need. As "large pharmaceutical companies continue to express no interest," Heise wrote in the New York Times in 2001, "government financing is critical."[26] Approximately $28 million of the $1.8 billion that the NIH invested in AIDS research in 1999 went to researching microbicides, compared to $180 million for vaccines.[27] As each clinical trial cost between $50 and $100 million to run, scientists demanded $1 billion for investment.[28]

At the 1998 conference in Geneva, Heise and others took matters into their own hands, founding the Global Campaign for Microbicides (GCM). Like other women AIDS activists who, in the words of BWH-BC's Jamie Penney, "did the work" that political and medical institutions refused to do, the GCM demanded greater political commitment to investing in and making available woman-controlled prevention methods, as well as actively engaging communities in the process of development.[29]

GCM won the support of sympathetic members of Congress. In 2000, Connie Morella (R-MD) and Nancy Pelosi (D-CA) introduced their Microbicide Development Act (MDA) in the House of Representatives to authorize $50–100 million annual investment in microbicides.[30] That same year, members of the GCM held the first international conference on the topic, Microbicides 2000, in Washington, DC, to raise funds and awareness in the field. Representatives introduced the MDA in Congress six times between 1999 and 2008. Although the bill never passed, federal funding for microbicides increased steadily between 2000 and 2010, more than tripling from $28 million in 1999 to $92 million in 2004.[31] Attesting to the power of grassroots and political coalitions, advocates succeeded in convincing the government to invest in what the pharmaceutical industry would not.

GCM contributed to a larger grassroots effort to increase government and nonprofit funding for microbicide research and development. In 2002, the microbiologist and epidemiologist Zeda Rosenberg quit her job as scientific director of the HIV Prevention Trials Network at Family Health International in North Carolina to start her own nonprofit organization dedicated to microbicide research, the International Partnership for Microbicides (IPM).[32] Echoing Gottemoeller and Watkins-Hayes, as well as birth control advocate Margaret Sanger, who, in the early twentieth century, promoted the vaginal diaphragm as a feminist contraceptive for its feel, efficacy, and ability to aid orgasms, Rosenberg emphasized the importance of context: "Nearly as important as whether it kills HIV is whether a microbicide feels acceptable, whether it can be used discreetly if necessary and how it is packaged and promoted." IPM first explored how to make the product appealing and useful to diverse groups of women before inventing its active ingredient.[33] Meanwhile, in 2004, GCM began a sponsor search.[34] Two years later, in 2006, Hillier launched the Microbicide Trials Network (MTN) with the NIH to support the process of licensing and approving microbicide products.[35] The Bill and Melinda Gates Foundation contributed millions to trials that sought to bring these products to market.[36]

Despite growing financial investment and political awareness, the "flip-flop world of microbicide research" was marked by scientific setbacks. Researchers trialed several other substances, hoping to "give women the power in the anti-AIDS war,"[37] but other gels proved ineffective or unsafe.[38] In the wake of disappointing results, women's health advocates such as Gottemoeller and Dr. Peter Piot, executive director of the United Nation's AIDS Program, attributed the struggle in microbicide research and development to a lack of resources.[39]

Rosenberg offered several explanations for the pharmaceutical industry's lack of enthusiasm for microbicides, including the fact that companies viewed vaccine development as more "glamorous" and prestigious work. Moreover, a product that put women's health and welfare needs before profit lacked private appeal.[40] IPM developed products primarily with funding from grants, thus, "unlike commercial pharmaceutical companies, IPM is not seeking to set a price designed to recoup investments in R&D [research and development]."[41] Researchers knew that they needed to make a microbicide product as inexpensive as possible due to the gendered elements of poverty and in order to "put prevention in the hands of women, more vulnerable both biologically and socially."[42] That meant that a microbicide product needed to cost less than an over-the-counter pill.

In addition to the question of profit, Rosenberg also attributed the lack of significant investment on the part of major pharmaceutical companies to a reluctance to develop a product that centered women's bodies and promoted women's sexual autonomy and agency: "Since this anti-AIDS strategy involves a product that needs to be used vaginally and is associated with sex, it had problems gaining acceptance. When you think about an HIV vaccine, you don't have to think about sex. It's a vaccine, like the one for influenza. When you think of a vaginal microbicide there's no way you can't think about sex. That makes some people very uncomfortable."[43]

The reticence of the pharmaceutical industry to fund a product that focused on women's sex acts and organs reflected the marginalization of women's sexual and reproductive health needs throughout the epidemic and continued the long history of government interference in the reproductive freedoms of women of color. Like the LAP with its explicit safer sex initiatives, microbicide advocates sought to promote women's safety through sexual, as well as economic, empowerment. They expressed this aim through promotional materials asserting, "With condoms, safer sex is his decision. We want to make it yours."[44] This message contrasted with the CDC and other public health agencies' tone-deaf safer sex publicity from the 1980s and 1990s that sought to give women verbal strategies to encourage men to engage in safer sex, but that still placed the burden of responsibility on them, such as, "If he doesn't have a condom, you just have to take a deep breath and tell him to go get one."[45] Advocates' efforts came up against not only the profiteering of drug companies reluctant to take a risk on a potentially unprofitable treatment designed primarily to benefit women but also a political agenda hostile to reproductive justice and dishonest about sexual assault by men.

Over the course of the next decade, the field of HIV prevention shifted away from microbicide research and toward the development of a daily pill to reduce the risk of contracting HIV through sex. Replicating women's underrepresentation in earlier HIV treatments, the clinical trials for this drug initially excluded cisgender women, and researchers knew little of women's interest in or ability to take the medication. Concerned that the rollout of the latest HIV treatment to come to market might marginalize women, advocates leading the field of microbicide turned their attention toward helping women prepare for the new medicine.

PREPARING WOMEN FOR THE PREVENTION AGENDA

After more than a decade of failed clinical trials, a breakthrough in the field of microbicide research came in 2008. A research team funded through the NIH reported that women could safely use a topical gel made with the antiretroviral drug tenofovir. The California-based pharmaceutical company, Gilead Sciences Inc., sold the drug under the brand name Viread. After proving that women could use the tenofovir gel—the first potential microbicide to use a licensed antiretroviral drug—safely, researchers needed to prove its effectiveness in preventing HIV transmission.[46] This breakthrough came in July 2010, when Dr. Salim S. Abdool Karim and Dr. Quarraisha Abdool Karim, who had led the clinical trial CAPRISA 004 in South Africa, confirmed that inserting a vaginal-gel version of tenofovir within twelve hours before and after sex reduced HIV incidence in women up to 54 percent.[47] Advocates at the 18th AIDS Conference in Vienna celebrated this potentially major development in women's health.[48]

A few months after the success of CAPRISA 004, a global trial in men who have sex with men and a small number of transgender women who have sex with men confirmed that, when taken daily, the pill version of tenofovir reduced new HIV infections by up to 92 percent.[49] The inclusion of transgender and the exclusion of cisgender women in the trial implied that pharmaceutical companies still put transgender women in the biological category of "men." Gilead also sold the pill version of tenofovir disoproxil fumarate (TDF) in combination with the drug emtricitabine under the brand name Truvada. In March 2012, the FDA approved Gilead's proposal to sell Truvada for HIV prevention. The FDA first approved Truvada for HIV treatment in 2004. In 2012, it became the first FDA-approved drug for the prevention of HIV and has dominated the field of prevention since.[50]

The rise of PrEP marked the decline of microbicides. Regulatory authorities approved Truvada for PrEP more quickly than a gel, because researchers proved them safe and effective for treatment first.[51] The relatively small size of the CAPRISA 004 trial and the fact that the tenofovir gel fell comparatively short of one hundred percent effectiveness convinced scientists and public health officials of the need for further trials before they campaigned for governments to approve them.[52]

Researchers struggled to raise enough money to fund further trials.[53] Studies that did secure funding found difficulty repeating the success of CAPRISA 004. Participants in a follow-up trial in South Africa, Uganda, and Zimbabwe faced challenges undertaking the daily regimen of gel application because the stigma associated with HIV and rumors of the medicine's harmful effects deterred them from using it. This underscored the need to develop medicines that not only worked but also acknowledged the social, economic, and interpersonal factors informing how and whether women took them.[54]

Women's health advocates continued to push for microbicides after the approval of PrEP because they acknowledged the need to develop tools from an intersectional feminist perspective. Women rely on public health insurance more than men, and women of color rely on it more than white women.[55] Moreover, a greater number of women with HIV live in poverty compared to HIV-positive men.[56] A gel costing about thirty cents to make that did not require a prescription had a better chance of reaching women with limited access to uninterrupted health care.[57] Pharmaceutical companies have the power to set and raise drug prices, and pills, in contrast to the gel, are enormously expensive. A prescription drug requiring regular laboratory tests to check for kidney function and bone density, Truvada is difficult to obtain without health insurance and consistent access to a doctor. Moreover, a gel that came in both a contraceptive and noncontraceptive form enabled women to protect themselves from HIV as well as other STDs like herpes, while deciding whether they also wanted protection from pregnancy—a dual benefit missed in other contraceptives like the oral pill. Only affecting a specific part of the body, relatively short-acting, and self-administered, a local gel involved lower risks of a user developing drug resistance and experiencing negative side effects.[58] Despite these benefits, economics hampered activist efforts. In 2012, GCM, an organization pivotal to pioneering prevention tools for women, closed because of a lack of money and support.[59]

Undeterred, feminist health advocates turned their attention toward helping women navigate Truvada for PrEP. Shortly before the FDA approved the drug, in March 2012, a group of women set up the US Women PrEP Working Group. Its members include Anna Forbes, the DC-based AIDS activist and former GCM co-founder, and Dázon Dixon Diallo, founder of the Atlanta-based AIDS organization Sister-Love, which provides Black women with tools and strategies to address the intersecting, structural oppressions that heighten their vulnerability in the epidemic.[60] Dixon Diallo drew parallels between the systemic challenges facing women navigating HIV/AIDS in the US with those confronting women in the Global South. Despite their different economies, she argued that the poverty, economic dependency, violence, and poor access to health care that arose from the US government's neoliberal, capitalist health agenda threatened women's health in both the US and countries like South Africa. As Dan Royles and Laura McTighe remind us, the advance of neoliberalism in the latter decades of the twentieth century blunted treatment access both domestically and globally.[61] Similar to other intersectional feminists who brought a human rights perspective to health activism—defining health not as the absence of disease but the presence of rights, equality, and financial security—Dixon Diallo pursued AIDS interventions that addressed the structural inequities that exacerbated HIV/AIDS in and beyond the US, including the prioritization of profit over public health.[62] Microbicides are one such intervention.

The concerns of Diallo, Forbes, and others that PrEP might not address the challenges women faced in navigating safe sex followed decades of failed attempts to provide women with a prevention tool that empowered them sexually and reproductively. Approved for sale in the US in May 1993, the female condom promised to give women greater control in protecting against pregnancy as well as STDs. In 1993, Cynthia A. Pearson of the National Women's Health Network celebrated the female condom for giving "women control over exposure to sexually transmitted disease" for the first time. Unfortunately, the initial optimism Pearson expressed about the product did not translate into sales. Women cannot hide its use from sexual partners, and some women who used it reported experiencing intimate partner violence.[63] Some also disliked its look and feel. The lack of an existing market and complexities in its manufacture resulted in the product selling at a much higher price than its alternative for men.[64] An intervention that advocates initially saw as a step forward for reproductive justice therefore missed decades of potential effectiveness. Ensuring that the roll out of PrEP did not replicate the problems of past interventions drove AIDS scientists and activists.

An early blow to the women's confidence in PrEP came as researchers announced that the method reduced the HIV infection rate in HIV-negative gay men and transgender women who have sex with men.[65] FEM-PrEP, a large-scale clinical trial of PrEP in cisgender women from Kenya, Tanzania, and South Africa, showed that PrEP did not prevent HIV in cis women. Researchers speculated whether the results arose from the fact that the drugs worked differently in cisgender women's bodies, from the differences in HIV exposure during vaginal or anal sex, or from the different levels of adherence that arose from negative side effects.[66] Whether rooted in biology, social context, or both, the disappointing results of FEM-PrEP underscored the limits of taking the results of clinical trials carried out in men and transgender women and applying them to cisgender women. In 2014, the CDC advised clinicians to provide PrEP to women "at substantial risk of HIV acquisition" before having assessed its safety and effectiveness among women in the US.[67] Although two studies from 2012 proved PrEP's effectiveness in reducing rates of infection in heterosexual women in countries in Africa, the first clinical trial to include cisgender women in US, the Sustainable Health Center Implementation PrEP Pilot (SHIPP) Study, did not begin until July 2014, underscoring the CDC's persistent exclusion of cis women.[68]

The marginalization of women in clinical research contrasted with the interference of the federal government in their reproductive lives. In 2017, President Trump reinstated a global version of the gag rule that President Reagan had introduced three decades earlier in 1984. Also known as the Mexico City Policy, it denied foreign aid to any non-governmental organizations (NGOs) that "perform or actively promote abortion as a method of family planning," forcing them to choose between providing comprehensive reproductive health care with their own money or forgoing financial support. Its domestic counterpart, the Hyde Amendment of 1981, already prevented federal money paying for abortions abroad.[69] The global gag rule also blocked funding to organizations that performed, advised on, or referred for legal abortions using their own funds. Reflecting its partisan nature, every Republican president since Reagan has implemented a version of the rule, and every Democratic president has overturned it. In 2017, Trump expanded its scope, banning funding to NGOs that provided, counseled, or advocated for the liberalization of abortion laws in their countries using their own funds. He also applied the ban to organizations that received funding through the President's Emergency Plan for AIDS Relief (PEPFAR), the largest US global health program, founded in 2003 by President George W. Bush.[70] PEPFAR, an initiative credited for its large contribution to global AIDS treatment and prevention, also uses foreign aid to promote the conservative tenets of abstinence and fidelity at the expense of more effective HIV-prevention options.[71] Trump's new policy further hampered the ability of organizations to provide key reproductive and sexual health tools such as contraceptives.[72] This, in turn, increased rates of unintended pregnancies and both legal and unsafe abortions, and undermined people's ability to access HIV testing, treatment, and prevention.[73] The negative consequences of Trump's global gag rule underline its intention to further an ideological rather than public health agenda. Since the 1980s, successive Republican governments have similarly used federal funding as a wedge to advance their misogynistic health agenda that seeks to limit women's reproductive rights and sexual freedoms and promote normative sex and gender roles in which sex and pregnancy takes place in heteronormative marriage.

Recent global and domestic policy practices that undermine women's health and rights are especially dangerous given the latest statistics on HIV. Women and girls, globally, make up more than half of all people living with HIV.[74] In the US, approximately twenty percent of new infections are in women.[75] Black women account for more than half of new HIV diagnoses in women, despite representing approximately fifteen percent of the female population, and one in forty-eight Black women is vulnerable to contracting HIV in their lifetime.[76] Nonetheless, PrEP use remains largely limited to white men aged 25 and over, and PrEP coverage is over twice as high among men as among women.[77] Forbes attributed this disparity partly to the original marketing of PrEP as a tool for men and debates around it, which, as Devon Betts noted, also centered whiteness and failed to consider how myths of Black promiscuity and hypersexuality fueled racial disparities in PrEP access.[78] When the CDC recommended its use among "at risk" women in 2014, women, overall, reported a low level of awareness of PrEP. Once informed, however, they expressed interest in using it.[79] Gilead released a study showing a twelve-fold increase in the numbers of women beginning PrEP between its approval in 2012 and 2017.[80] Nonetheless, only approximately ten percent of women the CDC estimates could benefit from PrEP received a prescription in 2019 and 2020.[81] With the power imbalance in condom negotiation and women's vulnerability to contracting HIV through unprotected vaginal sex with men, access to effective HIV prevention, including the option of PrEP, is crucial for women.[82]

The problems involved with PrEP, the global gag rule, and securing treatment for women are part of a larger problem with the political assault on Title X and Planned Parenthood. The Trump administration and the political right persistently worked to defund nonprofit health spaces, stopping them from receiving Medicaid reimbursement for the other preventative health services they provide, including hormone replacement therapy (HRT) for transgender patients, birth control, pregnancy care, cancer screenings, and, since the 1980s, HIV testing, treatment, and education services. Efforts to defund Planned Parenthood and other nonprofit treatment spaces are particularly harmful for the women who, due to the convergence of systemic barriers contributing to income inequality, lack access to private insurance. The preventative, persistent care offered at these nonprofit family-planning centers can mean the difference between life and death.

SAVING TITLE X IN THE FIGHT TO END AIDS

Guests at the Trump International Hotel in New York City on Thursday May 25, 2017, who looked out of their windows and onto Central Park West Street witnessed hundreds of women marching with tombstones that read "Died of AIDS" and "Died from Unsafe Abortion."[83] Cognizant of how attacks on reproductive health services hampered efforts to address HIV/AIDS, the marchers dramatized the threat Trump's recently announced global gag rule posed to people's lives. A few weeks earlier, people mobilized in states across the country to challenge Trump's efforts to repeal the ACA and block patients from accessing health services at Planned Parenthood centers.[84] The political assault on women's reproductive health services did not cease when the Senate blocked the repeal of ACA in July. Rather, one of the most recent and effective strategies conservatives have deployed in their ever-shifting attack on women's reproductive rights, including access to HIV/AIDS services, is the gutting of Title X.

Established in 1970, Title X of the Public Health Service Act is a federal grant program that gives funding to family-planning health centers. Title X–funded health centers provide regular, preventative care, including affordable birth control and reproductive health care, to people who are uninsured, low income, or seeking confidential services. They offer life-saving gynecological exams, contraceptives, and cancer and HIV/AIDS testing, treatment, and support. Crucially, Title X providers refuse no one care based on their ability to pay.[85] These sites are the only health-care option for many women. A 2016 survey reported that for sixty percent of patients, the Title X site they visited that year represented their only source of health care.[86]

Like Reagan's version of the domestic "gag rule" that preceded it, Trump's policy prohibited Title X funding for Planned Parenthood and other providers that did not physically and financially separate their abortion care from the services funded through other sources. Moreover, like its global counterpart, it prohibited doctors in the Title X program from performing abortions using other funds or referring patients to other abortion providers, even when patients requested them.[87]

Title X is a federal program designed to help low-income women access reproductive health services. Trump's Title X policy therefore targeted low-income women, and especially low-income women of color, who, because of decades of policies that have undermined their access to quality health care, already have worse health outcomes than white women with greater private insurance coverage.[88] HIV/AIDS is one such health disparity between women. Since the epidemic's outset, Black and Latina women have consistently experienced higher rates of and vulnerability to HIV.[89] Title X sites provide essential entry points for women who are uninsured or underinsured, providing HIV testing and immediate connection to care.[90] In 2017, during Trump's first year in office, more than sixty percent of the insured patients who visited a Title X site received coverage through Medicaid or other public sources. Moreover, of the approximately four million people who used a Title X provider, more than half either self-identified as non-white or Hispanic or Latinx.[91]

Mirroring other initiatives seeking to undermine legal abortion since the 1970s, the state of abortion funding and care underscored that a desire to punish women rather than address any scientific or social reality drove Trump's Title X policy. The Hyde Amendment already prevents women enrolled in Medicaid from using their insurance to pay for abortion services. Since its enactment in 1970, Title X has similarly prohibited federal funding for abortions.[92] Moreover, in 2018, the CDC reported that rates of abortion reached a historic low, calling into question the need for new policies that addressed its use.[93] In the 1980s, Reagan's evangelical Surgeon General Charles Everett Koop acknowledged abortion as a legal and medically viable, if morally undesirable, prevention option for perinatal HIV. In contrast to Koop's call for public health interventions that both prevented HIV as well as unwanted pregnancies, Republican officials in the twenty-first century have demonstrated how an uncompromising opposition to abortion and reproductive justice has shaped the Republican health agenda in the decades since. Republican conservatives such as Ohio governors John Kasich and his successor Mike DeWine persistently slashed public financing for Planned Parenthood clinics that also offer women non-abortion prevention and health services. These efforts led to the closure of two clinics in Ohio in 2019, neither of which provided abortions.[94]

The conservative strategy of targeting politically and economically marginalized women continues earlier antiabortion initiatives, such as the Hyde Amendment. As Congresswoman Katie Porter (D-CA) highlighted, the gendered aspects of poverty, such as the unpaid care work that women and girls disproportionately carry out, often leaves women unable to afford adequate medical care. Moreover, single mothers are more likely to lack insurance than those in two-parent households, which Black and Latina women are more likely than white women to head.[95] The new Title X policy therefore put preventative health services, such as screenings for the detection and treatment of STDs and reproductive cancers, further beyond the reach of women who, as a result of myriad systemic and policy factors, from a lack of access to adequate housing to a lack of insurance coverage, are disproportionately women of color and already facing delayed health diagnoses and higher rates of and mortality for cervical cancer, HIV, breast cancer, and other diseases.[96] Their experiences underscore how a capitalist health-care system leaves room for political exploitation and makes people sicker.

The twenty-year assault on Planned Parenthood has forced health clinics in states across the country to close, threatening women's health. In 2011, the Texas legislature slashed the state's family-planning budget and chose to forgo federal Medicaid funding rather than maintain its state contracts with Planned Parenthood clinics. As a result, eighty-two of the state's health clinics closed or stopped offering family-planning services, about a third of which belonged to Planned Parenthood.[97] Nearly thirty thousand fewer patients received reproductive health care, cancer screenings, STD tests, and other services as a result.[98] These closures also coincided with a doubling in maternal mortality rates that disproportionately involved Black women.[99] In 2011, under the direction of Mike Pence, the Indiana state government cut funding to Planned Parenthood, causing five clinics to close in the state, none of which provided abortion services. The closure of Planned Parenthood in Scott County left residents without access to HIV testing. High unemployment and poverty rates already limited people's access to health care in the state. The closure of Planned Parenthood clinics resulted in the worst HIV outbreak in Indiana history.[100]

Reflecting the conservative reliance on private solutions to public problems, as funding cuts have forced not-for-profit family-planning sites around the country to close, private retail companies such as CVS, Target, and Walgreens have opened alternative treatment sites within their drug stores to fill the gap.[101] Just as prison guards control access to health services for women in prison, retail clinics also have the power to remove women's freedom, placing their ability to access to primary care in the hands of individuals making value judgments about their bodies. Different states have different policies governing pharmacy practices. But, as private organizations, retail clinics can refuse to sell birth control without violating a woman's federal right to contraception and, in certain cases, pharmacists and sales associates are protected from serving a customer based on religious grounds.[102] Approximately forty percent of 67,000 pharmacies in the US are private retail companies with no obligation to offer reproductive health services.[103] That corporate leaders can choose not to guarantee women's access to contraception reveals the precarious state of women's health in a capitalist health-care system and the need for the government to protect women's uninterrupted access to health care.

The political right's efforts to make health care more privatized and politicized since the 1980s has culminated in the gutting of Title X and Planned Parenthood. Approximately one in four clinics receiving Title X funding left the program in 2019 to keep offering comprehensive health care, threatening the care of 1.6 million patients.[104] The dangerous consequence of privatized health care harms women needing access to regular care but who lack the means to pay for it, including low-income women with HIV. The deregulation of the pharmaceutical industry further compounds the challenges facing women trying to navigate an increasingly ideological health-care system, a situation that activists are currently working to resist.

TAKING ON BIG PHARMA

On May 8, 2019, at Gilead Sciences Inc.'s annual shareholder meeting in San Francisco, Emily Sanderson stood up in front of a panel of suited men and demanded that the company stop obstructing access to Truvada for PrEP. Sanderson, the national organizer of the international access organization Health GAP's Student Global AIDS Campaign, expressed her anger at "the fact that you would put profiteering ahead of the lives of people like me," and demanded to know the manufacturer's plan to make sure that every person in the US could access PrEP when they needed it.[105] Sanderson's protest did not mark the first time that the drug manufacturer faced criticism over the price of its HIV medicine. In 2013, following ACT UP/San Francisco's revival, the group organized a street action protesting the high price of Gilead's new drug, Stribild.[106] Six years later, Sanderson, acting on behalf of Health GAP, an organization founded in 1999 to protest President Clinton's policy of blocking countries outside of the US from manufacturing or acquiring generic versions of HIV medicines, repeated the call for widespread access to Gilead's prevention medication.[107] When the panelists pointed to the company's programs that defray co-pay costs as evidence of their efforts to make drugs affordable, another audience member interrupted, claiming that problems accessing these programs forced him off the medication.[108] That the rate of new HIV infections remained relatively stable at 40,000 per year between 2012 and 2016 suggests the drug's failure to reach all that might benefit from it.[109]

Despite the initial optimism over Truvada's potential to drastically curb the spread of HIV, many have struggled to access it. According to the CDC, twenty-five percent of the 1.2 million people who could benefit from PrEP received a prescription in 2020, an increase in recent years which saw the figure under ten percent. Nonetheless, gender, age, regional, and racial disparities persist in its use, especially among Black and Latinx American men, and women of all races.[110] Activists and epidemiologists have attributed people's difficulty in accessing the drug in part to its high cost, which, among other obstacles, has resulted in expensive out-of-pocket costs for patients, and which arise from Gilead's ability to set and raise the price.[111] The high cost of the medicine, combined with its negative side effects, the stigma of HIV/AIDS, and other challenges that hinder people's ability to take the medicine hampered efforts to control the virus for more than a decade and prove that biomedical interventions alone cannot curb diseases.[112]

Since the FDA approved Truvada for PrEP in 2012, Gilead has steadily raised the drug's price without making any therapeutic changes. When the FDA first approved Truvada for HIV treatment in 2004, Gilead charged $800 for a month's supply. In 2019, they charged $1,800. Since then, the company has increased the drug's price, earning Gilead approximately $36 billion in revenue.[113]

Truvada's high cost, which has put the drug beyond the reach of many, is a consequence of the particularities of the US health-care market and regulation. The question of how to maintain medical innovation while making drugs available, affordable, and accessible occupies debates over health care. The nature of that debate in the US differs from that of countries with nationalized health-care systems, as health care is treated as a privilege, not a right. This departure in values is not inevitable but a consequence of a series of political choices, including regarding the patent process and lack of bulk buying.[114]

Unlike in countries with a national health system, the US government does not systematically negotiate drug prices. Except for certain government agencies—such as the Veterans Administration (VA), which has the power to negotiate drug prices, resulting in lower costs—drug makers generally have freedom to set the price of their products.[115] In contrast, countries with nationalized health care can buy drugs in bulk and negotiate lower prices with drug manufacturers. In 2003, ostensibly to promote market competition, the Republican-controlled Congress prohibited the government from negotiating cheaper prices for prescription medicines through the new insurance plan for seniors, Medicare Part D.[116] Congress doubled down on restricting negotiation in the ACA of 2010.[117] President Joe Biden broke rank in August 2022, authorizing Medicare to negotiate the cost of certain drugs available on Parts B and D with the Inflation Reduction Act. As negotiation enables governments to maintain lower prices when a drug company has the exclusive rights to sell a product, restrictions on negotiation have resulted in unaffordable drug costs. In addition to bulk buying, the market exclusivity and the patent protection process also keep prices artificially high.

Patents typically last twenty years before a drug becomes generic. A drug that is FDA approved receives both a brand and generic name. The company responsible for developing the drug decides its brand name, and the drug's active ingredient becomes the generic name. During the period of patent protection, only the company that holds the drug's patent can manufacture, market, and profit from it. The drug manufacturer also receives a period of legally protected exclusivity during which to sell the medication under either its brand or generic name at a price of their choice. In allowing drug companies to set their own drug prices, the US health-care system is unique among industrialized nations.[118] During this period of market exclusivity, pharmaceutical companies effectively hold a monopoly on the drug, regardless of the human cost. As the development of new and improved medicines requires significant investment in research, patents ostensibly encourage drug companies to spend time and money developing a medicine they can profit from without the threat of competition. The drug industry claims that federal intervention in the marketplace would disincentivize them from funding the research of new and more effective medicines.[119]

Once the patent or period of market exclusivity ends, other drug manufacturers can apply to the FDA to sell generic versions of the brand-name drug. Without needing to recover investment in the drug's development, companies can sell the generic medication at a lower cost. Generic drugs, which contain the same active ingredient as the brand-name drug, therefore tend to cost much less than the original.

Since the Reagan era, lawmakers have relied on the availability of generic drugs to regulate drug prices without government intervention. The 1984 Hatch-Waxman Act, also known as the Drug Price Competition and Patent Term Restoration Act, sought to strike a balance between incentivizing innovation while making drugs more affordable through increased generic competition—extending the patents for brand-name drugs while making it easier for generic drugs to enter the market.[120] According to Robin Feldman and Evan Frondorf, drug manufacturers deployed several tactics to circumvent the new regulation. Brand-name companies brokered deals with generic companies to delay generic entry, and slightly altered the dosage of existing drugs, enabling them to add secondary patents to medicines with little therapeutic changes.[121] Steven W. Thrasher and others have challenged the industry argument that drug companies need large profits for research and development, finding that they spend more paying dividends to shareholders than on innovation.[122]

Although patents and profits are usually politically protected, the proactive steps the Eisenhower administration took to implement the polio vaccine in the 1950s proved that governments could go further to put access before corporate interests. In the mid-1950s, the scientist Jonas Salk chose not to patent his polio vaccine, likening it to patenting the sun. The decision not to patent the vaccine did not rest solely with Salk. The National Foundation for Infantile Paralysis, later called the March of Dimes, and the University of Pittsburgh also contributed to its development and considered but decided not to seek a patent as they and Salk did not think his methods original enough to qualify. Nonetheless, the lack of patent enabled the government to grant licenses to five companies to concurrently manufacture the drug.[123] Initially leaving the production and distribution of the vaccines to the March of Dimes and private drug companies, Eisenhower become more proactive after a series of scandals.[124] In 1955, he signed the Polio Vaccination Assistance Act, which directed Congress to appropriate $28 million to ensure that no child failed to receive vaccination "by reason of its cost."[125] Within three decades, the vaccination effort helped eliminate the polio virus from the US.[126] Unlike the relative speed with which the government addressed a disease that they originally associated with white children, typically cast as "innocent victims" in disease outbreaks, the government lacked urgency when tackling a disease associated with multiply marginalized groups.[127] The polio precedent has inspired AIDS activists.

In July 2018, the PrEP4ALL Collaboration, a multiracial, sex, and gender advocacy organization based in New York, released a forty-page agenda entitled "A National Action Plan for Universal Access to HIV Pre-Exposure Prophylaxis (PrEP) in the United States." Drawing on the polio precedent, it advocated widening access to available prevention medicine, outlining the steps the government could take to break Gilead's monopoly on Truvada. The Bayh-Dole Act of 1980 gave the government "march-in rights" to ignore the patent of a drug partly developed through federally funded research when a "health or safety" need exists and license other drug companies to manufacture it.[128] In 2019, the *Washington Post* revealed that the federal government issued $50 million in grants to researchers developing Truvada for PrEP and that following successful clinical trials the CDC filed patents on the treatment, which they secured in 2015.[129] As US taxpayers paid for Truvada for PrEP through the NIH, the public thereby retained the intellectual property rights to break Gilead's patent on the drug.

On May 9, 2019, the day after Sanderson protested Gilead's shareholder meeting in San Francisco, the company shared its plan to donate a free supply of Truvada to approximately 200,000 uninsured patients a year via the CDC through 2030. A day earlier, Gilead also announced its plan to let a generic version of Truvada come to the market in September 2020, a year earlier than it had agreed to under a patent settlement deal with Teva Pharmaceutical Industries Ltd., which won FDA approval of the lower-cost version in 2014.[130]

While Gilead's announcement demonstrated the power of activists to move drug companies to act, activists also highlighted the limited nature of this gesture. Aaron S. Lord, a member of PrEP4ALL and a physician at New York University School of Medicine, asked what, besides profit motive, stopped Gilead from releasing the rights to Truvada immediately.[131] Dr. Michael Saag, an HIV researcher at the University of Alabama and member of the Presidential Advisory Council on HIV/AIDS, also highlighted the inadequacy of Gilead's "nice gesture." Providing 200,000 people with the treatment fell short of the 1.2 million people that the CDC estimated could benefit from it. Industry-controlled charity relies on the benevolence of private companies and removes agency from individuals needing treatment. Moreover, charity care perpetuates tropes of who is deserving and undeserving of state support that have historically perpetuated race, class, and gender inequities in the US. Charity health care undermines the notion that everyone should have equal access to care and places people's health in the hands of private individuals or organizations that have the power to determine their worthiness for assistance.[132] Humane and compassionate health care requires equality, not charity. Private companies' desire for profit undermines access for all. To claim the free medicines, people still needed to undergo regular laboratory tests, the costs of which are not covered by the donation. Proving that offering medicines without ensuring people's ability to access them is insufficient, only 891 people benefited from this intervention as of June 2020.[133]

Gilead's gesture also failed to satisfy members of Congress. Following their announcement, the House Oversight and Reform Committee called Gilead CEO Daniel O'Day to a hearing before Congress to justify Truvada's cost. In 2015, a lack of competition enabled Turing Pharmaceuticals CEO Martin Shkreli to inflate the price of Daraprim pills, used to treat HIV and cancer, from $13.50 to $750 overnight.[134] On 16 May, Congresswoman Alexandria Ocasio-Cortez (D-NY) asked O'Day why Gilead sold Truvada for PrEP in the US for up to $2,000 a month in the US but as little as $6 in countries like South Africa. O'Day answered that unlike in other countries where the drug is generic, Gilead still held the patent on Truvada in the US, allowing the company to legally set and raise prices.[135] O'Day's comments highlighted the power of pharmaceutical companies to determine disease trajectories and underscored Thrasher's powerful statement that "those who controlled the means of pharmacological production controlled access to life itself."[136]

O'Day's testimony also failed to convince activists. The same week, Peter Staley, who joined ACT UP after testing positive for HIV in 1985 and who joined a breakaway organization, Treatment Action Group (TAG), in January 1992, Brenda Goodrow, an activist who has lived with HIV all her life, and several others filed a class-action antitrust lawsuit against Gilead Sciences Inc. and several of the nation's largest drug manufacturers, including Bristol-Myers Squibb (BMS) and the Johnson & Johnson subsidiary Janssen Pharmaceuticals.[137] Replicating the battles over the price of experimental drugs in the 1980s, the lawsuit, *Peter Staley, et al. v. Gilead Sciences, Inc., et al.*, is an example of women and men uniting around the common cause of securing health equality.[138] The case, filed in the US District Court for the Northern District of California in San Francisco, accuses Gilead of brokering deals that coerced other drug manufacturers to use Gilead's HIV medication, tenofovir disoproxil, in their combination pills, when cheaper, generic versions of the compound existed. In exchange, Gilead agreed not to market pills that competed with Bristol-Myers Squibb's and Janssen's HIV drugs after their patents expired. Plaintiffs claim that this agreement violated the Sherman Antitrust Act of 1890, enabling Gilead to maintain its monopoly in the HIV treatment market and charge "exorbitant, supracompetitive" prices for lifesaving medicine.[139] More than eighty percent of people starting HIV treatment, and one hundred percent of those who use PrEP, take a Gilead product. This lack of competition stunted the invention of new, safer, and more effective medicines, argued Staley.[140]

The complaint also accuses Gilead of keeping a safer formulation of tenofovir, tenofovir alafenamide (TAF), off market for more than a decade. The FDA approved Gilead's new drug, Descovy, containing TAF, in October 2019. Gilead charges around $2,000 per patient per month for Descovy, matching its pricing of brand-name Truvada.[141] Although generic versions of Truvada are now available in the US, the safer, patented PrEP drug is only available to those who can afford it. For cisgender women, Descovy is another new medicine with old problems. The FDA did not approve its use for cisgender women. Gilead excluded them from the clinical trials because of their struggle to find a "relevant female cohort" for study. As well as leaving unaddressed the economic and power issues that might impact women's ability or wish to use the drug, women must also pay out of pocket to buy the drug off-label, placing further economic obstacles in their path to treatment and prevention. Although women moved the FDA to change its guidance to broaden women's access to clinical research in 1993, drug manufacturers continue to privilege cisgender male bodies as normative to the detriment of women's health.[142]

In November 2019, the US government filed a lawsuit seeking $1 billion in damages for Gilead's alleged infringement of HHS's patents on PrEP therapy. Gilead rejected the government's charges, filing their own claim that successfully accused the federal government of violating research agreements by failing to give the manufacturer adequate notice of its patent applications.[143]

These patent battles continue. In April 2022, plaintiffs and Bristol-Myers Squibb reached an out-of-court settlement requiring the company to pay $10.8 billion that will reimburse the copayments paid on their HIV drug Evotaz. The jury trial for the suit involving Gilead and Janssen is set for May 2023. If the judge rules that the agreements reached between manufacturers to stunt competition are unconstitutional, the outcome could impact the cost of not only HIV medicine but other prescription drugs. Moreover, Gilead may yet have to license government patents for PrEP, depending on the outcome of the government's lawsuit against them. Activists want the government to put money won through the lawsuit back into widening access to PrEP.[144] The government's enforcement of its intellectual property rights is an unprecedented move that could set a model for future government action to hold drug companies accountable for their pricing of medicines.[145]

Activists have waged these battles with the understanding that the pharmaceutical industry cannot stop HIV with medicines alone. As Allan Brandt put it in 1985, drugs are not "magic bullets." Bringing the epidemic under control in its fifth decade requires confronting the systemic problems that keep women and all marginalized groups from seeking, securing, and staying in care, including not only the price of medicines but the unequal power dynamics in sexual relationships that available prevention methods fail to address.

CONCLUSION

The introduction of vaccines and cures did not signal the end of other infectious diseases. Similarly, the remarkable success of medical advances, spurred by activist interventions, in transforming an HIV infection from a "death sentence" to a chronic, manageable condition with medication by the close of the twentieth century should not give the impression that HIV is a problem of the past.

Ending the AIDS epidemic requires not only scientific breakthroughs but political choices. In addition to enforcing its patents on Truvada, the US government could take further action to reduce drug prices, for example, giving Medicare and Medicaid greater powers to negotiate costs or setting drug prices themselves.[146] The government could also broaden health-care access, expanding Medicaid in all fifty states and US territories, and work to address the poverty, educational and housing inequality, racism, sexism, homophobia, transphobia, ableism, and other social determinants that lead to worse health outcomes among people who are multiply marginalized, especially women of color.[147]

The urgency to address the intersections among poverty, racism, sexism, and health inequality has driven the action of this chapter. The imperative to address the structural inequities that exacerbate poor health outcomes is why organizations like Planned Parenthood decided to forgo Title X funding instead of adhering to Trump's regulations that denied full reproductive health services to everyone who required them, regardless of their ability to pay. It is why advocates also decried the restrictions Trump placed on foreign aid programs that undermined the ability for men and women in developing countries to protect themselves from HIV, other diseases, and unwanted pregnancies. It is why feminist scientists have worked tirelessly for more than three decades to bring to market a prevention tool specifically designed to meet women's interrelated sexual and economic health needs.

In December 2021, the IPM withdrew its application to license the dapivirine vaginal ring for HIV prevention among cisgender women from the FDA. Their withdrawal followed reports that the agency was unlikely to approve the ring because other prevention options are available to women.[148] Mirroring how the approval of a prevention pill eclipsed microbicide research a decade earlier, the government in 2021 approved a long-acting, injectable version of PrEP using the drug cabotegravir. While clinical trials have proven the success of injectable PrEP in preventing HIV among cisgender women, the ongoing struggle to make available a microbicide that gives women greater freedom over their sexual and reproductive health underscores the wider challenge that women faced in moving federal agencies and private companies to treat them as a group deserving of care throughout the epidemic.[149]

We do not know how current efforts to end the HIV epidemic will play out. Amid an evolving treatment and political landscape, poverty, sexism, ableism, homophobia, racism, and other vectors of discrimination continue to shape the trajectory of the epidemic and how people experience it. Activists for cheaper medicines have succeeded in keeping the AIDS epidemic in the public consciousness and moving the government to take the unprecedented action of suing a pharmaceutical company over the cost of its drugs. Feminist scientists will no doubt persist in their efforts to make microbicides a prevention option for women in the US. As with AIDS activism in the past, these activists and advocates may win specific gains that secure the approval of and widen access to new and innovative treatments. Nonetheless, without the introduction of universal health care, women's health and, indeed, the health of all, will remain precarious and subject to the ideological whims of lawmakers and political parties. As seen throughout US history, this reality will continue to most harm the disenfranchised and vulnerable in society, including women.

EPILOGUE

KIA LABEIJA LIES ON HER BACK on the floor of her bedroom in her Hell's Kitchen apartment in New York City. Wearing a red sequin dress and gold strappy heels, she turns her head toward the camera to stare frankly at the viewer. She hugs a framed photograph of herself and her mother, taken in 2014, called "Kia and Mommy: 24," one of a series of four self-portraits exploring what it was like growing up as an HIV-positive woman of color. "Twenty-four," her age at the time of the photograph, is also the title of her series that addresses her experience with the US health-care system. In "Mourning Sickness," she lies on the bathroom floor of her child-hood home in a floral bathrobe, again looking directly into the camera, her fuchsia lipstick matching her headscarf. The portrait addresses the violent side effects that come from taking a combination of antiretroviral drugs every day. The title, a play on words, connects the nausea from the HIV medication and the nausea experienced in pregnancy with the loss of her mother to AIDS.[1]

LaBeija was born Kia Michelle Benbow to a Black father and a Filipino mother in New York City in 1990. Following its first notice on AIDS among infants in December 1982 and the confirmation that women could transmit HIV during pregnancy, childbirth, and breast-feeding three years later, the CDC recommended that HIV-positive women "delay" pregnancy "until more is known about perinatal transmission of the virus." Most states followed suit. In 1987, New York State mandated that doctors offer counseling and voluntary HIV testing to all pregnant women and advise those who tested positive to postpone pregnancy.[2] Pregnant women who received a positive test result faced the dual burden of navigating a deeply stigmatized, life-threatening illness while resisting the threats posed to their ability to raise the children that some journalists, policymakers, and public health officials argued they should never have had. Women sometimes lost the battle to raise their own children, as well as the fight against HIV. In 2004, when LaBeija was fourteen, her mother, Kwan Bennett, an AIDS activist who founded the Asian and Pacific Islander Coalition on HIV/AIDS, died of AIDS-related complications.[3]

LaBeija's work attests to how developments in treatment regimens have led to the experiential shift from dying of AIDS to living with HIV within a generation. Not only did the introduction of ART in 1996 transform the meaning of HIV from a fatal disease to a chronic illness with consistent, uninterrupted access to medication, a greater variety of medicines now also exist to prevent the transmission of the virus. These medical developments, combined with the introduction of the Obama-era ACA in 2010, which saw ten million more adult women gain health coverage between 2010 and 2019, contributed to the six percent overall decrease in the number of women contracting HIV annually between 2015 and 2019.[4] Nonetheless, LaBeija's work also represents that of other activists seeking to keep what society perceives as the "end" of the HIV epidemic open, as people, especially those living at the intersection of multiple and mutually reinforcing oppressions, continue to navigate the systemic biases and structural inequalities that undermine their health and the efforts to bring the epidemic under control despite biomedical advances.[5] For instance, due to persistent socioeconomic inequalities, Black women continue to suffer disproportionately from HIV/AIDS compared to women from other racial and ethnic groups, they represent more than half of new HIV diagnoses in women despite making up approximately fifteen percent of the female population, and they have a one in forty-eight chance of contracting HIV in their lifetime.[6] Moreover, LaBeija's work powerfully defies those who continue to target women as the so-called guilty transmitters of HIV to innocent children.

In January 2008, police arrested thirty-seven-year-old Cecelia Ann Sliker, a white woman, in her home in Bradenton, Florida, on a charge of child neglect, a felony. Sliker pleaded guilty at the trial, and the Circuit Judge Debra Johnes Riva sentenced her to fifteen years in prison. As part of a plea deal, the judge reduced Sliker's sentence to two years' probation in Port Manatee jail. In the thirty-five states where HIV criminalization laws are still active, pregnant women like Sliker have a legal obligation to disclose their HIV status to a partner and seek medical treatment on behalf of their pregnancies.[7]

Authorities charged Sliker for failing to seek treatment to prevent perinatal transmission of HIV when she became pregnant in 2004. Sliker faced prosecution because the judge believed that improvements in treatment options for children left no excuse for her not to have pursued care.[8] Sliker reportedly knew of her HIV-positive status before giving birth to her first son in 2001, when she sought medical attention to successfully block transmission of the virus. Three years later, when she became pregnant again, she chose not to pursue medical care, keeping her HIV-positive status from her second son's father for fear of what he would do to her if he found out. Journalists did not explicitly state that Sliker was in an abusive relationship but her testimony, coupled with the fact she sought medical care for her first child but not her second, and the prevalent link between gender-based violence and HIV disclosure, suggests that fear of intimate partner violence informed her decision not to seek treatment.[9]

Sliker is one of many women who has carried the burden of the earlier moral panic over pregnant women infecting their children with HIV. In 2009, one year after Sliker's arrest, the US District Judge for Maine, John Woodcock, doubled the sentence of QLT, a twenty-eight-year-old, HIV-positive, five-month pregnant woman from Cameroon originally arrested for falsifying immigration documents. Woodcock explained that he detained QLT until she gave birth to ensure that she took her antiretroviral medication and stop her from "assault(ing)" her "unborn child" through HIV transmission, despite her having already arranged medical care in the US.[10]

Woodcock's ruling perpetuated several harmful misassumptions that have informed the mistreatment of HIV-positive women wishing to become pregnant and bring a pregnancy to term in medicine, policy, and law since the 1980s. These include the idea that women are the containers for fetuses who are already children with rights; second, that fetal health is distinct from women's health, and that women's bodies are harmful to developing pregnancies; third, that women, and, especially those deemed unworthy of the privileges of citizenship on account of their immigration or legal status, are incapable of making rational judgments about their medical needs; and, fourth, that the state is obliged to intervene in a woman's reproductive life to not only "protect" a fetus from the apparently harmful actions of its mother but society from the moral and financial cost of caring for the sick infant. QLT not only carried the burden of the earlier concern over the perceived "crisis" of women transmitting HIV to their fetus during pregnancy, but also the deeply racialized and xenophobic panic over people with HIV seeking residency and refuge in the United States.[11]

As Sliker's and QLT's arrests and detentions attest, these assumptions have become more institutionally entrenched since the 1980s. This entrenchment results partly from the medical advances that have empowered hostile law enforcement officers and judges to exercise their biases, challenging historians to resist neat endings following scientific discoveries. It also reflects how far coercion and punishment have come to shape the political approach to women's health since the Reagan era.

Ronald Reagan came to office in 1981 as policymakers, who were called to "get tough" on groups requiring government support, began winning the argument about what the state should prioritize in preserving public order. The Reagan administration advanced this emerging "law and order" agenda, promising to roll back recent advances in civil rights in part through the reestablishment of prescriptive normative sex and gender roles in what became known as the "family values politics" of the 1980s. Public figures leading the early AIDS response operated within a political context committed to upholding white, middle-class heteronormativity in ways that blunted effective, systematic measures to curb the epidemic. In the following decades, subsequent administrations continued to channel administrative energy and resources away from social welfare and towards law enforcement programs, pursuing increasingly punitive policies that harmed women as well as other vulnerable populations. These included measures on the obliteration of welfare, the expansion of prisons, and the failure to implement universal health care. The extreme anti-gay, anti-woman, anti-immigrant, and anti-welfare agenda of the Trump administration marked the culmination of a forty-year campaign on the part of conservative lawmakers and activists to restore white, heteronormative "traditional values" and punish those in opposition to them.[12]

The legacy of this assault on women's rights is evident in the gutting of the Title X program under Trump and the *Dobbs v. Jackson Women's Health Organization* (June 2022) ruling that the US Constitution does not confer a right to abortion.[13] *Dobbs* is devastating for reproductive rights. In addition to rendering abortion illegal or highly restricted in several states, the reversal of the *Roe v. Wade* decision raises the specter of the increased prosecution of people, including those with HIV, in relation to their pregnancies. In May 2022, State Representative Danny McCormick, a Republican, introduced a bill in the Louisiana State Legislature granting constitutional rights to "unborn children from the moment of fertilization" and classifying abortion as homicide. While McCormick withdrew his bill amid backlash, other state legislatures continued to debate laws seeking to grant fetuses rights and which equate abortion and murder.[14] Law enforcement officials in several states have already charged women with murder and manslaughter for miscarriages, stillbirths, and other pregnancy losses.[15] This criminalization in the name of fetal protection is not new. Since the 1970s, abortion opponents have promoted the notion that fetuses are human beings with rights akin to those of the women carrying them to erode women's rights. The National Advocates for Pregnant Women found at least 1,700 instances in which a woman has faced prosecution for an action that allegedly harmed her fetus between 1973 and 2020.[16] The testing, reporting, arrest, and detention of women in relation to their pregnancies has roots not only in the history of the war on drugs but also the AIDS epidemic. With the end of *Roe*, a pregnant person with HIV can face criminal charges both for seeking or having an abortion, as well as for having a baby, making clear how the recriminalization of abortion exacerbates existing threats to the reproductive lives of HIV-positive women. As Black women are more likely to seek an abortion, suffer from pregnancy-related complications, and contract HIV than white women, they experience this threat most harshly.

We know from the efforts of the women who fought to secure decent medical care in prison—as well as from Jessica Ordaz's research into the mistreatment of people with HIV/AIDS detained in immigration detention centers—that systems designed to punish cannot provide for people's even most basic medical needs.[17] As Laura McTighe asserted, "Prisons are no places to be sick."[18] The failure of many correctional facilities to uphold people in prison's constitutional right to medical treatment during the Covid-19 pandemic in early 2020 underscored the dangerous and often deadly health-care situation for women in prison. At CCWF, women's reports of mistreatment amid Covid-19 echoed the complaints women made more than thirty years before in relation to HIV/AIDS and other illnesses, namely, of staff responding inappropriately to the transmission of Covid-19 by confining women in proximity and failing to provide cleaning supplies, denying women access to medical care and daily prescribed medication, and belittling women who tested positive while punishing those who protested the life-threatening situation. As Stephen W. Thrasher aptly noted, despite their virological differences, the trajectory of Covid-19 in and beyond prison parallels that of HIV in that inequality rooted in capitalism, sexism, racism, ableism, and heterosexism has blunted efforts to tackle it, with society's most vulnerable, whom he argues are part of a "viral underclass," feeling its effects most starkly.[19] Nonetheless, stories of resistance also matched those of mistreatment, as women at CCWF joined with the CCWP and other advocates to demand improved conditions.[20] Although people in prison and activists have secured moderate gains in making state and federal prisons less inhumane in the decades since *Shumate v. Wilson* (1995), Woodcock and other judges who have detained pregnant women in prison for the sake of fetal health put these women, and their pregnancies, at risk.

The dangerous response to Covid-19 in prison and the end of *Roe* speak to several other legacies that emerge from the struggles between women demanding state recognition for access to lifesaving treatment and services while resisting punitive state intervention on behalf of the purported needs of fetuses, children, and the "general public," as documented throughout.

The federal response to Covid-19 revealed how multiply marginalized women continue to suffer from discriminatory economic and health policies that neglect their needs. Many domestic workers, most of whom are non-white women, did not qualify for the federal stimulus checks sent to workers to support them financially throughout the pandemic. Men of color, and women of all races, are more likely than white men to work at organizations that are exempt from Covid-19 paid-leave protections.[21] The increased burden of childcare during the pandemic also disproportionately fell to women, exacerbating existing inequities in job insecurity, access to health insurance, and paid family and sick leave. Gender inequities intersected with those of race and class, as Black and Latina women are more likely than white women to head single-parent households and engage in essential labor that both increased their chances of encountering Covid-19 and their need for childcare.[22] Deep-seated race, class, and gender disparities in employment underscore not only the inadequacy of a hybrid public-private, for-profit health system in which a person's job largely determines the care they receive and their entitlement to benefits, but also the recent proposals for private organizations to pay for their employee's abortion care.[23] Without universal health care, women, people of color, people living in poverty, and members of other marginalized groups will continue to suffer as a result of people in positions of authority making value judgments about their bodies and lives and their deservedness for support. Like HIV/AIDS, the uneven impact of Covid-19 across racial and ethnic groups underscores the urgent need to tackle the social and economic factors that lead to health disparities, and which are exacerbated by a capitalist health-care system.[24]

Contests over whose life is valuable also continue to play out in schools. On March 28, 2022, the Republican governor of Florida Ron DeSantis signed the Parental Rights in Education Law that restricts what teachers can say about gender and sexual orientation in the classroom. Several other states have followed suit, introducing bills aimed at controlling what teachers can say not only about sexuality and gender but also about race and racism.[25] Just as conservatives evoked the symbol of the child and the language of child protection to censor queer women's articulations of sexual health in the 1990s, Republican lawmakers are again purporting to act in the interest of children to maintain rigid boundaries around race, sex, and gender in society.

Moreover, the political campaign to censor references to women's sex acts and organs in the public sphere since the 1980s continues to blunt HIV-prevention efforts today. Throughout the epidemic, public health and cultural messaging advised women to abstain from sex or convince men to use condoms. The failed nonoxynol-9 microbicide trials of the 1990s showed that its use increased women's vulnerability to infection. The struggle of scientists like Dr. Sharon Hillier to bring to market a microbicide product developed from an intersectional feminist perspective in the US reflects the difficulty women have encountered in transcending their treatment as sexless mothers to center the diversity of their sexual lives and needs since the 1980s. The current battles over abortion, LGBTQ+ rights, criminal justice, and the health-care market are part of the legacy of the state neglecting women's health-care needs, censoring articulations of their nonnormative sexuality, and intervening into their bodies and lives on behalf of the symbolic needs of fetuses and children as seen throughout the AIDS epidemic.

History teaches us to interrogate things taken for granted. The increasingly privatized, politicized, and punitive treatment of women's health is not inevitable but a result of political choices that have exacerbated the harmful effects of HIV/AIDS in women. For instance, the reliance on criminalization to tackle HIV has not curbed intimate partner violence, economic inequality, or the other systemic factors that shape a woman's ability to address HIV. Rather, due to biases within the criminal justice system, these laws disproportionately harm people already vulnerable to police surveillance and who are also especially vulnerable to HIV, such as sex workers and Black men.[26] Women who disclose their status to avoid arrest may encounter interpersonal violence and abuse. They also risk losing their parental rights.[27] The disproportionate targeting of certain groups suggests that the purpose of these laws is to "protect" deserving citizens from the supposedly "immoral" actions of people who do not conform to social norms. Criminalization does not protect women. Rather, it entrenches the stigma and shame associated with HIV and deters women from testing, disclosing their status, and seeking treatment. It therefore fails as an effective, humane, and compassionate public health measure.[28]

The government could, and still can, chart an alternative path. They could stop criminalizing HIV transmission and exposure. They could broaden access to family planning, prenatal, maternal, and HIV health services and information. They could increase counseling and other support services for people with HIV. They could help foster a safer environment for HIV status disclosure by tackling the cultural and systemic roots of domestic violence and approve a cheap, widely available women-controlled microbicide product to give women greater power to engage in safe sex. Finally, they could tackle the roots of social inequality that result in disparate health outcomes in different communities, including in housing, education, employment, and health care.

Disease outbreaks call into question whose life is valued and on what terms. The steps lawmakers could take to end HIV require exploding the neglect-intervention dyad that shaped the experiences of women with HIV/AIDS and perpetuated gender inequality. This involves acting on a different vision of women's place in society, one in which the state recognizes them as a class of people deserving of state support on their own terms, free from prescription about their bodies and lives and the risk of punitive interference. *In Her Hands* documents women's struggle to achieve this vision. Despite setbacks, and operating within a political context increasingly hostile to their rights, women nevertheless secured gains, working in coalitions across identity categories and social status that combined diverse perspectives and harnessed different skills. Although gender continues to act as a vector of discrimination in US politics, activism waged from an intersectional perspective has the power to challenge the terms on which the state responds to women's demands. History teaches that realizing an alternative, more just and humane vision of society is always possible. HIV-positive women and advocates will no doubt continue fighting to secure this vision in the years to come.

Notes

INTRODUCTION

1. Kenneth B. Hymes et al., "Kaposi's Sarcoma in Homosexual Men—a Report of Eight Cases," *Lancet* 8247, no. 2 (March 1981): 598.

2. CDC, "Unexplained Immunodeficiency and Opportunistic Infections in Infants—New York, New Jersey, California," *MMWR* 31, no. 49 (December 17, 1982): 665–67; Randy Kennedy, "Elizabeth Glaser Dies at 47; Crusader for Pediatric AIDS," *New York Times*, December 4, 1994, Section 1, 58; Celeste Watkins-Hayes, *Remaking a Life: How Women Living with HIV-AIDS Confront Inequality* (Oakland: University of California Press, 2019), 1.

3. CDC, "Current Trends Update on Acquired Immune Deficiency Syndrome (AIDS)—United States," *MMWR* 31, no. 37 (September 24, 1982): 507–8, 513–14.

4. For analysis of the 4-H club and the treatment of AIDS as a disease of "deviant" behavior rather than systemic inequalities, see Evelynn Hammonds, "Race, Sex, AIDS: The Construction of 'Other,'" *Radical America* 20, no. 6 (1987), 31–32; Paula Treichler, "AIDS, Homophobia, and Biomedical Discourse: An Epidemic of

Signification," *October* 43 (Winter 1987): 44; Nancy Goldstein and Jennifer L. Manlowe, *The Gender Politics of HIV/AIDS in Women* (New York: New York University Press, 1997), 8; Treichler, *How to Have Theory in an Epidemic: Cultural Chronicles of AIDS* (Durham, NC: Duke University Press, 1999), 50–53. On the concept of private risk, see Melinda Cooper, *Family Values: Between Neoliberalism and the New Social Conservatism* (New York: Zone Books, 2017).

    5. Evelynn Hammonds, "Missing Persons: African American Women, AIDS, and the History of Disease," *Radical America* 21, no. 2 (1990): 17–18.

    6. Treichler, "AIDS, Homophobia, and Biomedical Discourse," 45–46; Cindy Patton, *Last Served? Gendering the HIV Pandemic* (London: Taylor & Francis, 1994), 4–5. On the racialized and gendered treatment of women as vectors of disease in other historical contexts, see Allan Brandt, *No Magic Bullet: A Social History of Venereal Disease in the United States Since 1980* (New York: Oxford University Press, 1987); Sander L. Gilman, "AIDS and Syphilis: The Iconography of Disease," *October* 43 (Winter 1987): 87–107; Katherine Beckett, "Fetal Rights and 'Crack Moms': Pregnant Women in the War on Drugs,' *Contemporary Drug Problems* 22 (Winter 1995): 587–612; Leslie J. Reagan, *Dangerous Pregnancies: Mothers, Disabilities, and Abortion in Modern America* (Berkeley: University of California Press, 2010).

    7. Hammonds, "Race, Sex, AIDS," 29. See, e.g., Charles Rosenberg, *The Cholera Years: The United States in 1832, 1849, and 1866* (Chicago: University of Chicago Press, 1962); Elizabeth Fee and Daniel M. Fox, eds., *AIDS: The Burdens of History* (Berkeley: University of California Press, 1988); Susan Sontag, *Illness as Metaphor and AIDS and Its Metaphors* (New York: Anchor Books, 1989); Marilyn Chase, *The Barbary Plague: The Black Death in Victorian San Francisco* (New York: Random House, 2003); Alice Wexler, *The Woman Who Walked into the Sea: Huntington's and the Making of a Genetic Disease* (New Haven: Yale University Press, 2008); Kathryn Olivarius, *Necropolis: Disease, Power, and Capitalism in the Cotton Kingdom* (Cambridge, MA: Harvard University Press, 2022); Steven W. Thrasher, *The Viral Underclass: The Human Toll When Inequality and Disease Collide* (New York: Macmillan, 2022).

    8. Patricia Hill Collins, *Black Feminist Thought: Knowledge, Consciousness, and the Politics of Empowerment* (New York: Routledge, 1991); Cathy J. Cohen, "Punks, Bulldaggers, and Welfare Queens: The Radical Potential of Queer Politics?" *GLQ* 3 (1997): 427–65; Dorothy E. Roberts, *Killing the Black Body: Race,*

Reproduction, and the Meaning of Liberty (New York: Vintage Books, 1999); Enid Logan, "The Wrong Race, Committing Crime, Doing Drugs, and Maladjusted for Motherhood: The Nation's Fury over 'Crack Babies,'" Social Justice 26, no. 1 (Spring 1999), 115–38; Gareth Davies, "The Welfare State," in The Reagan Presidency: Pragmatic Conservatism and Its Legacies, ed. W. Elliot Brownlee and Hugh David Graham (Lawrence: University Press of Kansas, 2003); Marisa Chappell, The War on Welfare: Family, Poverty, and Politics in Modern America (Philadelphia: University of Pennsylvania Press, 2010); Naomi Murakawa, The First Civil Right: How Liberals Built Prison America (Oxford: Oxford University Press, 2014); Julilly Kohler-Hausmann, Getting Tough: Welfare and Imprisonment in 1970s (Princeton: University of Princeton Press, 2017); Moya Bailey, Misogynoir: Black Women's Digital Resistance (New York: New York University Press, 2021).

9. My use of "multiply marginalized" was inspired by Darius Bost, "Black Lesbian Feminist Intellectuals and the Struggle against HIV/AIDS," Souls 21, nos. 2–3 (2019): 169–91; Watkins-Hayes, Remaking a Life, 24.

10. Many studies of the US AIDS epidemic focus predominantly on the 1980s and early-to-mid 1990s. See, e.g., Jennifer Brier, Infectious Ideas: U.S. Political Responses to the AIDS Crisis (Chapel Hill: University of North Carolina Press, 2009); Deborah Gould, Moving Politics: Emotion and ACT UP's Fight Against AIDS (Chicago: University of Chicago Press, 2009); Anthony M. Petro, After the Wrath of God: AIDS, Sexuality, and American Religion (New York: Oxford University Press, 2015); Richard A. McKay, Patient Zero and the Making of the AIDS Epidemic (Chicago: University of Chicago Press, 2017); and Karma R. Chávez, The Borders of AIDS: Race, Quarantine, and Resistance (Seattle: University of Washington Press, 2021).

11. Jonathan Bell, "Rethinking the 'Straight State': Welfare Politics, Health Care, and Public Policy in the Shadow of AIDS," Journal of American History 104, no. 4 (March 2018), 931–52; Sarah Schulman, Let the Record Show: A Political History of ACT UP New York, 1987–1993 (New York: Farrar, Straus and Giroux, 2021), 17–18.

12. Evelyn Brooks Higginbotham, Righteous Discontent: The Women's Movement in the Black Baptist Church (Cambridge, MA: Harvard University Press, 1993).

13. Jeanne Theoharis, Komozi Woodard, and Dayo F. Gore, eds., Want to Start to a Revolution? Radical Women in the Black Freedom Struggle (New York:

New York University Press, 2009); and Betty Luther Hilliman, "'The Most Pro-foundly Revolutionary Act a Homosexual Can Engage In': Drag and the Politics of Gender Presentation in San Francisco Gay Liberation Movement," *Journal of the History of Sexuality* 20, no. 1 (Jan. 2011), 153–81. On the relationship between AIDS and respectability politics, see Gould, *Moving Politics*; Ayana K. Weekley, "Saving Me through Erasure? Black Women, HIV/AIDS and Respect-ability," in *Black Female Sexualities*, ed. Joanna M. Braxton et al. (New Bruns-wick, NJ: Rutgers University Press, 2015); Kevin J. Mumford, *Not Straight, Not White: Black Gay Men from the March on Washington to the AIDS Crisis* (Chapel Hill: University of North Carolina Press, 2016); Jonathan Bell, "Between Pri-vate and Public: AIDS, Health Care Capitalism, and the Politics of Respectabil-ity in 1980s America," *Journal of American Studies* 54, no. 1 (2018): 159–83; Bost, "Black Lesbian Feminist Intellectuals and the Struggle against HIV/AIDS"; Daniel Royles, *To Make the Wounded Whole: The African American Struggle against HIV-AIDS* (Chapel Hill: University of North Carolina Press, 2021).

14. Hammonds, "Missing Persons," 7–22; Cathy Cohen, *The Boundaries of Blackness: AIDS and the Breakdown of Black Politics* (Chicago: University of Chi-cago Press, 1999), 175–78.

15. Cohen, "Punks, Bulldaggers, and Welfare Queens."

16. Carmen Retzlaff, "Can HIV Care Click in the Clink?" *POZ*, April 2004, 25.

17. Beatrix Hoffman, "Healthcare Reform and Social Movements in the US," *American Journal of Public Health* 93, no. 1 (2003): 69–79; and Hoffman, *Healthcare for Some: Rights and Rationing in the United States Since 1930* (Chicago: University of Chicago Press, 2012).

18. Neil Young, *We Gather Together: The Religious Right and the Problem of Interfaith Politics* (New York: Oxford University Press, 2016), 212.

19. Mary Ziegler, *Abortion and the Law in America: Roe v. Wade to the Present* (Cambridge: Cambridge University Press, 2020), 28–29.

20. See, e.g., *Webster v. Reproductive Health Services*, 492 US 490 (1989).

21. On the overlap between the fetal rights movement, the movement for reproductive justice, and the war on drugs, see Janet Golden, "'An Argument that Goes Back to the Womb': The Demedicalization of Fetal Alcohol Syn-drome, 1973–1992," *Journal of Social History* 33, no. 2 (Winter 1999): 269–98; Logan, "Wrong Race"; Rachel Roth, *Making Women Pay: The Hidden Costs of*

Fetal Rights (Ithaca: Cornell University Press, 2000); Sara Dubow, *Ourselves Unborn: A History of the Fetus in Modern America* (New York: Oxford University Press, 2011); Jennifer Nelson, *More than Medicine: A History of the Feminist Women's Health Movement* (New York: New York University Press, 2015); Johanna Schoen, *Abortion after Roe* (Chapel Hill: University of North Carolina Press, 2015); Jael Miriam Silliman, Marlene Gerber, and Loretta Ross, *Undivided Rights: Women of Color Organize for Reproductive Rights* (Chicago: Haymarket Books, 2016); Carol Mason, *Killing for Life: The Apocalyptic Narrative of Pro-Life Politics* (Ithaca: Cornell University Press, 2018); Laura Briggs, *Taking Children: A History of American Terror* (Oakland: University of California Press, 2020).

22. Kohler-Hausmann, "Getting Tough," 7; Nicholas F. Jacobs, Desmond King, and Sidney M. Milkis, "Building a Conservative State: Partisan Polarization and the Redeployment of Administrative Power," *American Political Science Association* 17, no. 2 (June 2019): 453.

23. Additional literature addressing the interconnections among criminal justice, welfare, family values politics, and neoliberalism at the end of the twentieth century include Loïc Wacquant, *Punishing the Poor: The Neoliberal Government of Social Insecurity* (Durham, NC: Duke University Press, 2009); Robert O. Self, *All in the Family: The Realignment of American Democracy Since the 1960s* (New York: Hill and Wang, 2012); Elizabeth Hinton, *From the War on Poverty to the War on Crime* (Cambridge, MA: Harvard University Press, 2016); Cooper, *Family Values*; Paul Renfro, *Stranger Danger: Family Values, Childhood, and the American Carceral State* (New York: Oxford University Press, 2020); Gary Gerstle, *The Rise and Fall of the Neoliberal Order* (New York: Oxford University Press, 2022).

24. See, e.g., Jenna M. Loyd and Alison Mountz, *Boats, Borders, and Bases: Race, the Cold War, and the Rise of Migration Detention in the United States* (Oakland: University of California Press, 2018); Trevor Hoppe, *Punishing Disease: HIV and the Criminalization of Sickness* (Oakland: University of California Press, 2018); Jessica Ordaz, "AIDS Knows No Borders," *Radical History Review* 140 (2021): 175–85; Chávez, *Borders of AIDS*.

25. Ida Susser, *AIDS, Sex, and Culture: Global Politics and Survival in Southern Africa* (Chichester: Wiley-Blackwell, 2009); Yana van der Meulen Rodgers, *The Global Gag Rule and Women's Reproductive Health: Rhetoric Versus Reality* (New York: Oxford University Press, 2018).

26. Kaiser Family Foundation, "Women's Health Insurance Coverage," December 21, 2022, https://www.kff.org/womens-health-policy/fact-sheet/womens-health-insurance-coverage/.

27. Jeremy A. Greene, *Generic: The Unbranding of Modern Medicine* (Baltimore: Johns Hopkins University Press, 2014); Robin Feldman and Evan Frondorf, *Drug Wars: How Big Pharma Raises Prices and Keeps Generics Off the Market* (Cambridge: Cambridge University Press, 2017).

28. Keeanga-Yamahtta Taylor, *Race for Profit: How Banks and the Real Estate Industry Undermined Black Homeownership* (Chapel Hill: University of North Carolina Press, 2019); Royles, *To Make the Wounded Whole*, chap. 7.

29. Historians have tended to treat AIDS and abortion politics as distinct subjects. Scholarship that deals with the government response to AIDS, especially within the Reagan administration, includes Cohen, *Boundaries of Blackness*; William B. Turner, "Mirror Images: Lesbian/Gay Civil Rights in the Carter and Reagan Administrations," in *Creating Change: Sexuality, Public Policy, and Civil Rights*, ed. John D'Emilio and William B. Turner (New York: St. Martin's Press, 2000); Amin Ghaziani, *The Dividends of Dissent: How Conflict and Culture Work in Lesbian and Gay Marches on Washington* (Chicago: University of Chicago Press, 2008); James T. Patterson, *Restless Giant: The United States from Watergate to Bush v. Gore* (New York: Oxford University Pres, 2005); Sean Wilentz, *The Age of Reagan: A History, 1974–2008* (New York: HarperCollins, 2008); Brier, *Infectious Ideas*; Doug Rossinow, *The Reagan Era: A History of the 1980s* (New York: Oxford University Press, 2015). For histories that deal with abortion politics in the same period, see note 21.

30. William C. Berman, *America's Right Turn: From Nixon to Clinton* (Baltimore: Johns Hopkins University Press, 1998); Lisa McGirr, *Suburban Warriors: The Origins of the New American Right* (Princeton: Princeton University Press, 2001); Self, *All in the Family*.

31. Kohler-Hausmann, *Getting Tough*, 6.

32. Theda Skocpol, *Protecting Soldiers and Mothers: The Political Origins of Social Policy in the United States* (Cambridge, MA: Belknap Press of Harvard University Press, 1992); Linda Gordon, *Pitied but Not Entitled: Single Mothers and the History of Welfare, 1890–1935* (New York: Free Press, 1994); Leslie J. Reagan, *When Abortion was a Crime: Women, Medicine, and Law in the United States, 1867–1973* (Berkeley: University of California Press, 1997); Rickie Solinger, *Wake Up*

Little Susie (New York: Routledge, 2000); Dorothy Roberts, *Shattered Bonds: The Color of Child Welfare* (New York: Basic Books, 2002); David K. Johnson, *The Lavender Scare: The Cold War Prosecution of Gays and Lesbians in the Federal Government* (Chicago: University of Chicago Press, 2004); Margot Canaday, *The Straight State: Sexuality and Citizenship in Twentieth-Century America* (Princeton: Princeton University Press, 2009); Reagan, *Dangerous Pregnancies*; Chappell, *War on Welfare*; Dorothy Sue Cobble, Linda Gordon, and Astrid Henry, *Feminism Unfinished: A Short, Surprising History of American Women's Movements* (New York: Liveright Publishing, 2014); Alix Genter, "Appearances Can be Deceiving: Butch-Femme Fashion and Queer Legibility in New York City, 1945–1969," *Feminist Studies* 42, no. 3 (2016): 604–31; Scott W. Stern, *The Trials of Nina McCall: Sex, Surveillance, and the Decades-Long Government Plan to Imprison "Promiscuous" Women* (Boston: Beacon Press, 2019).

33. Schulman, *Let the Record Show*, xiii.

34. Karlene Faith, *Unruly Women: The Politics of Confinement and Resistance* (Vancouver: Press Gang Publishers, 1993); Angela Y. Davis, *Are Prisons Obsolete?* (New York: Seven Stories Press, 2003); Juanita Diaz-Cotto, *Chicana Lives and Criminal Justice: Voices from El Barrio* (Austin: University of Texas Press, 2006); Ruth W. Gilmore, *Golden Gulag: Prisons, Surplus, Crisis, and Opposition In Globalizing California* (Berkeley: University of California Press, 2006); Victoria Law, *Resistance behind Bars: The Struggles of Incarcerated Women* (Oakland: PM Press, 2009); Heather Ann Thompson, "Why Mass Incarceration Matters: Rethinking Crisis, Decline, and Transformation in Postwar American History," *Journal of American History* 97, no. 3 (December 1, 2010): 703–34; Michelle Alexander, *The New Jim Crow: Mass Incarceration in the Age of Colorblindness* (New York: New Press, 2012); Beth E. Richie, *Arrested Justice: Black Women, Violence, and America's Prison Nation* (New York: New York University Press, 2012); Murakawa, *First Civil Right*; Hinton, *From the War on Poverty to the War on Crime*; Scott De Orio, "The Invention of Bad Gay Sex: Texas and the Creation of a Criminal Underclass of Gay People," *Journal of the History of Sexuality* 26, no. 1 (January 2017): 53–87; Emily L. Thuma, *All Our Trials: Prisons, Policing, and the Feminist Fight to End Violence* (Urbana: University of Illinois Press, 2019).

35. Nelson, *More Than Medicine*, 195.

36. Leslie J. Reagan, "Crossing the Border for Abortions: California Activists, Mexican Clinics, and the Creation of a Feminist Health Agency in the

1960s," *Feminist Studies* 26, no. 2 (Summer 2000), 323–48; Naomi Rogers, "'Caution: The AMA May be Dangerous to your Health': The Student Health Organizations (SHO) and American Medicine, 1965–1970," *Radical History Review* 80 (Spring 2001): 5–34; Ann Cvetkovich, *An Archive of Feelings: Trauma, Sexuality, and Lesbian Public Cultures* (Durham, NC: Duke University Press, 2003); Jennifer Nelson, *Women of Color and the Reproductive Rights Movement* (New York: New York University Press, 2003); Harriet A. Washington, *Medical Apartheid: The Dark History of the Medical Experimentation on Black Americans from Colonial Times to the Present* (New York: Doubleday, 2006); Amber Jamilla Musser, "From Our Body to Yourselves: The Boston Women's Health Book Collective and the Changing Notions of Subjectivity, 1969–1973," *Women's Studies Quarterly* 35, no. 1/2 (2007): 93–109; Deidre Cooper Owens, *Medical Bondage: Race, Gender, and the Origins of American Gynecology* (Athens: University of Georgia Press, 2017); Wendy Kline, *Bodies of Knowledge: Sexuality, Reproduction, and Women's Health in the Second Wave* (Chicago: University of Chicago Press, 2010); Alondra Nelson, *Body and Soul: The Black Panther Party and the Fight against Medical Discrimination* (Minneapolis: University of Minnesota Press, 2011); Nelson, *More Than Medicine*; Katie Batza, "From Sperm Runners to Sperm Banks: Lesbians, Assisted Conception, and Challenging the Fertility Industry, 1971–1983," *Journal of Women's History* 23, no. 2 (2016), 82–102; Batza, *Before AIDS: Gay Health Politics in the 1970s* (Philadelphia: University of Pennsylvania Press, 2018); Wendy Kline, *Coming Home: How Midwives Changed Birth* (Oxford: Oxford University Press, 2019); Schulman, *Let the Record Show*.

37. On women as the supports and caregivers of men, see Sara M. Evans, *Tidal Wave: How Women Changed America at Century's End* (New York: The Free Press, 2003); Ghaziani, *Dividends of Dissent*; Victoria Noe, *Fag Hags, Divas, and Moms: The Legacy of Straight Women in the AIDS Community* (Chicago: King Company Publishing, 2019); Ruth Coker Burks, *All the Young Men* (London: Trapeze, 2021). On women's exclusion from the initial medical response to HIV/AIDS, see Brier, *Infectious Ideas*, 171–79; Alexis Shotwell, "'Women Don't Get AIDS, They Just Die From It': Memory, Classification, and the Campaign to Change the Definition of AIDS," *Hypatia* 29, no. 2 (Spring 2014): 509–25; Tamar W. Carroll, *Mobilizing New York: AIDS, Antipoverty, and Feminist Activism* (Chapel Hill: University of North Carolina Press, 2015); Bell, "Rethinking the 'Straight State,'" 947. On histories exploring HIV-positive women and activists' organiz-

ing, see Nelson, *More Than Medicine*; Sara Matthiesen, "Equality versus Reproductive Risk: Women-and-AIDS Activism and False Choice in the Clinical Trials Debate," *Signs* 41, no. 3 (2016): 579–601; Jennifer Brier, "'I'm Still Surviving': Oral Histories of Women Living with HIV/AIDS in Chicago," *The Oral History Review* 45 (2018): 68–83; Bost, "Black Lesbian Feminist Intellectuals"; Royles, *To Make the Wounded Whole*; Schulman, *Let the Record Show*; and Margot Canaday, *Queer Career: Sexuality and Work in Modern America* (Princeton: Princeton University Press, 2022). Key sociological and ethnographical accounts of women and HIV/AIDS include Treichler, *How to Have Theory in an Epidemic*; Gena Corea, *The Invisible Epidemic: The Story of Women with AIDS* (New York: HarperCollins, 1992); Patton, *Last Served?*; Beth E. Schneider and Nancy E. Stoller, *Women Resisting AIDS: Feminist Strategies of Empowerment* (Philadelphia: Temple University Press, 1995); Goldstein and Manlowe, *Gender Politics*; Nancy E. Stoller, *Lessons from The Damned: Queers, Whores, and Junkies Respond to AIDS* (New York: Routledge, 1998); Watkins-Hayes, *Remaking a Life*.

38. See, e.g., articles in *Radical History Review* 140 (2021); Royles, *To Make the Wounded Whole*; Schulman, *Let the Record Show*; Thrasher, *Viral Underclass*.

39. For a definition of moral panic, see Renfro, *Stranger Danger*, 5.

40. Cultural accounts of the epidemic that do foreground women include Jim Hubbard's documentary *United in Anger* (2012) and Harriet Hirshorn's *Nothing Without Us: The Women Who Will End AIDS* (2017).

CHAPTER 1

1. Don Colburn, "'I Just Started Crying': People with AIDS Struggle to Live in the Shadow of Death," *Washington Post*, September 4, 1985, H8; Bart Barnes, "AIDS Counselor Sonya Sherman Dies," *Washington Post*, August 12, 1986, B6; Sandra G. Boodman, "Covering the AIDS Beat," *Washington Post*, August 14, 1988, 37.

2. CDC, "Current Trends Update on Acquired Immune Deficiency Syndrome (AIDS)—United States," *MMWR* 31, no. 37 (September 24, 1982): 507–8, 513–14.

3. CDC, "Unexplained Immunodeficiency and Opportunistic Infections in Infants," 665–67.

4. On the historical treatment of women as the vectors of disease in men and children, see Introduction, n. 6.

5. For scholarship on the regulation of women's reproduction under Reagan, see Introduction, n. 8.

6. Cooper, *Family Values*, 169.

7. Jeanie Russell Kasindorf, "The Plague," *New York Magazine*, undated; box 1, folder Clippings & Articles, RE 11, 1964–1993, Linda Laubenstein Papers, MC 891, Arthur & Elizabeth Schlesinger Library on the History of Women in America, Radcliffe Institute, Harvard University, Boston (hereafter, Schlesinger Library).

8. Siddhartha Mukherjee, *The Emperor of all Maladies: A Biography of Cancer* (London: Fourth Estate, 2011), 315.

9. Meryl Gordon, "The Woman Who 'Discovered' AIDS," *McCall's* (May 1993): 112.

10. Steven Epstein, *Impure Science: AIDS, Activism, and the Politics of Knowledge* (Berkeley: University of California Press, 1996), 45–46.

11. CDC, *"Pneumocystis* pneumonia—Los Angeles," *MMWR* 30, no. 21 (June 5, 1981): 250–52.

12. Bost, "Black Lesbian Feminist Intellectuals," 179.

13. CDC, *"Pneumocystis* pneumonia," 250–52.

14. Hymes et al., "Kaposi's Sarcoma in Homosexual Men," 598–600.

15. Cooper, *Family Values*, 204–5.

16. Bost, "Black Lesbian Feminist Intellectuals" 179.

17. CDC, "Current Trends Update on Acquired Immune Deficiency Syndrome (AIDS)," 507–8, 513–14.

18. Cindy Patton, *Inventing AIDS* (New York: Routledge, 1990), 128; Cooper, *Family Values*, 204–205.

19. Chris Norwood, "Alarming Rise in Deaths: Are Women Showing New AIDS Symptoms?" *Ms.* (July 1988): 65.

20. Treichler, *How to Have Theory in an Epidemic*, 46.

21. CDC, "Epidemiologic Notes and Reports Update on Kaposi's Sarcoma and Opportunistic Infections in Previously Healthy Persons—United States," *MMWR* 31, no. 22 (June 11, 1982): 294, 300–1.

22. CDC, "Current Trends Update on Acquired Immune Deficiency Syndrome (AIDS)," 507–8, 513–14.

23. For more on the significance of the 4-H categories, see Introduction, n. 4.

24. CDC, "AIDS Weekly Surveillance Report—United States," *MMWR* (December 22, 1983): 1.

25. Larry Doyle, "Study: Inner City Pregnant Women Latest AIDS Victims," *New Pittsburgh Courier*, December 5, 1987, 1.

26. CDC, "Unexplained Immunodeficiency and Opportunistic Infections in Infants," 665–67.

27. CDC, "Epidemiologic Notes and Reports Immunodeficiency among Female Sexual Partners of Males with Acquired Immune Deficiency Syndrome (AIDS)—New York," *MMWR* 31, no. 52 (January 7, 1983): 697–98.

28. CDC, "Current Trends Revision of the Case Definition of Acquired Immunodeficiency Syndrome for National Reporting—United States," *MMWR* 34, no. 25 (June 28, 1985): 373–75.

29. Cooper, *Family Values*, 205–6.

30. Theresa McGovern, "S. P. v. Sullivan: The Effort to Broaden the Social Security Administration's Definition of AIDS," *Fordham Urban Law Journal* 21, no. 4 (1994): 1083.

31. Brier, *Infectious Ideas*, 173.

32. Hammonds, "Missing Persons," 8, 16.

33. WHAM!, "Consensus Statement Regarding the CDC AIDS Definition," 1–2, box 1, folder CDC HIV/AIDS Protest, Women's Health Action and Mobilization (WHAM!) records, Tamiment Library, New York University.

34. Risa Denenberg, "Pregnant Women and HIV," in Marion Banzhaf et al., *Women, AIDS, and Activism by the ACT UP/NY Women and AIDS Handbook Group* (Boston: South End Press, 1999), 31.

35. McGovern, "S. P. v. Sullivan," 1085–86. On AIDS and disability politics, see Bell, "Rethinking the 'Straight State,'" and Canaday, *Queer Career*.

36. Terry McGovern interview by Sarah Schulman, May 25, 2007, transcript, 24, interview 076, *ACT UP Oral History Project*.

37. Chris Norwood, "The Silent Minority," *The Discovery Channel*, February 1990, 13, folder Women and AIDS Articles, Subject file: AIDS, Lesbian Herstory Archive, Brooklyn, New York. Hereafter, LHA.

38. McGovern interview by Schulman, 25.

39. Hoffman, *Healthcare for Some*, 170–71.

40. CDC, "1987 Revision of Case Definition for AIDS for Surveillance Purpose," *MMWR* 36, no. 1S (August 14, 1987), 3S-15S.

41. Norwood, "Silent Minority," 13; CDC, "Current Trends Update: Acquired Immunodeficiency Syndrome—United States, 1981–1988," *MMWR* 38, no. 14 (April 14, 1989): 229–32, 234–36.

42. Bell, "Rethinking the 'Straight State,'" 948; Kimberly Christensen, "Vessels, Vectors, and Vulnerability: Women in the U.S. HIV/AIDS Epidemic," in *Beyond Reproduction: Women's Health, Activism, and Public Policy*, ed. Karen L. Baird (Madison, NJ: Fairleigh Dickinson University Press, 2009), 65.

43. John Langone, "AIDS: The Latest Scientific Facts," *Discover*, December 1985, quoted in Treichler, "AIDS, Homophobia, and Biomedical Discourse," 37.

44. Lawrence K. Altman, "Heterosexuals and AIDS: New Data Examined," *New York Times*, January 22, 1985; Sara Rimer, "Fear of AIDS Grows among Heterosexuals," *New York Times*, August 30, 1985, A1; Erik Eckholm, "Heterosexuals and AIDS: The Concern is Growing," *New York Times*, October 28, 1986, C7.

45. Treichler, "AIDS, Homophobia, and Biomedical Discourse," 45–46; Jane Gross, "Bleak Lives: Women Carrying AIDS," *New York Times*, August 27, 1987, quoted in Hammonds, "Missing Persons," 9.

46. Weekley, "Saving Me Through Erasure?," 184.

47. Hammonds, "Missing Persons," 17–20.

48. ACT UP Women's Caucus, "Action at Cosmopolitan Magazine January 15, 1988," in *The ACT UP Women's Caucus Women and AIDS Handbook*, ed. Maria Maggenti (March 1989), 91–92. Version of the handbook in box 3, folder ACT UP Women's Caucus and AIDS Handbook 1989, WHAM! records, Tamiment Library; Carol Brennan, "Cosmopolitan," last updated January 2018, https://www.encyclopedia.com/literature-and-arts/literature-english/american-literature/cosmopolitan.

49. Sydney Bryn Austin, "AIDS and Africa: United States Media and Racist Fantasy," *Cultural Critique* 14 (Winter 1989–90): 129.

50. Christensen, "Vessels, Vectors, and Vulnerability," 57.

51. Michael S. Serill, "AIDS: In the Grip of the Scourge," *Time*, February 16, 1987; John C. Caldwell and Pat Quiggin, "The Social Context of AIDS in Sub-Saharan Africa," *Population and Development Review* 15, no. 2 (June 1989): 185–234; Eileen Stillwaggon, "Racial Metaphors: Interpreting Sex and AIDS in Africa," *Development and Change* 34, no. 5 (2003): 812–14; Adrian Flint and Vernon Hewitt, "Colonial Tropes and HIV/AIDS in Africa: Sex, Disease, and Race," *Commonwealth and Comparative Politics* 53, no. 3 (2015), 302–3.

52. Women and AIDS Resource Network, "The Problem," 1, box AIDS, folder Women and AIDS Articles, LHA.

53. Goldstein and Manlowe, *Gender Politics*, 5.

54. Hammonds, "Missing Persons," 11.

55. Jean Carlomusto interview by Sarah Schulman, December 19, 2002, interview 005, transcript, 21, *ACT UP Oral History Project*.

56. Brier, *Infectious Ideas*, 171.

57. Cvetkovich, *An Archive of Feelings*, 174–75; Schulman, *Let the Record Show*, 20.

58. Schulman, *Let the Record Show*, 31.

59. Carlomusto interview by Schulman, 11–12; Maria Maggenti interview by Sarah Schulman, January 20, 2003, interview 010, transcript, 30–31, *ACT UP Oral History Project*.

60. Schulman, *Let the Record Show*, xvi.

61. Bost, "Black Lesbian Feminist Intellectuals," 183.

62. Maggenti interview by Schulman, 25–30; Maxine Wolfe, interview by Jim Hubbard, February 19, 2004, interview 043, transcript, *ACT UP Oral History Project*, 57–62; ACT UP/NY, "Action at Cosmopolitan Magazine January 15, 1988," 91–92.

63. ACT UP flyer, "Don't Go To Bed With *Cosmo*," undated, box 3, folder ACT UP Women's Caucus Women and AIDS Handbook 1989, WHAM! records, Tamiment Library.

64. McGovern, "S. P. v. Sullivan," 1090–91, 1095–96.

65. McGovern, "S. P. v. Sullivan," 1084, 1087–88, 1089.

66. McGovern interview by Schulman, 23; Brier, *Infectious Ideas*, 173.

67. Brier, *Infectious Ideas*, 174.

68. Corea, *Invisible Epidemic*, 251–52; Carlomusto interview by Schulman, 29–30.

69. "Women Don't Get AIDS, They Just Die From It," Gran Fury Collection, Manuscripts and Archives Division, The New York Public Library, https://digitalcollections.nypl.org/items/510d47e3-5399-a3d9-e040-e00a18064a99.

70. Nina Reyes, "Hundreds of Women Storm CDC Over AIDS Definition," *Outweek*, December 19, 1990, 16; Royles, *To Make the Wounded Whole*, 203; Nelson, *More Than Medicine*, 163–64.

71. Maggenti interview by Schulman, 27–28.

72. Reyes, "Hundreds of Women Storm CDC Over AIDS Definition"; Royles, *To Make the Wounded Whole*, 204.

73. McGovern interview by Schulman, 21.

74. CDC, "1993 Revised Classification System for HIV Infection and Expanded Surveillance Case Definition for AIDS Among Adolescents and Adults," *MMWR* 41, no. RR-17 (December 18, 1992).

75. McGovern, "S.P. v. Sullivan," 1094–95; Cooper, *Family Values*, 208.

76. Wolfe, "CDC Campaign, 9/92–12/92," box 4, folder 24, Maxine Wolfe papers, LHA; CDC "Current Trends Update: Impact of the Expanded AIDS Surveillance Case Definition for Adolescents and Adults on AIDS Case Reporting—United States, 1993," *MMWR* 43, no. 9 (March 11, 1994): 160–61, 167–70; Brier, *Infectious Ideas*, 175.

77. Marion Banzhaf, Tracy Morgan, and Karen Ramspacher, "Reproductive Rights and AIDS: The Connections," in Banzhaf et al., *Women, AIDS, and Activism*, 207.

78. Banzhaf, Morgan, and Ramspacher, "Reproductive Rights and AIDS," 207.

79. Golden, "An Argument that Goes Back to the Womb," 273.

80. Matthiesen, "Equality versus Reproductive Risk," 585.

81. Epstein, *Impure Science*, 259–60; William M. Miley, *The Psychology of Well Being* (Westport, CT: Greenwood Publishing, 1999), 192–93.

82. Christensen, "Vessels, Vectors, Vulnerability," 61–62.

83. NOW Legal Defense and Education Fund, "Facts on Women and AIDS," June 1988, 2, box 139, folder 14, BWHBC records.

84. Christensen, "Vessels, Vectors, Vulnerability," 61.

85. Susan Okie, "Stopping it at the Source: Researchers Plan to Test AIDS During Pregnancy," *Washington Post*, October 10–16, 1988, 39.

86. Banzhaf, Morgan, and Ramspacher, "Reproductive Rights and AIDS," 206; Emily Hobson, *Lavender and Red: Liberation and Solidarity in the Gay and Lesbian Left* (Berkeley: University of California Press, 2016), 171–72.

87. Marion Banzhaf interview by Sarah Shulman, April 18, 2007, interview 070, transcript, 56–57, *ACT UP Oral History Project*.

88. Carrie Wofford, "Sitting at the Table," *Outweek*, April 3, 1991, 22.

89. Epstein, *Impure Science*, 259.

90. James J. Jones, *Bad Blood: The Tuskegee Syphilis Experiment* (New York: Free Press, 1981).

91. Laura Briggs, *Reproducing Empire: Race, Sex, Science, and U.S. Imperialism in Puerto Rico* (Berkeley: University of California Press, 2002), 111. For the impact of past medical exploitation on the Black community's response to AIDS, see Royles, *To Make the Wounded Whole*, 106–8.

92. Banzhaf interview by Shulman, 56–63; Gould, *Moving Politics*, 365; Brier, *Infectious Ideas*, 162, 164.

93. Banzhaf interview by Shulman, 57–58, 59–60; Schulman, *Let the Record Show*, 565, 572.

94. Wofford, "Sitting at the Table," 22.

95. Gould, *Moving Politics*, 356; Schulman, *Let the Record Show*, 569.

96. Banzhaf interview by Shulman, 61.

97. Wofford, "Sitting at the Table," 23.

98. Marcia Angell, "The Ethics of Clinical Research in the Third World," *New England Journal of Medicine* 337, no. 12 (1997): 847–48.

99. Edward M. Connor et al., "Reduction of Maternal-Infant Transmission of Human Immunodeficiency Virus Type 1 with Zidovudine Treatment," *New England Journal of Medicine* 331, no. 18 (November 3, 1994): 1173.

100. CDC, "Recommendations of the U.S. Public Health Service Task Force on the Use of Zidovudine to Reduce Perinatal Transmission of Human Immunodeficiency Virus," *MMWR* 43, no. RR-11 (August 5, 1994): 1–20.

101. Hoppe, *Punishing Disease*, 7. On the construction of the "general population," see Treichler, "AIDS, Homophobia, and Biomedical Discourse," 43–44.

102. Brandt, *No Magic Bullet*, 195.

103. Ruth C. Engs, *The Progressive Era's Health Reform Movement: A Historical Dictionary* (Westport, CT: Praeger, 2003), 345.

104. Cindy Patton, "Feminists Must Oppose Widespread Testing," *Sojourner: The Women's Forum*, July 1987, 3.

105. See, e.g., Alan M. Dershowitz, "Crucial Steps in Combatting the AIDS Epidemic," *New York Times*, March, 16, 1986, Section A, 27; Julie Rovner, "AIDS Fiery Debate, Senate Passes AIDS Bill," *CQ Health*, April 30, 1988, 1167–69, box 2, folder AIDS Summary 1987, K. Kae Rairdin files, RRPL, Simi Valley; "When to Test for AIDS," *New York Times*, May 12, 1987; "Bush Appoints Dannemeyer Spokesman on AIDS," *New York Native*, October 10, 1988, box 148, folder 42, C. Everett Koop papers, National Library of Medicine, Bethesda, Maryland, hereafter NLM.

106. Petro, *After the Wrath of God*, 1–2; Hoppe, *Punishing Disease*, 1–2; Chávez, *Borders of AIDS*, 12.

107. William Buckley, "Crucial Steps in Combating the Aids Epidemic; Identify All the Carriers," *New York Times*, March 18, 1986.

108. Schulman, *Let the Record Show*, 101, 238.

109. Loyd and Mountz, *Boats, Borders, and Bases*, 154–74; Chávez, *Borders of AIDS*, 11–12.

110. Chávez, *Borders of AIDS*, 14.

111. Margaret Engel, "Many Prostitutes Found to be AIDS Carriers," *Washington Post*, September 20, 1985, A1; Susan Okie and Linda Wheeler, "D.C. Prostitutes Show a 50 Pct. AIDS Virus Rate," *Washington Post*, March 4, 1987, A9.

112. Hoppe, *Punishing Disease*, 112.

113. Jeanne DeQuine, "Prostitute Who Told Customers She was Healthy Dies of AIDS," *USA Today*, October 19, 1988, box 148, folder 42, Koop papers, NLM.

114. Bruce Lambert, "AIDS Among Prostitutes Not as Prevalent as Believed, Studies Show," *New York Times*, September 20, 1988; Hoppe, *Punishing Disease*, 116.

115. Brandt, *No Magic Bullet*, 21, 31–32, 94; Stern, *Trials of Nina McCall*, 5; Hammonds, "Missing Persons," 16–31; Hoppe, *Punishing Disease*, 4–5.

116. Carola Marte and Kathryn Anastos, "Women—The Missing Persons in the AIDS Epidemic Part II," *Health/PAC Bulletin* (Spring 1990): 12; Zoe Leonard, "HIV-Antibody Testing and Legal Issues for HIV-Positive People," in Banzhaf et al., *Women, AIDS, and Activism*, 60.

117. Brandt, *No Magic Bullet*, 147–51.

118. Domestic Policy Council to the President, "AIDS Testing," May 27, 1987, 6, box 1, folder 2, T. Kenneth Cribb, Jr. files, RRPL, Simi Valley; Heather Shannon, House Committee on Health Care, Committee on Health Care Bill No.: S.432, S.435. Title: "An Act Relative to Testing for the Human Immunodeficiency Virus of Persons Filing Their Intentions to Marry." Sponsor: Sen. Kirby. Hearing Date: March 7, 1988, box 2, folder AIDS (4), Rairdin files, RRPL.

119. Phillip M. Boffey, "Reagan Urges Wide AIDS Testing but Does Not Call for Compulsion," *New York Times*, June 1, 1987.

120. Frank Donatelli, "Proposed Telegram to Governor Sununu," 1–2, May 18, 1987, box 1, folder AIDS (2 of 4), Cribb, Jr. files, RRPL, Simi Valley.

121. Paul D. Cleary et al., "Compulsory Premarital Screening for the Human Immunodeficiency Virus: Technical and Public Health Considerations," *JAMA* 258, no. 13 (October 2, 1987): 1757; "Analysis of Key AIDS-Related Legislative Proposals," April 1986, 2, AIDS Coalition to Identify Orange County Needs, box 15, Coyote records, Schlesinger Library.

122. Sandra G. Boodman, "Premarital AIDS Testing Annoying Many in Illinois," *Washington Post*, July 30, 1988; Edward Walsh, "Facing HIV Test for Marriage License, Illinois Couples Voted with their Feet," *Washington Post*, September 19, 1991, A3; Isabel Wilkerson, "Prenuptial Tests for AIDS Repealed," *New York Times*, June 24, 1989, 6.

123. Washington, *Medical Apartheid*, 192, 202–3.

124. Randall Hansen and Desmond King, *Sterilized by the State: Eugenics: Race, and the Population Scare in Twentieth-Century North America* (Cambridge: Cambridge University Press, 2013), 249.

125. Briggs, *Reproducing Empire*, 111; Nelson, *More than Medicine*, 204.

126. Danielle McGuire, *At the Dark End of the Street: Black Women, Rape, and Resistance; A New History of the Civil Rights Movement from Rosa Parks to the Rise of Black Power* (New York: Alfred A. Knopf, 2010), 191–92; Rosalyn Baxandall and Linda Gordon, "Second Wave Feminism," in *A Companion to American Women's History*, ed. Nancy Hewitt (Malden, MA: Blackwell Publishing, 2002), 420.

127. Barbara Santee and Carol Leigh, "HIV-Positive Women Have Rights Too—and They're Often Denied," *On the Issue*, 1988, 11, box 139, folder 10, BWHBC.

128. Dick Thompson, "Packing Protection in a Purse: Condoms are Becoming a Part of a Woman's Sexual Survival Kit," *Time Magazine Health & Fitness*, September 15, 1988; Lisa Sabbage, "Fighting for Our Lives: Women & AIDS," *Broadsheet* (March 1989): 21; Warren E. Leary, "Female Condom is Approved," *New York Times*, May 11, 1993.

129. Roth, *Making Women Pay*, 2; Cooper, *Family Values*, 167–75.

130. Beckett, "Fetal Rights and 'Crack Moms,'" 595–97.

131. Centers for Disease Control, Atlanta, GA, 1990, NLM, https://stacks .cdc.gov/view/cdc/34465.

132. Reagan, *Dangerous Pregnancies*, 186–202.

133. Centers for Disease Control, Atlanta, GA, 1983, NLM, https://stacks .cdc.gov/view/cdc/34804.

134. Chris Norwood, "Is Preventing AIDS the Responsibility of Women? The Media Seem to Think So," *Glamour*, July 1987, 18.

135. Robin Warshaw, *I Never Called It Rape: The Ms. Report on Recognizing, Fighting, and Surviving Date and Acquaintance Rape* (New York: Harper and Row, 1988).

136. Esther R. Rome, "Are Women Responsible for AIDS Prevention?," 2, undated, box 25, folder 21, BWHBC records.

137. Laura Giges, "AIDS: A Woman's Issue," *The Santa Cruz Women's Health Center*, reprinted in *Women Wise*, 1985/86, box 140, folder 1; Esther R. Rome, "AIDS Burden Falls on Women," *Middlesex News*, June 8, 1987, 1, box 139, folder 10; "Tests Confirm Condoms Block AIDS Virus," *Medical World News*, January 27, 1986, box 140, folder 2; Anna Quindlen, "Life in the 30's: For women, the condom campaign is slightly tardy," *New York Times*, Jun. 17, 1987; Carol Emert, "Women and AIDS: The New Sexual Responsibility," *Second Century Radcliffe News*, June 1988, 8, box 140, folder 1, BWHBC records.

138. Zoe Leonard, "Prostitutes and HIV Infection," in Banzhaf et al., *Women, AIDS, and Activism*, 182.

139. Norwood, "Silent Minority,"13.

140. Kathryn Anastos and Carola Marte, "Women—The Missing Persons in the AIDS Epidemic," *Health/PAC Bulletin*, Winter 1989, 22, box 139, folder 14, BWHBC records.

141. Marion Banzhaf et al., "Preface," *Women, AIDS, and Activism*, vii.

142. Kat Doud, "Demanding a Condom," in Banzhaf et al., *Women, AIDS, and Activism*, 191.

143. Ntozake Shange, *for colored girls who have considered suicide/when the rainbow is enuf* (New York: Scribner, ca. 1977, 2010), 76; Emma Day, "Native Women, AIDS Activism, and the Coatlicue Theatre Company in the United States," *The Theatre Annual: A Journal of Theatre and Performance of the Americas*, 71 (2018): 43–61.

144. Our Bodies, Ourselves: The Nine U.S. Editions, https://www .ourbodiesourselves.org/publications/the-nine-u-s-editions/; and Publications, https://www.ourbodiesourselves.org/about-us/our-history/publications/.

145. Musser, "From Our Body to Yourselves," 94–95.

146. Quickening, "ACNM Thanks Patricia Loftman, CNM, FACNM, MS, LM for a Decade of Service as Chair of the Midwives of Color Committee and

Service on the Board of Directors," *American College of Nurse-Midwives*, November 4, 2019, https://quickening.midwife.org/acnm-news/acnm-thanks-patricia-loftman-cnm-facnm-ms-lm-for-a-decade-of-service-as-chair-of-the-midwives-of-color-committee-and-service-on-the-board-of-directors/.

147. Boston Women's Health Book Collective, *New Our Bodies, Our Selves: A Book by and for Women* (New York: Simon & Schuster, 1992), 11.

148. BWHBC, *New Our Bodies, Our Selves*, 9–10, 337–38.

149. Risa Denenberg interview by Sarah Schulman, July 11, 2008, interview 093, transcript, 5, 9, *ACT UP Oral History Project*.

150. Denenberg, "Pregnant Women and HIV," in Banzhaf et al., *Women, AIDS, and Activism*, 159–60.

151. Banzhaf, Morgan, and Ramspacher, "Reproductive Rights and AIDS," in Banzhaf et al., *Women, AIDS, and Activism*, 207.

152. BWHBC, *New Our Bodies, Our Selves*, 336.

153. Denenberg, "Pregnant Women and HIV," 160, 163.

154. Hobson, *Lavender and Red*, 183.

155. Royles, *To Make the Wounded Whole*, 208–9.

156. International Working Group on Women and AIDS, "An Open Letter to the Planning Committees of the International Conference on AIDS," distributed at AIDS Conference in Washington, DC, June 1, 1987, 1, box 139, folder 10, BWHBC records.

157. International Working Group on Women and AIDS, "An Open Letter to the Planning Committees of the International Conference on AIDS," Distributed at AIDS Conference in Washington, DC, June 1, 1987, 1–2, box 139, folder 10, BWHBC records.

158. John O'Connor, "Us Social Welfare Policy: The Reagan Record and Legacy," *Journal of Social Policy* 7, no. 1 (1998): 40; Gareth Davies, "The Welfare State," in *The Reagan Presidency: Pragmatic Conservatism and Its Legacies*, ed. W. Elliot Brownlee and Hugh David Graham (Lawrence: University Press of Kansas, 2003), 211–12, 225–27.

159. Jamie Penney, "Women & AIDS," July 1992, 1–2, here 2, box 79, folder 21, BWHBC.

160. Penney, "Women & AIDS," 2.

161. McGovern, "S. P. v. Sullivan," 1093–94; Wolfe, "CDC Campaign, 9/92–12/92," box 4, folder 24, Maxine Wolfe papers, LHA.

162. Christensen, "Vessels, Vectors, and Vulnerability," 67–69; Matthiesen, "Equality versus Reproductive Risk," 589–90. For more on WHAM!'s AIDS activism, see Carroll, *Mobilizing New York*.

163. HHS, "Guideline for the Study and Evaluation of Gender Differences in the Clinical Evaluation of Drugs: Notice," *Federal Register* 58, no. 139 (July 1993): 39406–16.

164. "S.1—103rd Congress (1993–1994): National Institutes of Health Revital-ization Act of 1993," June 10, 1993, 133–35, https://www.congress.gov/103/statute /STATUTE-107/STATUTE-107-Pg122.pdf; Katherine A. Liu and Natalie A. Dipietro Mager, "Women's Involvement in Clinical Trials: Historical Perspec-tive and Future Implications," *Pharmacy Practice* 14, no. 1 (2016): 708.

165. HHS, "Guideline for the Study and Evaluation of Gender Differences," 39408.

166. Matthiesen, "Equality versus Reproductive Risk," 592–93, 595.

167. Christensen, "Vessels, Vectors, and Vulnerability," 69–73.

168. Schulman, *Let the Record Show*, xxiii.

169. Hoffman, "Healthcare Reform and Social Movements in the US," 79.

CHAPTER 2

1. Memorandum from Donald A. Clarey to Nancy J. Risque, "Dr. Koop's Speech at the Press Club," March 24, 1987, box 1, folder "AIDS—HHS/Koop" (1 of 2), T. Kenneth Cribb, Jr. files, Ronald Reagan Presidential Library (RRPL).

2. "Pre-Pregnancy AIDS Test Urged," *AP-NY*, March 25, 1987, 1, box 1, folder "AIDS—HHS/Koop" (1 of 2), Cribb files, RRPL.

3. Jack Fowler, "Koop Report to Find No Proof of Abort Damage to Women," *Lifeletter*, no. 4, March 1988, 2, box 14, series II, Nancy Risque files, RRPL.

4. "Pre-Pregnancy AIDS Test Urged," 1.

5. Margaret Engel, "An AIDS 'Epidemic' in Babies," *Washington Post*, May 27, 1985; "High Costs Cited for AIDS Boarder Babies," *New York Times*, October 9, 1988, 34; Peri Klass, "AIDS," *New York Times*, June 18, 1989; CDC, "AIDS Weekly Surveillance Report," *HIV/AIDS Weekly Surveillance Report*, December 28, 1987, 1.

6. Thrasher, *Viral Underclass*, 182.

7. Jennifer Brier, "Reagan and AIDS," in *A Companion to Ronald Reagan*, ed. Andrew L. Johns (Malden, MA: Wiley Blackwell, 2015), 230–33; Petro, *After the Wrath of God*, 90.

8. Kimberley Kelly, "The Spread of 'Post Abortion Syndrome' as Social Diagnosis," *Social Science & Medicine* 102 (2014): 18; Ellie Lee, *Abortion, Motherhood, and Mental Health: Medicalizing Reproduction in the United States and Great Britain* (Hawthorne, NY: Aldine de Gruyter, 2003), 22–24.

9. Petro, *After the Wrath of God*, 71–72; William Martin, *With God on Our Side: The Rise of the Religious Right in America* (New York: Broadway Books, 1996), 240–41; William B. Turner, "'Adolph Reagan?' Ronald Reagan, AIDS, and Lesbian/Gay Civil Rights," July 13, 2009, 15–16, https://ssrn.com/abstract=1433567; Patterson, *Restless Giant*, 180.

10. Ellen Bilofsky, "The Coercion of Carol Doe," in *Health/PAC Bulletin* (Spring 1990): 16, box 139, folder 14, BWHBC, Schlesinger Library.

11. Maxwell Gregg Bloche, "Beyond Autonomy: Coercion and Morality in Clinical Relationships," *Health Matrix* 6, no. 229 (1996): 229–304, 231–32.

12. *Doe v. Jamaica Hospital*, 608 N.Y.S.2d 518 (N.Y.App.Div. 1994).

13. Henri E. Norris, Esq., "Women and Reproductive Rights," 1987, Carton II, box 538, folder Women's AIDS Network, Coyote Records, 1-2; Canaday, *Queer Career*, 208. See also Micki Siegel, "Children with AIDS: The Youngest Victims," *Good Housekeeping* (August 1988): 110.

14. Brandt, *No Magic Bullet*, 19; Washington, *Medical Apartheid*, 191.

15. Beth Widmaier Capo, *Textual Contraception: Birth Control and Modern American Fiction* (Columbus: Ohio State University Press, 2021), 111.

16. Wexler, *Woman Who Walked into the Sea*.

17. Reagan, *Dangerous Pregnancies*, 6.

18. Howard L. Minkoff and Richard H. Schwarz, "AIDS: Time for Obstetricians to Get Involved," *Obstetrics and Gynecology* 68, no. 2 (August 1986): 267.

19. See, e.g., Anthony J. Pinching and Donald J. Jeffries, "AIDS and HTLV-III/LAV Infection: Consequences for Obstetrics and Perinatal Medicine," *Obstetrical and Gynecological Survey* 92, no. 1211 (1985): 569–70; Minkoff and Schwarz, "AIDS: Time for Obstetricians to Get Involved," 267; Donald P. Francis and James Chin, "The Prevention of Acquired Immunodeficiency Syndrome in the United States: An Objective Strategy for Medicine, Public Health, Business, and the Community," *JAMA* 257, no. 10 (March 1987): 1361.

20. CDC, "Current Trends Recommendations for Assisting in the Prevention of Perinatal Transmission of Human T-Lymphotropic Virus Type III/Lymphadenopathy-Associated Virus and Acquired Immunodeficiency Syndrome," *MMWR* 34, no. 48 (December 6, 1985): 721–26, 731–32.

21. Bloche, "Beyond Autonomy," 323.

22. Wexler, *Woman Who Walked Into the Sea*, 162–163; Reagan, *Dangerous Pregnancies*.

23. Marte and Anastos, "Women—The Missing Persons in the AIDS Epidemic Part II," 11, 14, 16.

24. Nelson, *Women of Color*, 65.

25. Brier, "Reagan and AIDS," 226.

26. Jacobs, King, and Milkis, "Building a Conservative State," 456–61; Hoffman, *Healthcare for Some*, 170–71.

27. Fern Schumer Chapman, "Official Advocates AIDS Testing of Pregnant Women," *Washington Post*, September 20, 1988; Susan Y. Chu et al., "Impact of the Human Immunodeficiency Virus Epidemic on Mortality in Women of Reproductive Age, United States," *JAMA* 264, no. 2 (July 1990): 225–26; Susan Y. Chu et al., "Impact of the Human Immunodeficiency Virus Epidemic on Mortality in Children, United States," *Pediatrics* 87, no. 6 (June 1991): 807.

28. Carl T. Rowan, "Children with AIDS," *Washington Post*, September 10, 1988.

29. Douglas Pike, "In Search of Answers on the Abortion Issue," *Philadelphia Inquirer*, August 8, 1988.

30. Wexler, *Woman Who Walked Into the Sea*; Reagan, *Dangerous Pregnancies*.

31. Wendy Chavkin, "Preventing AIDS, Targeting Women," *Health/PAC Bulletin* (Spring 1990): 22.

32. Cindy Patton, "Feminists Must Oppose Widespread Testing," *Sojourner: The Women's Forum* (July 1987): 12–13; Risa Denenberg, "Pregnant Women and HIV," in Banzhaf et al., *Women, AIDS, and Activism*, 159.

33. Denenberg, "Pregnant Women and HIV"; Zoe Leonard, "HIV-Antibody Testing and Legal Issues for HIV-Positive People," in Banzhaf et al., *Women, AIDS, and Activism*, 159, 62; and Marte and Anastos, "Women—The Missing Persons in the AIDS Epidemic Part II," 11.

34. Jeffrey L. Reynolds, "Keep Policy on Newborns' HIV Test," *Viewpoints*, June 2, 1994, 105.

35. Marte and Anastos, "Women—The Missing Persons in the AIDS Epidemic Part II," 12; Chavkin, "Preventing AIDS, Targeting Women," 20.

36. Lawrence Feinberg, "D.C. to Test Newborns, Clinic Patients for AIDS," *Washington Post*, August 18, 1988; "Testing for AIDS," *Washington Post*, August 25, 1988.

37. Marte and Anastos, "Women—The Missing Persons in the AIDS Epidemic Part II," 11–12.

38. "It's a Baby, Not a Statistic, Stupid. News from Assemblywoman Nettie Mayersohn," July 1993, 1–3, here 2; "Mayersohn Makes a Statewide Appeal; Says Babies' Lives are at Stake. News from Assemblywoman Nettie Mayersohn," December 28, 1993, http://www.columbia.edu/itc/hs/pubhealth/p9740/readings /blindedseropervalence_mayersohn-2.pdf; James Dao, "Mothers to Get AIDS Test Data Under Accord," *New York Times*, October 10, 1995, A1.

39. "It's a Baby, Not a Statistic, Stupid," 2–3.

40. Reynolds, "Keep Policy on Newborns' HIV Test," 105; Nettie Mayersohn, "The 'Baby AIDS' Bill," *Fordham Urban Law Journal* 24, no. 4 (1997): 726.

41. Timothy Ross and Anne Lifflander et al., "The Experiences of New York City Foster Children in HIV/AIDS Clinical Trials," *Vera Institute of Justice* (January 2009); 48, 88–89, 65.

42. Hoppe, *Punishing Disease*, 4–5, 116, 126–27.

43. "Text—S. 2240—101st Congress (1989–1990): Ryan White Comprehensive AIDS Resources Emergency Act of 1990," August 18, 1990, 603, accessed January 2022, https://www.congress.gov/101/statute/STATUTE-104/STATUTE-104-Pg576.pdf.

44. Corea, *Invisible Epidemic*, 48; Aziza Ahmed, "HIV and Women: Incongruent Policies, Criminal Consequences," *Yale Journal of International Affairs* 6, no. 1 (Winter 2011): 37.

45. Ahmed, "HIV and Women," 38–39.

46. Logan, "Wrong Race," 134–35; Roberts, *Killing the Black Body*, 3.

47. Briggs, *Taking Children*, 12.

48. Washington, *Medical Apartheid*, 215, 212.

49. Logan, "Wrong Race," 124.

50. Roth, *Making Women Pay*, 146–47.

51. Washington, *Medical Apartheid*, 212; Golden, "'An Argument that Goes Back to the Womb,'" 281.

52. Mason, *Killing for Life*, 90–91; Ross and Lifflander et al., "Experiences of New York City Foster Children in HIV/AIDS Clinical Trials," 65.

53. Mason, *Killing for Life*, 94, 91, 97; Roth, *Making Women Pay*, 21.

54. "Pre-Pregnancy AIDS Test Urged," 1.

55. My thanks to Manon Parry for her help in developing this argument.

56. Memorandum from Gary L. Bauer to Marlin Fitzwater, "Dr. Koop and AIDS Question," March 25, 1987, 1–2, box 1, folder AIDS—HHS/Koop (1 of 2), Cribb files, RRPL.

57. Mary Ziegler, After Roe: The Lost History of the Abortion Debate (Cambridge, MA: Harvard University Press, 2015), 66–68.

58. Guttmacher Institute, "State Funding of Abortion under Medicaid," last updated July 1, 2022, https://www.guttmacher.org/state-policy/explore/state-funding-abortion-under-medicaid.

59. Schoen, *Abortion After Roe*, 157.

60. Rachel Louise Moran, "A Woman's Health Issue? Framing Post-Abortion Syndrome in the 1980s," *Gender & History* 33, no. 3 (2021): 790.

61. Dubow, *Ourselves Unborn*, 66.

62. Margaret Carlson, "A Doctor Prescribes Hard Truth: C. Everett Koop, America's Surgeon General, Has an Opinion on Everything Healthful, But He Nonetheless Enjoys Meat and Martinis," *Time* (April 24, 1989): 82, box 148, folder 43, Koop papers, NLM.

63. Committee on Labor and Human Resources, "Nomination: Hearing Before the Committee on Labor and Human Resources," October 1, 1981, 134–37, 176–85, http://hdl.handle.net/2027/pur1.32754076791106; Remarks of Chairman Henry A. Waxman Before Planned Parenthood, May 29, 1981, 5, box 2, folder Planned Parenthood Federation of America, Inc., Mary Elizabeth Quint files, RRPL.

64. "Senate Confirms Koop, 68–24," *New York Times*, November 17, 1981, A14.

65. C. Everett Koop, *The Memoirs of America's Family Doctor* (Grand Rapids, MI: Zondervan Publishing, 1992), 248–49.

66. Carlson, "A Doctor Prescribes Hard Truth," 82.

67. Petro, *After the Wrath of God*, 61–64.

68. Koop, "Introduction to the AIDS Archive," 1–2, box 148, folder 32, Koop papers, NLM.

69. Brier, "Reagan and AIDS," 231.

70. Koop, *Memoirs*, 261; Koop, "Introduction to the AIDS Archive," 3–4, 5–6, box 148, folder 32, Koop papers, NLM.

71. Koop, "Statement by C. Everett Koop, M.D. Surgeon General U.S. Public Health Service," October 22, 1986, Washington DC, 2–6, box 1, folder AIDS Education—Koop Statement, Davis files, RRPL.

72. Koop, *Memoirs*, 279–80.

73. Deborah Steelman, "Memorandum to the Director, DPC Meeting on AIDS Education—Background," January 13, 1987, 2, box 11, folder DPC Meeting re: AIDS Education, Sprinkel files, RRPL.

74. DHHS, "Information/Education Plan to Prevent and Control AIDS in the United States," January 1, 1987, 18, box 1, folder AIDS—II, Davis files; Edwin Meese III, "Memorandum for the Domestic Policy Council. Subject: AIDS Education," February 11, 1987, box 5, folder 1, Klenk files, RRPL; Koop *Memoirs*, 281.

75. Koop, *Memoirs*, 276–77.

76. Letter from Gil Gerald, National Coalition of Black Lesbians and Gays, to C. Everett Koop, October 24, 1986, folder Scrapbook, Koop papers, NLM.

77. Letter from Gary B. MacDonald, AIDS Action Council, to C. Everett Koop, October 22, 1986, folder Scrapbook, Koop papers, NLM.

78. Letter from Craig B. Leman, M.D., to C. Everett Koop, April 17, 1987. For other letters of support, see AIDS folder, Koop papers, box 149, NLM.

79. Letter to the editor, "A Doctor's Good Advice," *Washington Post*, October 24, 1986, A.

80. Priscilla Alexander, "The A(IDS) Word," AIDS 0787.3, undated, box 1, folder 34, Coyote records, Schlesinger Library; "Flying the Koop," *Washington Times*, October 27, 1986.

81. Mason, *Killing for Life*, 114–18.

82. Sandra G. Boodman, "How C. Everett Koop Shook up His Former Allies on the Right and Surprised His New Friends on the Left," *Washington Post*, November 15, 1987.

83. Mason, *Killing for Life*, 80; Dubow, *Ourselves Unborn*, 161; Moran, "A Woman's Health Issue?" 790–91.

84. Koop, *Memoirs*, 334, 348.

85. Faye Wattleton, *Life on the Line* (New York: Ballantine Books, 1996), 355.

86. Suzanne Staggenborg, "The Survival of the Pro-Choice Movement," *Journal of Policy History* 7, no. 1 (1995): 164–68; Schoen, *Abortion After Roe*, 181; Nelson, *More Than Medicine*, chapter 4; Ziegler, *Abortion and the Law in America*, 31; Marianne Szegedy-Maszak, "Calm, Cool and Beleaguered: Faye Wattleton Mobilizes Planned Parenthood for the Next Abortion-Rights Campaign," *New York Times*, August 6, 1989, SM16.

87. Silliman, Gerber, and Ross, *Undivided Rights*, 43.

88. Memorandum from Robert W. Sweet, Jr., to Ralph C. Bledsoe, "Surgeon General's Report on Abortion," March 25, 1988, box 14, folder Dr. Koop (Abortion & AIDS), Risque files.

89. Koop, *Memoirs*, 305.

90. Moran, "A Woman's Health Issue?," 790–91, 794–98.

91. O'Connor, "Us Social Welfare Policy," 40.

92. Letter from Margaret J. Atwood to President Reagan, printed on a letter from Faye Wattleton to President Reagan, undated, box 9, folder 6, Sweet files, RRPL.

93. Emphasis in the original. Letter from Pandora M. Cooke to President Reagan, May 18, 1987, box 9, folder 6, Sweet files, RRPL.

94. Critchlow, "Mobilizing Women: The 'Social' Issues," in Brownlee and Graham, *Reagan Presidency*, 301–2; Lawrence J. McAndrews, *What They Wished For: American Catholics and American Presidents, 1960–2004* (Athens: University of Georgia Press, 2014), 230–31.

95. Memorandum, "Actions on the Anniversary of *Roe v. Wade*," January 23, 1987, box 1, folder Abortion Memo 01/23/1987, Davis files, RRPL. Emphasis in the original.

96. Young, *We Gather Together*, 212.

97. Ziegler, *Abortion and the Law in America*, 28–29.

98. Prudence Flowers, "'Voodoo Biology': The Right-to-Life Campaign against Family Planning Programs in the United States in the 1980s," *Women's History Review* 29, no. 2 (2020): 331, 348–49.

99. Robert E. Windom to Joanne Gasper, "Reprimand," January 23, 1987, 1, folder Abortion, Davis files, RRPL; Flowers, "Voodoo biology," 347–48.

100. Nancy Risque to Senator Baker, Will Ball, "Jo Ann Gasper," March 10, 1987, box 1, folder Abortion, Davis files, RRPL.

101. Koop, *Memoirs*, 347–48.

102. Charlie Jeffries, "Adolescent Women and Antiabortion Politics in the Reagan Administration," *Journal of American Studies* 52, no. 1 (2018): 193–94.

103. Koop, *Memoirs*, 348.

104. Koop, *Memoirs*, 349.

105. Wattleton, *Life on the Line*, 354.

106. D.P. Swartz, M.D., and M.K. Pananjpe, M.D., "Abortion: Medical Aspects in a Municipal Hospital," *Bulletin of the New York Academy of Medicine* 47, no. 8 (August 1971): 846; Wattleton, *Life on the Line*, 94; Reagan, *When Abortion Was a Crime*, 209.

107. Wattleton, *Life on the Line*, 353.

108. Letter to the Editor, "A Doctor's Good Advice," *Washington Post*, October 24, 1986, Section A.

109. Jack Fowler, "Koop Report to Find No Proof of Abort Damage to Women," *Lifeletter*, no. 4, March 1, 1988, box 14, folder Dr. Koop (Abortion & AIDS), Risque files, RRPL; Warren E. Leary, "Koop Says Abortion Report Couldn't Survive Challenge," *New York Times*, March 17, 1989; Koop, *Memoirs*, 349.

110. McGuire, *At the Dark End of the Street*, xx. My thanks to Nonie Kubie for highlighting this point.

111. Koop, *Memoirs*, 349; Memorandum from Robert W. Sweet, Jr., to Nancy Risque, "Washington Post Article—'The Ex-Abortionists'/Koop Report," April 1, 1988, box 14, folder Dr. Koop (Abortion & AIDS), Risque files, RRPL.

112. Sweet, Jr., to Risque, "Washington Post Article."

113. Memorandum for the DPC, "National AIDS Mailing," 1, March 25, 1988, box 5, folder CDC AIDS Mailer (1), Klenk files, RRPL.

114. Annotated copy of DHHS, *Understanding AIDS: A Message from the Surgeon General*, 1988, 2, box 5, folder CDC AIDS Mailer (1), John Klenk files, RRPL.

115. Memorandum from Sweet, Jr., to Bledsoe, "Surgeon General's Report on Abortion"; Karen Newman, *Fetal Positions: Individualism, Science, Visuality* (Stanford, CA: Stanford University Press, 1996), 19–21.

116. Koop to President Ronald Reagan, January 9, 1989, reprinted in "Medical and Psychological Impact of Abortion: "Hearing Before the Human Resources and Intergovernmental Relations Subcommittee of the Committee on Government Operations, House of Representatives, One Hundred First Congress, First

Session. Vol. 4. March 16, 1989. U.S. Government Printing Office, 1989. Digitized July 10, 2012," http://hdl.handle.net/2027/pur1.32754076877616, 68–71.

117. Sweet, Jr., to Risque, "Washington Post Article."

118. Memorandum from Risque to the President, "Surgeon General's Update on Health Effects of Abortion Study," January 9, 1989, box 14, folder Dr. Koop (Abortion & AIDS), Risque files, RRPL.

119. Michael Specter, "Koop Won't Issue Report on Abortion: Studies of Effects Called Inconclusive," *Washington Post*, January 10, 1989; Martin Tolchin, "Koop's Stand on Abortion's Effect Surprises Friends and Foes Alike," *New York Times*, January 11, 1989.

120. Nada L. Stotland, M.D., "The Myth of the Abortion Syndrome," *JAMA* 268, no. 15 (October 1992): 2078.

121. Koop, *Memoirs*, 334; *Webster v. Reproductive Health Services*, 492 US 490 (1989).

122. Ziegler, *Abortion and the Law*, 104–5.

123. *Planned Parenthood v. Casey*, October 1991, 834, 837, https://tile.loc.gov /storage-services/service/ll/usrep/usrep505/usrep505833/usrep505833.pdf.

124. Moran, "A Women's Health Issue?" 800–801.

125. Nelson, *More Than Medicine*, 144; Silliman, Gerber, and Ross, *Undivided Rights*, 35; Schoen, *Abortion After Roe*, 160, 180.

126. Self, *All in the Family*, 403.

127. Petro, *After the Wrath of God*, 65–66; Jennifer Brier, "'Save Our Kids, Keep AIDS out': Anti-AIDS Activism and the Legacy of Community Control in Queen's New York," *Journal of Social History* 39, no. 4 (Summer 2006): 965–87.

128. David Michaels, "Estimates of the Number of Motherless Youth Orphaned by AIDS in the United States," *JAMA* 268, no. 24 (December 1992): 3456; Ross and Lifflander et al., "Experiences of New York City Foster Children in HIV/AIDS Clinical Trials," 48, 78–79, 83–84, 88–89.

129. Ann P. Meredith, "The San Francisco AIDS Foundation's Women and AIDS Support Group," 1987, from the collection *Until That Last Breath!*, Ann P. Meredith papers, box 45, folder 3, Schlesinger Library.

130. Cynthia Chris, "Reviews: Women and AIDS," *Afterimage* 17, no. 1 (January 1989): 17; Suvan Geer, "Exhibit Gives AIDS Human Face—A Woman's," *Los Angeles Times*, July 28, 1989; Kay Longcope, "A Wide-Angle View of AIDS:

Exhibit Sheds Light on Women, the Epidemic's 'Invisible Population,'" *Boston Globe*, April 12, 1990; Ann P. Meredith, "Women and AIDS: A Document," 13, Meredith papers, box 45, folder 47.1, Schlesinger Library.

131. Norwood, "Silent Minority," 13.

132. Adam Gershenson, "The Neediest Cases; Giving Solace to Children Made Orphans by AIDS," *New York Times*, December 13, 1998, 52; Brian Weil, *Every Seventeen Seconds: A Global Perspective on the AIDS Crisis* (New York: Aperture, 1992), 13–31.

133. Crystal Nix, "Infants Linger in Hospitals, Awaiting Foster Homes," *New York Times*, December 12, 1986, A1; Sandra Boodman, "Covering the AIDS Beat," *Washington Post*, August 14, 1988, 37; Pia McKay, "'Little Miss Smith,' You're Not Alone: Perhaps We Who've Been Homeless Too Can Help Save the Boarder Babies," *Washington Post*, November 12, 1989, D1; Roberts, *Shattered Bonds*, 179; Solinger, *Wake Up Little Susie*, 34.

134. Bernard Weinraub, "Reagan Cut Held to Affect 20% of Welfare Families," *New York Times*, March 24, 1981; Spencer Rich, "Reagan Welfare Cuts Found to Worsen Families' Poverty," *Washington Post*, July 29, 1984; Roberts, *Shattered Bonds*, 181.

135. Renfro, *Stranger Danger*.

136. Silliman, Gerber, and Ross, *Undivided Rights*, 25–50.

137. Marlene Gerber Fried, "Abortion in the United States—Legal but Inaccessible," in *Abortion Wars: A Half Century of Struggle, 1950–2000*, ed. Rickie Solinger (Berkeley: University of California Press, 1998), 201–11.

138. Chavkin, "Preventing AIDS, Targeting Women," 20.

139. Schoen, *Abortion After Roe*, 169.

140. Corea, *Invisible Women*, 51.

141. Carol Schlesinger, "A Program to Aid 'Boarder Babies,'" *New York Times*, June 28, 1998, NJ17.

142. Rickie Solinger, *Beggars and Choosers: How the Politics of Choice Shapes Adoption, Abortion, and Welfare in the United States* (New York: Farrar, Straus and Giroux, 2002), 118, 132; Renfro, *Stranger Danger*, 177.

143. "Scandal at Hale House," *New York Times*, May 20, 2001.

144. Stephen W. Nicholas and Elaine J. Abrams, "Boarder Babies with AIDS in Harlem: Lessons in Applied Public Health," *American Journal*

of Public Health 92, no. 2 (February 2002): 163, https://dx.doi.org/10.2105/ajph.92.2.163.

145. Washington, *Medical Apartheid*, 213.

146. "Human Resources, Still Reeling," *New York Times*, October 6, 1989, Section A, 30.

147. James D. Hegarty et al., "The Medical Care Costs of Human Immunodeficiency Virus-Infected Children in Harlem," *JAMA* 260, no. 13 (October 7, 1988): 1901; "Cost for Child with AIDS: $90,347," *Richmond Times-Dispatch*, October 7, 1988.

148. Nicholas and Abrams, "Boarder Babies with AIDS in Harlem: Lessons in Applied Public Health," *American Journal of Public Health* 92, no. 2 (February 2002): 163, https://dx.doi.org/10.2105/ajph.92.2.163.

149. Ross and Lifflander et al., "Experiences of New York City Foster Children in HIV/AIDS Clinical Trials," 48–49; Cooper, *Family Values*, 203.

150. Koop, "Introduction to the AIDS Archive: AIDS Lecture April 6, 1987," 1, Koop papers, NLM.

151. Nicholas and Abrams, "Boarder Babies with AIDS in Harlem," 163–65.

152. "Text—S.945—100th Congress (1987–1988): Abandoned Infants Assistance Act of 1988." October 18, 1988, 2533.

153. Ross and Lifflander et al., "Experiences of New York City Foster Children in HIV/AIDS Clinical Trials," 65.

154. Nicholas and Abrams, "Boarder Babies with AIDS in Harlem," 164.

155. Jacqueline B. James, "Too Much Love for One Place: Second 'Grandma's House' to Care for Babies with AIDS Virus," *Washington Post*, September 28, 1989, 1, 3, here 1.

156. Lois Romano, "The Hug That Says it All: Barbara Bush Visits AIDS Infants," *Washington Post*, March 23, 1989, D2.

157. Sandra G. Boodman, "Easing a Short but Difficult Journey: 'Grandma's House' Keeps AIDS-Infected Babies from Languishing in Hospital," *Washington Post*, May 12, 1988, B1.

158. Weil, *Every Seventeen Seconds*, 37.

159. Janet Mitchell, "What About the Mothers of HIV infected Babies?" *NAN Multi-Cultural Notes on AIDS Education and Service* 1, no. 10 (April 1988): 1, folder Women and AIDS Articles, LHA.

160. Dorothy E. Roberts, "Punishing Drug Addicts Who Have Babies: Women of Color, Equality, and the Right to Privacy," in Solinger, *Abortion*

Wars, 149; Logan, "Wrong Race," 132; Dubow, *Ourselves Unborn*, 104; Silliman, Gerber, and Ross, *Undivided Rights*, 34.

161. Douglas Crimp, "How to have Promiscuity in an Epidemic," *October* 43, AIDS: Cultural Analysis/Cultural Activism (Winter, 1987), 263.

162. CDC, "Recommendations of the Public Health Service Task Force on the Use of Zidovudine to Reduce Perinatal Transmission of Human Immuno-deficiency Virus."

163. CDC, "Achievements in Public Health: Reduction in Perinatal Transmission of HIV Infection—United States, 1985–2005," *MMWR* 55, no. 21 (June 2, 2006): 592–97. For an overview of the debates over trial 076, see Chapter 1.

164. Catherine Hanssens, Alison Mehlman, and Margo Kaplan, "Pregnancy and HIV: Medical and Legal Considerations for Women and their Advocates," *The Center for HIV Law and Policy* (December 2009): 12–13.

165. For a more detailed discussion of HIV criminalization during pregnancy, see the Epilogue.

166. Marte and Anastos, "Women—The Missing Persons in the AIDS Epidemic Part II," 14.

167. See, for instance, Koop, "AIDS Lecture May 26, 1987," 1–4, here 3; "AIDS Lecture July 11, 1987," 1–3, here 1–2, box 148, folder "Introduction to the AIDS Archive," Koop files, NLM.

168. Lynn M. Paltrow and Jeanne Flavin, "Arrests of and Forced Interventions on Pregnant Women in the United States, 1973–2005: Implications for Women's Legal Status and Public Health," *Journal of Health Politics, Policy and Law* 38, no. 2 (April 2013): 315, 316; Michele Goodwin, "How the Criminalization of Pregnancy Robs Women of Reproductive Autonomy," *The Hastings Center Report* 47, no. S3 (November–December 2017): S19, S24, https://www.newyorker.com/magazine/2022/07/04/we-are-not-going-back-to-the-time-before-roe-we-are-going-somewhere-worse.

169. See, e.g., S.B. No.8. (2021), 1–2, https://capitol.texas.gov/tlodocs/87R/billtext/pdf/SB00008H.pdf

170. Roth, *Making Women Pay*, 151–59; Logan, "Wrong Race," 126; Ralf Jürgens et al., "Ten Reasons to Oppose the Criminalization of HIV Exposure or Transmission," *Reproductive Health Matters* 17, no. 34 (2009): 168–69.

171. Brier, "I'm Still Surviving," 78; Watkins-Hayes, *Reclaiming a Life*, 68.

CHAPTER 3

1. Lesbian Avengers, "Don't Let Them Rest in Peace. Avenge the Oregon Martyrs," box 7, folder 10, WAC records, NYPL; Kelly Cogswell, *Eating Fire: My Life as a Lesbian Avenger* (Minneapolis: University of Minnesota Press, 2014), 19.

2. Initiative Petition submitted by the Oregon Citizens Alliance, Oregon History Society Research Library, accessed April 2022, https://www.oregon encyclopedia.org/articles/oregon_citizens_alliance/#.Ymj6yy1Q2X1.

3. Anna Quindlen, "Public & Private: Putting Hatred to a Vote in Oregon," *New York Times*, October 28, 1992; Bettina Boxall, "Battle Lines Drawn Over Oregon's Anti-Gay Measure," *Los Angeles Times*, October 22, 1992.

4. The Lesbian Avengers, "An Incomplete History," accessed April 2022, http://www.lesbianavengers.com/about/history.shtml.

5. Cogswell, *Eating Fire*, 21.

6. See, e.g., instance Jim Downs's discussion of the arson attack on the UpStairs Lounge in New Orleans in June 1972 in his *Stand by Me: The Forgotten History of Gay Liberation* (New York: Basic Books, 2016).

7. Cogswell, *Eating Fire*, 23.

8. The founding members of the Lesbian Avengers were already influential AIDS organizers. For instance, Maxine Wolfe helped found the ACT UP/NY Women's Caucus. Cvetkovich, *An Archive of Feelings*, 175; Brier, *Infectious Ideas*, 171. On the Dyke March, see Cogswell, *Eating Fire*, 49–51.

9. Lesbian Avengers, *Communiqué: From the Frontline. New York: Lesbian Avengers*, no. 3 (June 1993): 1, BWHBC, Schlesinger Library.

10. Verta Taylor and Leila J. Rupp, "Women's Culture and Lesbian Feminist Activism: a Reconsideration of Cultural Feminism," *Signs* (1993): 32–61; Becky Thompson, "Multiracial Feminism: Recasting the Chronology of Second Wave Feminism" *Feminist Studies* (Summer 2002): 336–60; Gould, *Moving Politics*, 391–92.

11. Self, *All in the Family*, 6; Gerstle, *Rise and Fall of the Neoliberal Order*, 14.

12. Laurie Fitzpatrick, "Lesbians and AIDS," *A&U: America's AIDS Magazine* 30 (March/April 1997): 22–24, box 47, folder 3, Ann P. Meredith papers, Schlesinger Library.

13. Corea, *Invisible Epidemic*, 45–51; Treichler, *How to Have Theory in an Epidemic*, 54.

14. Taylor and Rupp, "Women's Culture and Lesbian feminist Activism," 32–61; Rachel Corbman, "Remediating Disability Activism in the Lesbian Feminist Archive," *Continuum: Journal of Media & Cultural Studies* 32, no. 1 (2017): 18–28.

15. Amber Hollibaugh, *My Dangerous Desires: A Queer Girl Dreaming Her Way Home* (Durham, NC: Duke University Press, 2000), 187–91.

16. Gould, *Moving Politics*, 257–63.

17. For examples, see Introduction, n. 32.

18. Bell, "Between Private and Public," 164–65; Canaday, *Queer Career*, 225.

19. Gould, *Moving Politics*, 157.

20. Alice Terson, "Positively Lesbian," *LAP Notes* 1 (April 1993): 3, BWHBC records.

21. Hollibaugh, *My Dangerous Desires*, 191.

22. Lillian Faderman, *Surpassing the Love of Men: Romantic Friendship and Love between Women from the Renaissance to the Present* (New York: Morrow, 1981); John D'Emilio and Estelle B. Freedman, *Intimate Matters: A History of Sexuality in America*, 3rd ed. (Chicago: University of Chicago Press, 2012); Elizabeth Lapovsky Kennedy and Madeline D. Davis, *Books of Leather, Slippers of Gold: The History of a Lesbian Community* (New York: Routledge, 1993); Estelle B. Freedman, "The Prison Lesbian: Race, Class and the Construction of the Aggressive Female Homosexual, 1915–1965," *Feminist Studies* 22, no. 2 (Summer 1996): 397–415; Canaday, *Straight State*, 174–213.

23. Taylor and Rupp, "Women's Culture and Lesbian Feminist Activism," 33.

24. Radical Lesbians, "The Woman-Identified-Woman," 1970, 1-4, Women's Liberation Movement Print Culture Digital Collection, https://idn.duke.edu/ark:/87924/r3gx1t; Adrienne Rich, "Compulsory Heterosexuality and Lesbian Existence," *Signs* 5, no. 4 (Summer 1980): 648–49; Cheryl Clarke, "Lesbianism: An Act of Resistance," in *This Bridge Called My Back: Writings by Radical Women of Color*, ed. Cherríe Moraga and Gloria Anzaldúa (Watertown, MA: Persephone Press, c. 1981); Sarah Lucia Hoagland, "Lesbian Separatism: An Empowering Reality," *Sinister Wisdom* 34 (Spring 1988): 23–33, LC Periodical PS 508 W7 S54.

25. Barbara Smith, "Response to Adrienne Rich's 'Notes from Magazine: What does Separatism Mean?'" in *Sinister Wisdom* 20 (1982): 101, LC Periodical PS 508 W7 S54; Barbara Smith and Beverly Smith, "Across the Kitchen Table: A

Sister-to-Sister Dialogue," in Moraga and Anzaldúa, *This Bridge Called My Back* (Albany: State University of New York Press, c. 2015), 118–21.

26. Deirdre English, Amber Hollibaugh, and Gayle Rubin, "Talking Sex: A Conversation on Sexuality and Feminism," *Feminist Review* 11 (Summer 1982): 43.

27. Lorna Norman Bracewell, "Beyond Barnard: Liberalism, Antipornography Feminism, and the Sex Wars," *Signs* 42, no. 1 (Autumn 2016): 26–27; SaraEllen Strongman, "'Creating Justice Between Us': Audre Lorde's Theory of the Erotic as Coalitional Politics in the Women's Movement," *Feminist Theory* 19, no 1 (2017): 45–47.

28. Ann Ferguson, "Sex War: The Debate between Radical and Libertarian Feminists," *Signs* 10, no. 1 (Autumn 1984): 107; Judith Grant, "Andrea Dworkin and the Social Construction of Gender: A Retrospective," *Signs* 31, no. 4 (Summer 2006): 969.

29. Bracewell, "Beyond Barnard," 35–36, 41; Elisa Glick, "Sex Positive: Feminism, Queer Theory, and the Politics of Transformation" *Feminist Review* 64 (Spring 2000): 21.

30. Self, *All in the Family*, 209.

31. Gould, *Moving Politics*, 66, 67.

32. Hollibaugh, *My Dangerous Desires*, 189–92, 196, 207.

33. Anne Harris interview with Amber Hollibaugh, "Invisibility of Lesbians with AIDS," undated, box Lesbians—AIDS, LHA; Hollibaugh, *My Dangerous Desires*, 196.

34. Gould, *Moving Politics*, 193.

35. Cvetkovich, *An Archive of Feelings*, 191–93; Zoe Leonard interview with Sarah Schulman, January 13, 2010, interview no. 106, transcript, 11–12, *ACT UP Oral History Project*.

36. Polly Thistlethwaite interview by Sarah Schulman, January 6, 2013, interview 154, transcript, 27–32, *ACT UP Oral History Project*; Maxine Wolfe interview by Jim Hubbard, February 19, 2004, interview 043, transcript, 72–73, *ACT UP Oral History Project*.

37. Patton, *Last Served?* 69, 50.

38. Amber Hollibaugh, "Notes from LAP," and Cynthia S. Madansky, "In the Beginning," *LAP Notes* 1 (April 1993): 1, 2, BWHBC records, Schlesinger Library.

39. Catherine Saalfield, "Coming to Safer Sex," *LAP Notes* 2 (Spring 1994): 13, BWHBC, Schlesinger Library.

40. Hobson, *Lavender and Red*, 191.

41. Hollibaugh, *My Dangerous Desires*, 206.

42. Gould, *Moving Politics*, 66.

43. Hollibaugh, *My Dangerous Desires*, 206, 209; Gould, *Moving Politics*, 67

44. Brier, *Infectious Ideas*, 172; Harris interview with Hollibaugh.

45. Anne Harris, "The Invisibility of Women with AIDS," undated, box 9, folder 280, Judy Greenspan papers, LGBT archive, New York; Rebecca Cole and Sally Cooper, "Lesbian Exclusion from HIV/AIDS Education: Ten Years of Low-Risk Identity and High-Risk Behavior," *SIECUS Report* (December 1990/ January 1991): 19, Subject file: AIDS, LHA.

46. Hollibaugh, *My Dangerous Desires*, 207–8.

47. Ann P. Meredith, "Women and AIDS: A Document," undated, 14, box 45, folder 47.1, Meredith papers, Schlesinger Library.

48. Hollibaugh, *My Dangerous Desires*, 209.

49. Hollibaugh, *My Dangerous Desires*, 203, 208; Kristin G. Esterberg, "From Accommodation to Liberation: A Social Movement Analysis of Lesbians in the Homophile Movement," *Gender and Society* 8, no. 3 (September 1994): 430.

50. Cole and Cooper, "Lesbian Exclusion from HIV/AIDS Education," 18.

51. Naja Sorella, "A/part of the Community," *Sinister Wisdom* 39 (Winter 1989–90), 104–7, 53–63, LC Periodical PS 508 W7 S54. See also Jackie Winnow, "Lesbians Evolving Health Care: Cancer and AIDS," *Feminist Review* 41 (Summer 1992): 68–76; June Jordan, *Some of Us Did Not Die: New and Selected Essays* (New York: Basic Books, 2002), 94–100.

52. GMHC, "HIV Counseling, Testing & Prevention Initiative," 6–7, box 400, folder 7, GMHC records, NYPL; Patton, *Last Served?* 72.

53. AIDS: News and Information. City and County of San Francisco Department of Public Health, "Two New Surveys Show that Lesbians and Bisexual Women are at Risk for HIV Infection," October 19, 1993, 1, box 2, folder Centers for Disease Control/Lesbians Get AIDS Protest, August 1994, Lesbian Avenger Records, Gay Lesbian Bisexual Transgender (GLBT) Historical Society Archives & Special Collections, San Francisco. On AIDS cases in San Francisco, see CDC, *HIV/AIDS Surveillance Report* 5, no. 4 (1994): 7; on San Francisco's activist history, see Hobson, *Lavender and Red*.

54. Terry A. Maroney, "Lesbians, HIV & Violence," *LAP Notes* 2 (Spring 1994): 10, BWHBC records.

55. Meredith, "Women and AIDS: A Document," 14.

56. Lesbian Avengers et al., "Lesbians Don't Die of AIDS. Do They? This One Did," Flyer, undated, box 2, folder Political Funeral for Joan Baker, October 23, 1993. See other leaflets, posters, and miscellaneous ephemera in box 2, folder Political Funeral for Joan Baker, October 23, 1993, Lesbian Avengers, GLBT.

57. Leaflets in box 2, folder Centers for Disease Control/Lesbians Get AIDS protest, August 1994, Lesbian Avenger records, GLBT.

58. Press Release, "Lesbian Avengers Target the CDC's AIDS Policies," August 1994, box 2, folder Centers for Disease Control/Lesbians Get AIDS protest, August 1994, Lesbian Avenger records, GLBT Archives.

59. CDC, "HIV/AIDS Surveillance Report" January 1992, 20, accessed April 2022, https://www.cdc.gov/hiv/pdf/library/reports/surveillance/cdc-hiv-surveillance-report-1991-vol-4.pdf.

60. GMHC, "HIV Counseling, Testing & Prevention Initiative," 6–7; Deborah Bybee, "Michigan Lesbian Health Survey Results Relevant to AIDS," undated, vi, LHA.

61. Cole and Cooper, "Lesbian Exclusion from HIV/AIDS Education," 18. See the CDC reports listed in footnote 71, below, for examples.

62. Patton, *Last Served?* 66; Gould, *Moving Politics,* 357; Safer sex pamphlet, 15, folder 00630, LHA.

63. Patton, *Last Served?* 6.

64. See, e.g., CDC, "HIV/AIDS Surveillance Report," January 1991, 9, https://www.cdc.gov/hiv/pdf/library/reports/surveillance/cdc-hiv-surveillance-report-1990-vol-3.pdf.

65. Maria T. Sabatini et al., "Kaposi's Sarcoma and T-Cell Lymphoma in an Immunodeficient Woman: A Case Report," *AIDS Research* 1, no. 2 (1984): 135–37; Michael Marmor et al., "Possible Female-to-female Transmission of Human Immunodeficiency Virus [letter], *Annals of Internal Medicine* 105, no. 6 (December 1986): 969; Josiah D. Rich et al., "Transmission of HIV Presumed to Have Occurred via Female Homosexual Contact," *Clinical Infectious Diseases* 17, no. 6 (1993): 1003–5.

66. Lisa Winters, "In Memory of Cookie, 9/19/60–6/25/93," *LAP Notes* 2 (Spring 1994): 9, BWHBC records.

67. CDC Division of HIV/Prevention, "Minutes of Lesbian HIV Issues Meeting," March 6, 1996, 7, box 401, folder 1, GMHC, NYPL.

68. Treichler, *How to Have Theory in an Epidemic*, 54.

69. Hammonds, *Missing Persons*; Brandt, *No Magic Bullet*; Reagan, *Dangerous Pregnancies*.

70. Susan Y. Chu et al., "Epidemiology of Reported Cases of AIDS in Lesbians, United States 1980–89," *American Journal of Public Health* 80, no. 11 (November 1990): 1381.

71. CDC, "AIDS Weekly Surveillance Report," December 29, 1986, 1, https://www.cdc.gov/hiv/pdf/library/reports/surveillance/cdc-hiv-surveillance-report-1986.pdf. See, e.g., the listing of multiple exposure categories in: CDC, "HIV/AIDS Surveillance Report," January 1989, 19, https://www.cdc.gov/hiv/pdf/library/reports/surveillance/cdc-hiv-surveillance-report-1988-vol-1.pdf.

72. Leonard interview with Schulman, 48. On drug use among WSW, see Meaghan B. Kennedy et al., "Assessing HIV Risks among Women Who Have Sex with Women: Scientific and Communication Issues," *Journal of the American Medical Women's Association* (May/August 1995): 104; on Leonard's needle-exchange activism, see Schulman, *Let the Record Show*, 292–94; and perspective on safer sex, see Leonard, "Lesbians in the AIDS Crisis," in Banzhaf et al., *Women, AIDS, and Activism*, 116.

73. Esterberg, "From Accommodation to Liberation"; Hilliman, "'The Most Profoundly Revolutionary Act,'" 156; Christina B. Hanhardt, *Safe Space: Gay Neighborhood History and the Politics of Violence* (Durham, NC: Duke University Press, 2013), 4.

74. Quoted in Leonard, "Lesbians in the AIDS Crisis," 113.

75. Emily M. Coleman et al., "Arousability and Sexual Satisfaction in Lesbian and Heterosexual Women," *Journal of Sex Research* 19, no. 1 (February 1983): 58.

76. Royles, *To Make the Wounded Whole*, 199–201.

77. Workshop Facilitator: Marianela Virella, Negotiating Safer Sex Workshop, Safer Sex Workshops, and Feeling Good All Over Workshop, and various other guides, box 401, folder 8, 9, 15, 16, GMHC, NYPL.

78. Douglas Crimp, "How to have Promiscuity in an Epidemic," in "AIDS: Cultural Analysis/Cultural Activism," special issue, *October* 43 (Winter 1987): 253; Batza, *Before AIDS*, 119.

79. Petro, *After the Wrath of God*, 89–90.

80. Cynthia Madansky, "fierce fists," in *Gendered Epidemic: Representations of Women in the Age of AIDS*, ed. Nancy L. Roth and Katie Hogan (New York: Routledge, 1998), 83.

81. Genter, "Appearances Can be Deceiving," 605, 616–18.

82. Canaday, *Straight State*, 12–13, 177.

83. Madansky, "fierce fists," 83, 87; The Galaei Project, *Let's Talk AIDS*, leaflet, 1995, box 401, folder 1, GMHC records, NYPL. For examples of other lesbian safer sex posters, see Stoller, *Lessons from the Damned*, 56.

84. LAP, *The Safer Sex Handbook for Lesbians* (1993), Subject file: AIDS, LHA.

85. Madansky, "fierce fists," 83.

86. Jennifer L. Kaplan, "Focus Group Evaluation of the *Safer Sex Handbook for Lesbians*," Department of Evaluation Research at the Gay Men's Health Crisis, Inc., August 11, 1994, 1–19, here 1, box 400, folder 6, GMHC.

87. Kaplan, "Focus Group Evaluation," 5–6, 7–8, 9, 12.

88. Gillian Frank, "'The Civil Rights of Parents': Race and Conservative Politics in Anita Bryant's Campaign against Gay Rights in 1970s Florida," *Journal of the History of Sexuality* 22, no. 1 (January 2013): 132, 138, 143–45.

89. Simon Hall, "Americanism, Un-Americanism, and the Gay Rights Movement," *Journal of American Studies* 47 (2013): 1117–18.

90. For a definition of the concept of moral panic, see Renfro, *Stranger Danger*, 5.

91. John D'Emilio and Estelle B. Freedman, "Foreword," in Allan Berube, *Coming Out Under Fire: The History of Gay Men and Women in WWII* (Chapel Hill: University of North Carolina Press, 2010), xi–xiii.

92. H.R. 3396—104th Congress: Defense of Marriage Act of 1996, https://www.govtrack.us/congress/bills/104/hr3396.

93. Chappell, *War on Welfare*, 1–2.

94. Steven Lee Myers, "How a 'Rainbow Curriculum' Turned into Fighting Words," *New York Times*, December 13, 1992, Section 4, 6; Robert D. McFadden, "Bishop Assails School Leaders Over Lessons on Homosexuals," *New York Times*, December 28, 1992, Section B, 8.

95. Lally Weymouth, "Mrs. Cummins's Triumph," *Washington Post*, January 8, 1993, A19; Myers, "How a 'Rainbow Curriculum' Turned into Fighting Words."

96. Steven Lee Myers, "Few Using Curriculum in Dispute: 'Children of the Rainbow' is Staying on the Shelf," *New York Times*, December 6, 1992, Section 1, pg. 49.

97. Myers, "Few Using Curriculum in Dispute"; McFadden, "Bishop Assails School Leaders."

98. Sam Dillon, "Board Removes Fernandez as New York Schools Chief After Stormy 3-Year Term," *New York Times*, February 11, 1993.

99. Cogswell, *Eating Fire*, 12, 14–15.

100. Frank, "'Civil Rights of Parents,'" 159–60.

101. Jason Deparle, "111 Held in St. Patrick's AIDS Protest," *New York Times*, December 11, 1989. See also Adrienne E. Christiansen and Jeremy J. Hanson, "Comedy as Cure for Tragedy: ACT UP and the Rhetoric of AIDS," *Quarterly Journal of Speech* 82, no. 2 (1996): 157; Carroll, *Mobilizing New York*, 20–21.

102. Christine Russell, "AIDS Report Calls for Sex Education: Surgeon General Urges End to 'Silence,' Opposes Compulsory Testing," *Washington Post*, October 23, 1986, A1.

103. Janice M. Irvine, *Talk About Sex: The Battles over Sex Education in the United States* (Berkeley: University of California Press, 2002), 1, 88–89.

104. Madansky, "fierce fists," 86.

105. Mary Otto, "Rallying Cry is a Perceived Gay Threat to Kids," *The Mercury News*, September 6, 1994; Madansky, "fierce fists," 86.

106. Otto, "Rallying Cry."

107. Madansky, "fierce fists," 86; Lynda Richardson, "Cortines, Upset, Moves Student AIDS Center," *New York Times*, March 23, 1994.

108. Madansky, "fierce fists," 89.

109. Richardson, "Cortines, Upset, Moves Student AIDS Center."

110. "Lesbian Safer Sex Handbook Under Attack," *LAP Notes* 2 (Spring 1994): 13; Madansky, "fierce fists," 85, 87, 89.

111. Madansky, "fierce fists," 85.

112. Neil Genzlinger, "Louis Sheldon, Anti-Gay Minister with Political Clout, Dies at 85," *New York Times*, June 5, 2020.

113. Matt Schudel, "Louis P. Sheldon, Inflammatory Anti-Gay Crusader of 'Traditional Values,' Dies at 85," *Washington Post*, June 6, 2020; David D. Dunlap, "Hearing Held on Gay Issues in the Schools: A Debate on Values Moves to Capitol Hill," *New York Times*, December 10, 1995, 31.

114. Otto, "Rallying Cry."

115. Exchange in Amber Hollibaugh, "Seducing Women into a 'Lifestyle of Vaginal Fisting,'" in *Policing Public Sex: Queer Politics and the Future of AIDS Activism*, ed. Alison Redick et al. (Boston: South End Press, 1996), 321–23.

116. Kevin Merida, "Republicans' Showing in Elections Renews Gay Rights Debate," *Washington Post*, November 25, 1994, A33.

117. *Congressional Record* 133, no. 20, October 14, 1987, 27766–71.

118. *Congressional Record* 140, no. 103, August 1, 1994; Katharine Q. Seelye, "Senate Backs Cuts for Schools that Endorse Homosexuality," *New York Times*, August 2, 1994.

119. CDC Division of HIV/Prevention, "Minutes of Lesbian HIV Issues Meeting," 4.

120. Helene D. Gayle, letter to meeting participants, 8 March 1996; Division of HIV/Prevention, "Minutes of Lesbian HIV Issues Meeting," 4.

121. CDC, "Report on Lesbian HIV Issues Meeting, Apr. 20–21, 1995," undated, 3, box 401, folder 1, GMHC; Eileen Hansen, "Woman-To-Woman HIV Transmission Finally Acknowledged," *LAP Notes* 3 (Summer 1995): 20, BWHBC records, Schlesinger Library.

122. "Minutes of Lesbian HIV Issues Meeting," 5–6, 9–10.

123. Chu et al., "Epidemiology of Reported Cases of AIDS in Lesbians," 1381.

124. Kennedy et al., "Assessing HIV Risk," 103.

125. See the CDC HIV Surveillance reports, https://www.cdc.gov/hiv/library/reports/hiv-surveillance-archive.html#1989–1982-Reports.

126. Dázon Dixon, "Facing Reality: AIDS Education and Women of Color," in Banzhaf et al., *Women, AIDS, and Activism*, 228.

127. Bybee, "Michigan Lesbian Health Survey."

128. Hoffman, *Healthcare for Some*, 169.

129. David W. Dunlap, "From AIDS Conference, Talk of Life, Not Death," *New York Times*, July 15, 1996, Section A, 7.

130. Madansky, "fierce fists," 85.

131. Hollibaugh, "Seducing Women into a 'Lifestyle of Vaginal Fisting,'" 334.

132. Hall, "Americanism, Un-Americanism, and the Gay Rights Movement," 1127; Cooper, *Family Values*, 210.

133. *Planned Parenthood of Southeastern Pennsylvania v. Casey*, 505 U.S. 841 (1992).

134. Mason, *Killing for Life*, 80–81.

135. Lesbian Avengers, "Prison Officials Called to Task for Medical Neglect: Demonstrations at Chowchilla Bear Witness to Suffering of Women Prisoners," July 8, 1995, box 2, folder Chowchilla Demonstration for medical care for women prisoners, Lesbian Avengers records, GLBT.

CHAPTER 4

1. Noelle Hanrahan, "To Die in Chowchilla," *San Francisco Bay Guardian*, January 26, 1994, 9; Gilmore, *Golden Gulag*, 88–89, 106.

2. Hanrahan, "To Die in Chowchilla," 9; Barbara Bloom, Barbara Owen, and Stephanie Covington, "Women Offenders and the Gendered Effects of Public Policy," *The Policy Studies Association* 21, no. 1 (2004): 35; Lawrence A. Greenfeld and Tracy L. Snell, *Women Offenders*, special report for the Department of Justice, December 1999, 5; Elizabeth Swavola et al., *Overlooked: Women and Jails in an Era of Reform* (New York: Vera Institute of Justice, 2016), 23.

3. Sandra G. Boodman, "HIV in Prison: Is Isolation Cruel or Prudent? Alabama Sued Over Testing, Segregating Those with AIDS Virus," *Washington Post*, April 29, 1989, A1.

4. Joann Walker, "Medical Treatment at Chowchilla," undated, box 5, folder 179, JGP, LGBT Community Center National Archive, New York.

5. Laura McTighe, "Our Relationships Carry the Movement," *Radical History Review* 140 (May 2021): 186.

6. Perry F. Smith, MD, et al., "HIV Infection among Women Entering the New York State Correctional System," *American Journal of Public Health* 81, suppl. (May 1, 1991): 35, https://doi.org/10.2105/AJPH.81.Suppl.35; Allen Beck et al., "Survey of State Prison Inmates, 1991," U.S. Department of Justice: Bureau of Justice Statistics (March 1993), 25, https://bjs.ojp.gov/content/pub/pdf/SOSPI91.PDF; Anne S. De Groot, M.D., "Alarming Statistics about Incarcerated Women," *Positively Aware: The Journal of Test Positive Aware Network* (July–August 2001): 19, box 8, folder 247, JGP; Akilah Wise, "In Prison, Women are 9 Times More Likely to be HIV-Positive," *The Nation*, November 24, 2017, https://www.thenation.com/article/in-prison-women-are-9-times-more-likely-to-be-hiv-positive/.

7. Dan Berger, *Captive Nation: Black Prison Organizing in the Civil Rights Era* (Chapel Hill: The University of North Carolina Press, 2014); Heather Ann

Thompson, *Blood in the Water: The Attica Prison Uprising of 1971 and Its Legacy* (New York: Pantheon Books, 2016).

8. Nelson, *More Than Medicine*, 202; Royles, *To Make the Wounded Whole*, 198, 200, 205, 214.

9. Law, *Resistance behind Bars*; Thuma, *All Our Trials*. On the history of women's prison activism, see Faith, *Unruly Women*; Davis, *Are Prisons Obsolete?* 60–83; Diaz-Cotto, *Chicana Lives and Criminal Justice*; and Stern, *Trials of Nina McCall*.

10. Coalition to Support Women Prisoners at Chowchilla (CSWPC), "Chowchilla Prison: A Medical Hellhole," undated leaflet, 5; Corey Weinstein, M.D., and Catherine Campbell, CCWF Medical Interviews, "AIDS/HIV Care with Joann Walker and Brenda Lee Ivy," undated, 1, box 5, folder 179; Paul Collins to Brenda Lee Ivy, August 2, 1993; Judy Greenspan to Joann Walker, July 1, 1993, box 5, folder 181, JGP.

11. See, e.g., *Gates v. Deukmejian*, 1987 (CA), *Doe v. Meachum*, 1988 (CT), *Harris v. Thigpen*, 1990 (AL), and *Austin v. Pennsylvania Dept of Corrections*, 1990 (PA). Reagan, "Crossing the Border for Abortions"; Rogers, "'Caution: The AMA May be Dangerous to your Health.'"

12. Regina Kunzel, *Criminal Intimacy: Prison and the Uneven History of Modern American Sexuality* (Chicago: University of Chicago Press, 2008), 228–29, 235.

13. Alexander, *New Jim Crow*; Hinton, *From the War on Poverty to the War on Crime*; Kohler-Hausmann, *Getting Tough*; Richie, *Arrested Justice*.

14. Angela Y. Davis and Cassandra Shaylor, "Race, Gender, and the Prison Industrial Complex: California and Beyond," *Meridians* 2, no. 1 (2001): 1–25; Law, *Resistance behind Bars*.

15. Mary E. Odem, *Delinquent Daughters: Protecting and Policing Adolescent Female Sexuality in the United States, 1885–1920* (Chapel Hill: University of North Carolina Press, 2000).

16. Kate Manne, *Down Girl: The Logic of Misogyny* (New York: Oxford University Press, 2018), 21.

17. Bailey, *Misogynoir*, 1.

18. Nina Siegal, "Dying behind Bars: Women in California Prisons are Facing Death Sentences for Lack of Basic Health Care," *San Francisco Bay Guardian*, February 5, 1997, 17, box 8, folder Shumate healthcare access report, Nancy E. Stoller Papers Concerning Prison Inmate Health, University of California San Francisco Archives, San Francisco, CA (hereafter, Stoller Papers).

19. Washington, *Medical Apartheid*, 65; Owens, *Medical Bondage*, 3.

20. Gilmore, *Golden Gulag*, 93.

21. Diaz-Cotto, *Chicana Lives and Criminal Justice*, 266.

22. Gilmore, *Golden Gulag*.

23. Thomas Ferrick Jr. and Michael B. Coakley, "City Says No to Condoms for Inmates," *Philadelphia Inquirer*, August 23, 1988, 1A; Charles W. Colson, "Condoms: No Way to Control AIDS in Prison," *Washington Post*, June 26, 1991, A18; Matthew Purdy, "As AIDS Increases behind Bars, Costs Dim Promise of New Drugs," *New York Times*, May 26, 1997, 1–2; Memorandum from Otis R. Bowen to Beryl W. Sprinkel, Chairman, Council of Economic Advisors from the Secretary, "Assessing the Benefits of Testing for AIDS," July 20, 1987, 1–2, box 11, folder 2, Beryl W. Sprinkel Files, RRPL. For more on HIV testing in prisons, see Kunzel, *Criminal Intimacy*, 230–32.

24. Brier, *Infectious Ideas*, 158; Brian G Williams et al., "Modelling the Impact of Antiretroviral Therapy on the Epidemic of HIV," *Current HIV Research* 9, no. 6 (2011): 367–82, here 367.

25. Albert R. Jonsen and Jeff Striker, eds., *The Social Impact of AIDS in the United States* (Washington, DC: National Academies Press, 1993), 182.

26. Purdy, "As AIDS Increases behind Bars," 1.

27. John Zeh, "The Agony of AIDS Inside and Out," *Studies on the New Left* 14, nos. 1–2 (Spring-Summer 1989): 146–52, here 151.

28. Amy Goldstein, "AIDS Plan Creates Prison Paradox: Issues Collide in D.C. Proposal to Distribute Condoms to Inmates," *Washington Post*, May 19, 1992, D6.

29. Hoffman, *Healthcare for Some*, 177–78, 182; Schulman, *Let the Record Show*, 542.

30. Kunzel, *Criminal Intimacy*, 234; Laurie Fitzpatrick, "Lesbians and AIDS," 22–24, box 47, folder 3, Meredith Papers.

31. Kelly Safreed Harmon, "HIV Incarcerated Women," *Positively Aware: The Journal of Test Positive Aware Network* (July–August 2001): 18–21, here 21, box 8, folder 247, JGP.

32. Letter from P.A./Albion Correctional Facility to the LAP, reprinted in *LAP Notes* 1 (April 1993): 12, Periodicals.

33. Siegal, "Dying behind Bars," 17.

34. Nena Messina and Christine Grella, "Childhood Trauma and Women's Health Outcomes in a California Prison Population," *American Journal of Public Health* 96, no. 10 (October 2006): 1842.

35. Nancy E. Stoller, "Project Title: Declining Health Conditions in U.S. Prisons for Women: A Twenty-five-year Perspective," 1998–99, 3, box 8, folder Lawsuit for women prisoners in California, 1999–2000, Stoller Papers.

36. Legal Services for Prisoners with Children (LSPC), "Protecting Basic Human Rights," Vol. 2, Spring 1997, 1, box 2, folder Newsletters/Publications, Stoller Papers; Siegal, "Dying behind Bars," 17.

37. On institutional sexism in medicine, see Introduction, n. 36.

38. Siegal, "Dying behind Bars," 19.

39. Nena Messina and Christine Grella, "Childhood Trauma and Women's Health Outcomes," *American Journal of Public Health* 96, no. 10 (October 2006): 1842.

40. Nancy Stoller, "Improving Access to Health Care for California Women's Prisoners," report submitted to California Program on Access to Care, California Policy Research Center, University of California, Office of the President, January 2001, 18, https://www.prisonlegalnews.org/media/publications/improving_health_care_for_ca_women_prisoners_2001.pdf.

41. Pew Charitable Trusts, "Prison Health Care: Costs and Quality: How and Why States Strive for High-performing Systems," 2017, 29, http://www.pewtrusts.org/~/media/assets/2017/10/sfh_prison_health_care_costs_and_quality_final.pdf; Chad Kinsella, "Corrections Health Care Costs," 2004, 2, https://www.prisonpolicy.org/scans/csg/Corrections+Health+Care+Costs+1-21-04.pdf.

42. Retzlaff, "Can HIV Care Click in the Clink?" 25; Amy Pétre Hill, "Death through Administrative Indifference," *Hastings Women's Law Journal* 13, no. 2 (Summer 2002): 229–30; Gilmore, *Golden Gulag*, 95.

43. Charisse Shumate et al., Plaintiffs, v. Pete Wilson, et al., Defendants, "Class Action Complaint," April 4, 1995, 12, https://www.clearinghouse.net/chDocs/public/PC-CA-0011-0001.pdf.

44. Retzlaff, "Can HIV Care Click in the Clink?" 23–25; Allen J. Beck and Paige M. Harrison, *Prisoners in 2000* (Washington, DC: Bureau of Justice Statistics, 2001), 5.

45. Retzlaff, "Can HIV Care Click in the Clink?" 24–25; Safreed Harmon, "HIV Incarcerated Women," 18; Beverly Henry, quoted in Judy Greenspan, "Positive Women Prisoners Speak Out," *Positively Aware: The Journal of Test Positive Aware Network* (July-August 2001): 25–26, box 8, folder 247, JGP.

46. Laura M. Maruschak, Marcus Berzofsky, and Jennifer Unangst, *Medical Problems of State and Federal Prisoners and Jail Inmates, 2011–2012* (Washington, DC: Bureau of Justice Statistics, 2015; revised 2016); and International Committee of the Red Cross, "Health in Prison: Looking after Women in a Man's World," February 27, 2009, https://www.icrc.org/en/doc/resources/documents/interview/women-health-prison-interview-020309.htm.

47. Members of ACE Program at Bedford Hills, *Breaking the Walls of Silence: AIDS and Women in a New York Maximum Security Prison* (New York: Overlook Press, 1998); Kathy Boudin and Judith Clark, "Community of Women Organize Themselves to Cope with the AIDS Crisis: A Case Study from Bedford Hill Correctional Facility," *Social Justice* 17, no. 2 (Summer 1990): 90.

48. Bruce Shapiro, "Kathy Boudin's Prison Odyssey," *The Nation*, March 20, 1995, 380–82, here 381–82; Law, *Resistance behind Bars*, 37; Tom Robbins, "Judith Clark's Radical Transformation," *New York Times Magazine*, January 15, 2012, 28; "Nothing Without Us: The Women Who Will End AIDS' Chronicles Black Women's Silent Plight with HIV/AIDS," *Vibe* (online), December 1, 2017.

49. Mireya Navarro, "An AIDS Activist Who Helped Women Get Help Earlier," *New York Times*, November 15, 1992, E9; McGovern, "S. P. v. Sullivan," 1092; Schulman, *Let the Record Show*, 240–41.

50. The Women of the ACE Program of the Bedford Hills Correctional Facility, New York, in *Wall Tappings: An International Anthology of Women's Prison Writings, 200 to the Present*, ed. Judith A. Scheffler (New York: Feminist Press at CUNY, 2002), 28–35.

51. Boudin and Clark, "Community of Women Organize Themselves," 92.

52. Boudin and Clark, "Community of Women Organize Themselves," 93.

53. Katrina Haslip, "A Community of Women: Living with AIDS," in Scheffler, *Wall Tappings*, 28–29. For more on the ACE program, see Kathy Boudin et al., "Voices," in Banzhaf et al., *Women, AIDS, and Activism*, 143–55; Boudin and Clark, "Community of Women Organize Themselves," 90–109; Schulman, *Let the Record Show*, 241–42, 396–98.

54. Thuma, *All Our Trials*, chap. 2; and Law, *Resistance behind Bars*, 11–13.

55. Faith, *Unruly women*, chap. 7.

56. Marilyn Kalman and Rachel Lederman, "Talking with Three Lesbian Political Prisoners," *Sinister Wisdom* 37 (Spring 1989): 100–110; Law, *Resistance behind Bars*, 23.

57. Felicia Crowe, "Women Prisoners at Niantic, Ct.," *Women Alive* (Autumn 1995): 8, Subject file AIDS, LHA, 8.

58. Law, *Resistance behind Bars*, 6–11; Thuma, *All Our Trials*, 56, 59–60.

59. California Department of Corrections, Department Operations Manual, 2022, 402–3, https://www.cdcr.ca.gov/regulations/wp-content/uploads/sites /171/2022/03/CDCR-DOM_2022.pdf.

60. Linda Eagerton, "Dianna Reyes," May 21, 1994, 1–2, box 5, folder 181, JGP.

61. Hobson, *Lavender and Red*, 159, 190–91; Cooper, *Family Values*, 188–94, 209–14; Renfro, *Stranger Danger*, 177.

62. Violent Crime Control and Law Enforcement Act of 1994, Public Law 103–322, 103rd Congress, September 13, 1994, 1815–17, https://www.congress .gov/103/statute/STATUTE-108/STATUTE-108-Pg1796.pdf.

63. By 1997, twenty-six states and the federal government had enacted some form of a "three strikes" law. James Austin, John Clark, Patricia Hardyman, and D. Alan Henry, "Three Strikes and You're Out: The Implementation and Impact of Strike Laws," NCJ 181297, National Criminal Justice Reference Service Virtual Library, U.S. Department of Justice, March 6, 2000, 1–108, here 1, https://www.ojp.gov/pdffiles1/nij/grants/181297.pdf.

64. Gilmore, *Golden Gulag*, 49, 93, 104, 107–9.

65. Robyn L. Cohen, "Prisoners in 1990," *U.S. Department of Justice: Bureau of Justice Statistics Bulletin* (January 25, 1993): 1–10, here 4, https://bjs.ojp.gov/content /pub/pdf/p90.pdf.

66. Stoller, "Improving Access to Health Care," 19–20; Gilmore, *Golden Gulag*, 7.

67. Thrasher, *Viral Underclass*, 160.

68. Elizabeth Swavola et al., "Overlooked," 23; Briggs, *Taking Children*, 14.

69. Greenfeld and Snell, *Women Offenders*, 5; Victoria Law, "How Many Women are in Prison for Defending Themselves Against Domestic Violence?" *BitchMedia*, September 16, 2014, https://www.bitchmedia.org/post/women-in-prison-for-fighting-back-against-domestic-abuse-ray-rice.

70. Peter Applebome, "Women in U.S. Prisons: Fast-Rising Population," *New York Times*, June 16, 1987, A16; Hill, "Death through Administrative Indifference," 231. For more on the rise and persistently high rates of women's incarceration since the 1980s, see Wendy Sawyer, "The Gender Divide: Tracking

Women's State Prison Growth," *Prison Policy Initiative*, January 9, 2018, https://www.prisonpolicy.org/reports/women_overtime.html; Aleks Kajstura, "Women's Mass Incarceration: The Whole Pie 2019," October 29, 2019, https://www.prisonpolicy.org/reports/pie2019women.html.

71. CDCR, "Central California Women's Facility (CCWF): Details and History," undated, https://www.cdcr.ca.gov/facility-locator/ccwf/.

72. On the growth of California prisons in this period, including the opening of CCWF and VSPW, see Davis, *Are Prisons Obsolete?* 11–13.

73. Stoller, "Improving Access to Health Care," 166.

74. Weinstein and Campbell, Interviews with Women at Chowchilla (CCWF) on 8/19/93, 1 and on 8/20/93, 1, box 5, folder 179, JGP.

75. "Chowchilla Prison: A Medical Hellhole," 1, 4–5.

76. PEN § 5007.5 (1994).

77. Shumate et al. v. Wilson et al., "Class Action Complaint," 2–3, 5–6, 14.

78. Stoller, "Improving Access to Health Care," 27, 29.

79. Shumate et al. v. Wilson et al., "Class Action Complaint," 12.

80. Hill, "Death by Administrative Indifference," 229.

81. CSWPC, "Stop the Murder of Women Prisoners with AIDS at Chowchilla!" poster, 1994, and Joann Walker, "From a Woman's Point of View," undated, 1–2, here 2, box 5, folder 179, JGP.

82. CSWPC, "Editorial Response to February 1 Opinion Page article, 'Inmates are out of line,'" 1–2, box 6, folder 186, JGP; Hanrahan, "To Die in Chowchilla"; Judy Greenspan to James Gomez, 1–2, here 1, August 13, 1993, box 6, folder 186, JGP.

83. Judy Greenspan, "Voices from the Chowchilla Women's Prison," *Prison Legal News*, March 1994, 12.

84. "Chowchilla Prison: A Medical Hellhole," 4.

85. Siegal, "Dying behind Bars," 19.

86. Nelson, *Body and Soul*, 115–16.

87. CCWP, "Tribute to Charisse Shumate," *The Fire Inside* 4 (May 1997): 1, box 8, folder 237, JGP.

88. Between 1994 and 2003, the State of California granted compassionate release to 196 of the 634 people who applied for it. "Charisse Shumate: Fighting for Our Lives," produced by Freedom Archives and CCWP, 2004, video, 40:08, https://vimeo.com/19050308.

89. Urszula Wislanka, "Mail Restrictions Raise the Question: What Makes Us Human?" *The Fire Inside* 6 (May 1997): 5, box 8, folder 237, JGP.

90. Paul Collins to Brenda Lee Ivy, August 2, 1993, box 5, folder 181, JGP.

91. Details of who Caruso was writing to are not included in the letter. Gina Marie Caruso, "Help!", undated, box 5, folder 181, JGP.

92. LSPC, "Shumate v. Wilson," 1, box 8, folder Lawsuit for women prisoners in California, 1999–2000, Stoller Papers.

93. Twillah Wallace to Barbara Lee, undated, box 5, folder 179, JGP.

94. See, e.g., Joann Walker to Doctor Nadin Khoury, April 1, 1994; Joann Walker to Assembly Committee on Public Safety, April 7, 1994; Paula Keola to Assembly Persons, April 14, 1994, box 5, folder 179; LSPC, "Shumate v. Wilson," 1.

95. Stoller, "Improving Access to Health Care," 7.

96. Judy Greenspan to California State Assembly Committee on Public Safety, March 8, 1994; Interviews with Women at Chowchilla (CCWF) on 8/19/93 by Corey Weinstein, M.D., and Catherine Campbell, 1–10 & on 8/20/93, 1–7, box 5, folder 179; and Elizabeth Alexander to James Gomez, October 3, 1994, box 5, folder 181, JGP.

97. Judy Greenspan, "Women Prisoners with AIDS Fight for Quality Medical Care," September 22, 1994, 1–3, here 1, box 5, folder 180, JGP.

98. Judy Greenspan, "Struggle for Compassion: The Fight for Quality Care for Women with AIDS at Central California Women's Facility," *Yale Journal of Law & Feminism* 6, no. 2 (1993): 383–95, here 383; JGP, "History or Bio," LGBT Community Center, https://gaycenter.org/archive_item/judy-greenspan-papers/.

99. Joann Walker praised Judy Greenspan's advocacy work in Walker, "Joint Venture Victory at Chowchilla," January 5, 1994, box 6, folder 185, JGP.

100. Mike McKee, "State Settles Suit Over Prison Medical Care," *The Recorder* 146, July 30, 1997, 1–2, here 2, box 8, folder Lawsuit for women prisoners in California, 1999–2000, Stoller Papers; and CSWP, "Women Prisoners with AIDS Face Death and Abuse," in *Newsline*, ed. People with AIDS Coalition (PWAC) NY, undated, 38–39, here 39, box 5, folder 179, JGP.

101. Judi Parks, "Protest on Behalf of Women Prisoners with HIV this Saturday," *Bay Area Reporter*, January 27, 1994, 11, box 5, folder 179, JGP.

102. Judy Greenspan, "Joann Walker—A Fighter and a Legend in Her Time," undated, 1–4, here 1, box 5, folder 179; Deborah Paul, Balagno, and Joann Walker, "HIV/AIDS Task Force Proposal," March 19, 1993, 1–2, box 5, folder 181, JGP.

103. "Chowchilla Prison: A Medical Hellhole," 1–5; Walker, "From a Woman's Point of View," 1; Greenspan, "Joann Walker," 1.

104. Hanrahan, "To Die in Chowchilla," 9.

105. CCWF Medical Interviews, "AIDS/HIV Care with Joann Walker and Brenda Lee Ivy," 1.

106. Greenspan, "Joann Walker," 1; Greenspan to Gomez, 1.

107. Greenspan, "Joann Walker," 1.

108. Greenspan to Gomez, 1–2.

109. Greenspan, "Joann Walker," 2.

110. Judy Greenspan to William Brady, December 7, 1993, box 6, folder 190; "Send Betty Jo Ross Home for Christmas," flyer, box 5, folder 180, JGP.

111. James Gomez to Teena Farmon, October 28, 1993, box 6, folder 185, JGP.

112. ACT UP/San Francisco, "Prisoners and AIDS Activists Demand Compassionate Release for Woman Prisoner at Chowchilla," November 8, 1993, box 5, folder 180; Greenspan, "Joann Walker," 1–3, here 2, JGP.

113. "Send Betty Jo Ross Home for Christmas," flyer; Mike Shriver to James Gomez, January 3, 1994, box 6, folder 185, JGP.

114. Greenspan, "Joann Walker," 2.

115. Out of Control—Lesbian Committee to Support Women Political Prisoners & Joann Walker, "Letter from Chowchilla PWA," and Jennie / LAGAI, "Medical Neglect at Chowchilla–Demo Jan. 29," published in *Out of Time* 21 (January 1994): 1, box 5, folder 179, JGP. For more on the protest, see Robert R. Phipps, "Prison's Medical Care Protested," *Merced Sun-Star*, January 29, 1994, A3; Robert R. Phipps, "Protesters Will Decry Treatment of Inmates," *Madera Tribune*, January 29–30, 1994, 1–2; and Judi Parks, "Activists Rally at Chowchilla for Better Prisoner Healthcare," *Bay Area Reporter*, February 3, 1994, 11, box 5, folder 179, JGP.

116. Parks, "Protest on Behalf of Women Prisoners," 11.

117. Nancy Moniz for the Board of Resist to Judy Greenspan, January 28, 1994, box 6, folder 185, JGP.

118. Joann Walker, "Medical Treatment at Chowchilla," undated, box 5, folder 179, JGP.

119. Walker, "Letter from Chowchilla PWA."

120. Greenspan, "Joann Walker," 2; and Hanrahan, "To Die in Chowchilla," 9.

121. Joann Walker to Ellen M. Barry, April 14, 1994, box 5, folder 179, JGP.

122. Phipps, "Prison's Medical Care Protested," A3.

123. CSWPC, "Editorial Response," 1–2.

124. Greenspan, "Struggle for Compassion," 385, 393; Joann Walker, "Dropping Like Flies," undated, 1, box 5, folder 180, JGP.

125. CSWP, "Women Prisoners with AIDS Face Death and Abuse," in *Newsline*, ed. People with AIDS Coalition NY, undated, 38–39, here 38, box 5, folder 179, JGP.

126. Catherine Campbell, "Interview with Joann Walker on 4/22/94 in the Merced Community Hospital," April 25, 1994, 2–4, box 5, folder 180, JGP.

127. CCWP members, "Tribute to Joann Walker," *The Fire Inside* 1 (June 1996): 1, box 8, folder 237; Miriam Berman, "Joann Walker, Prison Organizer, Granted Compassionate Release," undated, box 5, folder 179, JGP.

128. Twillah Wallace, "A Tribute to Joann Walker, A Dear Friend," undated, box 6, folder 187, JGP.

129. On references to Walker in the media, see, e.g., Marx Arax, "Prison Releases Woman Dying of AIDS," *Los Angeles Times*, A3, January 6, 1994; Joann Walker, "Dropping Like Flies: Another Death at the Central California Women's Facility," in *Newsline*, ed. People with AIDS Coalition NY, 41. On Walker's influence on other inmates in and beyond CCWF, see Frederick Carl Beasley, "Come to the Edge," undated, box 5, folder 179, JGP; and quote from Charisse Shumate in Diana Block, "Legislative Hearings: Women Prisoners Tell it Like it is," *The Fire Inside* 16 (December 2000), https://www.womenprisoners.org/fire/000223.html.

130. Greenspan, "Struggle for Compassion," n. 23, 385.

131. Judy Greenspan to Amnesty Representative, March 31, 1994, JGP; Judy Greenspan to Richard Waters, April 13, 1994, box 5, folder 181, JGP.

132. Judy Greenspan to Susan Sward, March 22, 1994; Judy Greenspan and Rachel Lederman, general letter to the press, March 10, 1994, box 5, folder 180, JGP.

133. Merrily A. Friedlander to Judy Greenspan, February 3, 1995, box 5, folder 181, JGP.

134. Judy Greenspan to Twillah Wallace, June 10, 1994, box 5, folder 181, JGP; Judy Greenspan to Judith M. Dodd, June 29, 1994, box 5, folder 181, JGP.

135. LSPC draft copy of the class-action complaint, September 23, 1–8; Elizabeth Alexander to James Gomez, October 3, 1994, 1–5, box 5, folder 181, JGP.

136. Hill, "Death through Administrative Indifference," 225.

137. ACLU, "About the National Prison Project," undated, https://www.aclu.org/other/about-aclu-national-prison-project.

138. *Estelle v. Gamble*, 429 U.S. 97, here 104–5 (1976).

139. McKee, "State Settles Suit," 2.

140. Shumate et al. v. Wilson et al., "Class Action Complaint," 1.

141. Shumate et al. v. Wilson et al., "Class Action Complaint," 2, 18.

142. "Charisse Shumate: Fighting for Our Lives."

143. Shumate et al. v. Wilson et al., "Class Action Complaint," 11–18.

144. Siegal, "Dying behind Bars," 17.

145. E.g., see *Gates v. Deukmejian*, 1987 (CA), *Doe v. Meachum*, 1988 (CT), *Harris v. Thigpen*, 1990 (AL), and *Austin v. Pennsylvania Dept of Corrections*, 1990 (PA).

146. Judy Greenspan to Lynn McCoy, November 30, 1997, box 10, folder 280, JGP.

147. Judy Greenspan, "Women Campaign for Better Medical Care," *The Fire Inside* 6 (December 1997), https://www.womenprisoners.org/fire/000460.html.

148. Dorsey Nunn and Karen Shain to Judy Greenspan, March 14, 1995, box 5, folder 181, JGP.

149. Law, *Resistance behind Bars*, 132, 140–41; CCWP, "The Fire Inside," https://womenprisoners.org/the-fire-inside-archive/; CCWP, "Our Story," https://womenprisoners.org/about-us/.

150. Charisse Shumate, "The Pros and Cons of Being a Lead Plaintiff," *The Fire Inside* 6 (December 1997): 2, box 8, folder, 237, JGP.

151. Shumate et al. v. Wilson, "Class Action Complaint," 2–3.

152. Charisse Shumate, "The Battle Must Go On!" *The Fire Inside* 4 (May 1997): 1, box 8, folder 237, JGP.

153. Karen Shain, "'Women Prisoners Win Shumate Case!' Demonstration for Rights of Women Prisoners Set for October 4th," *The Fire Inside* 5 (September 1997), https://www.womenprisoners.org/fire/000474.html; Civil Rights Litigation Clearinghouse Case Profile, "Shumate v. Wilson," last updated December 3, 2022, https://clearinghouse.net/case/582/.

154. Charisse Shumate et al., Plaintiffs, v. Wilson, et al., Defendants, "Settlement Agreement," September 9, 1997, 8–9, 14, https://www.clearinghouse.net/chDocs/public/PC-CA-0011-0004.pdf.

155. Shain, "Women Prisoners Win Shumate Case!"

156. Civil Rights Litigation Clearinghouse Case Profile, "Shumate v. Wilson."

157. Shumate et al. v. Wilson, "Settlement Agreement," 4–7.

158. Law, *Resistance behind Bars*, 118–19.

159. Civil Rights Litigation Clearinghouse Case Profile, "Shumate v. Wilson." https://clearinghouse.net/doc/2830/; https://clearinghouse.net/doc/2830/.

160. Civil Rights Litigation Clearinghouse Case Profile, "Shumate v. Wilson," https://www.clearinghouse.net/detail.php?id=582; Law, *Resistance behind Bars*, n. 155, 247.

161. Charisse Shumate, et al., Plaintiffs, v. Pete Wilson, et al., Defendants, "Order," August 8, 2000, 1–5, here 2–3, https://www.clearinghouse.net/chDocs /public/PC-CA-0011-0011.pdf; and Order of Dismissal, August 21, 2000, 1–3, https://www.clearinghouse.net/chDocs/public/PC-CA-0011-0008.pdf; S.866— Prison Litigation Reform Act of 1995.

162. Greenspan, "Positive Women Prisoners Speak Out," 25–26.

163. Safreed Harmon, "HIV Incarcerated Women," 18; Law, *Resistance behind Bars*, 40.

164. Diana Block and Donna Willmott, "Legislative Hearings: Speaking Truth to Power," *The Fire Inside* 16 (December 2000), https://www.womenprisoners.org /fire/000224.html.

165. Janice Jordan, "Legislative Hearings: Battered Women Speak," *The Fire Inside* 16 (December 2000), https://www.womenprisoners.org/fire/000222 .html.

166. Block and Willmott, "Legislative Hearings."

167. Katie Szymanski, "Medical Conditions Worsen inside State Prison for Women," *Bay Area Reporter*, December 14, 2000, 18, box 6, folder 185, JGP.

168. CCWP members, "Women Sue for Healthcare," *The Fire Inside* 1 (Summer 1996), https://www.womenprisoners.org/fire/000816.html.

169. Jim Davis, "3 Prison Deaths Questioned: An Independent Inquiry is Sought at Chowchilla Facility," *Fresno Bee*, December 20, 2000, A1, box 6, folder 185, JGP.

170. Judy Greenspan, "Notes on the Death of Another Women Prisoner at the Central California Women's Facility," 1–2, here 1, box 6, folder 185, JGP.

171. Davis, "3 Prison Deaths"; Amnesty International Press Release, "USA: Independent Investigation into Deaths at California Prison Urgently Needed," December 21, 2000, 1–2, box 6, folder 185, JGP.

172. Davis, "3 Prison Deaths"; Eric Baily and Mark Arax, "Deaths of Women in State Prison Probed," *Los Angeles Times*, December 20, 2000, A3; Sabin Russell, "State Probing 5 Recent Deaths of Female Inmates at Chowchilla," *San*

Francisco Chronicle, December 13, 2000, A6; and Sabine Russell, "2 More Die at Women's Prison in Chowchilla: 3 of 7 Recent Deaths under Investigation," *San Francisco Chronicle*, December 20, 2000, A3.

173. Amnesty International, "USA: Independent investigation."

174. Davis, "3 Prison Deaths," A1; Russell, "2 More Die at Women's Prison," A3; CCWP, "Dedication to Twillah Wallace," *The Fire Inside* 19 (Fall 2001), https://www.womenprisoners.org/fire/000183.html.

175. Law, *Resistance behind Bars*, 39–40.

176. CCWP, "Charisse Shumate, A Warrior, a Friend, an Inspiration," *The Fire Inside* (Fall 2001), https://www.womenprisoners.org/fire/000182.html (accessed December 2021); The Freedom Archives, "Charisse Shumate—Fighting for Our Lives," undated, http://www.freedomarchives.org/Charisse.html.

177. Thuma, *All Our Trials*, 4.

178. LSPC, "Protecting Basic Human Rights," 1.

179. History of CCWP and *Charisse Shumate: Fighting for our Lives*, film, August 15, 2003, CCWP, http://womenprisoners.org/about/000085.html.

180. *Brown v. Plata*, 563 U.S. 493 (2011), 1.

181. McTighe, "Our Relationships Carry the Movement," 192.

182. CCWP, "Women Prisoners Will Have Their Day in Court," *The Fire Inside* 4 (May 1997): 1, box 8, folder 237, JGP.

183. Law, *Resistance behind Bars*, 28.

CHAPTER 5

1. Sharon Hillier et al., "In Vitro and in Vivo: the Story of Nonoxynol 9," *Journal of Acquired Immune Deficiency Syndromes* 39, no. 1 (May 2005): 1–8, https://doi.org/10.1097/01.qai.0000159671.25950.74.

2. Susan Okie, "AIDS Study Prompts New Look at Prevention," *Washington Post*, August 14, 2000, A3.

3. Sharon Lerner, "Product to Protect Women from H.I.V. Is Elusive," *New York Times*, July 3, 2001, F6; Jordan Lite, "New Push for Woman-Controlled AIDS Prevention," *Women's Enews*, May 19, 2002, https://womensenews.org/2002/05/new-push-woman-controlled-aids-prevention/.

4. Royles, *To Make the Wounded Whole*, 166, 169.

5. Robert H. Goldstein and Rochelle P. Walensky, "Where Were the Women? Gender Parity in Clinical Trials," *New England Journal of Medicine* 381, no. 26 (2019): 2491–93.

6. Devon Betts, "Who Gets to be a TruvadaWhore: Promiscuity, Race, and Queer Politics," *Radical History Review* 140 (May 2021): 158–59.

7. Watkins-Hayes, *Remaking a Life*, 179–80.

8. David W. Dunlap, "From AIDS Conference, Talk of Life, Not Death," *New York Times*, July 15, 1996; Brier, *Infectious Ideas*, 158.

9. Lawrence K. Altman, "Failed Tests on Monkeys Frustrates Hopes for AIDS Vaccine," *New York Times*, July 3, 1998, A15.

10. Rupa Chinai, "Cocktail of Drugs' Yields Positive Results on HIV," *The Times of India*, August 3, 1996, 13.

11. Dunlap, "From AIDS Conference."

12. Lawrence K. Altman, "AIDS Meeting Ends with Little Hope of Breakthrough: Emphasis on Prevention," *New York Times*, July 5, 1998, 1; Claudia Dreifus, "A Conversation with Zeda Rosenberg; Agency Seeks a Virus-Killer for Women to Help Control the Spread of AIDS," *New York Times*, July 29, 2003, https://www.nytimes.com/2003/07/29/health/conversation-with-zeda-rosenberg-agency-seeks-virus-killer-for-women-help.html.

13. Bachi Karkaria, "Bedfellows for the Condom: Global Strategists Help Find New Prevention Tools for AIDS," *Times of India*, November 4, 2006.

14. CDC, "HIV/AIDS Surveillance Report: U.S. HIV and AIDS Cases Reported through June 2000," *MMWR* 12, no. 1 (June 2000): 3.

15. Denis McClean, "£30m AIDS Fund Contribution Praised: Denis Mcclean Reports from the 15th International AIDS Conference in Bangkok," *Irish Times*, July 13, 2004; Royles, *To Make the Wounded Whole*, 208.

16. Zena Stein, "HIV Prevention: The Need for Methods Women Can Use," *American Journal of Public Health* 80, no. 4 (1990): 460–62.

17. Marea Murray, "An Activist Perspective on the First National Women and HIV Conference," *Gay Community News*, January 7–13, 1990, 10.

18. Dinsa Sachan, "Zeda Rosenberg: Determined to Empower Women to Prevent HIV Infection," *The BMJ* 359 (October 2, 2017), https://doi.org/10.1136/bmj.j4424.

19. Kounteya Sinha, "Ahead of World AIDS Day, Hope Rides on Push for Prevention & Drug Dole: Bid to keep out HIV during Sex," *Times of India*, November 30, 2006.

20. Megan Gottemoeller, "Empowering Women to Prevent HIV: The Microbicide Advocacy Agenda," in "AIDS: Global Concerns for Women," special issue, *Agenda: Empowering Women for Gender Equity* 16, no. 44 (2000): 36.

21. Fernando Notario-Pérez et al., "Historical Development of Vaginal Microbicides to Prevent Sexual Transmission of HIV in Women: From Past Failures to Future Hopes," *Drug Design, Development, and Therapy* 11 (June 15, 2017): 1767–87, https://doi.org/10.2147/DDDT.S133170.

22. Jane K. Stoever, "Stories Absent from the Courtroom: Responding to Domestic Violence in the Context of HIV and AIDS," *North Carolina Law Review* 87, no. 4 (May 2009): 1173, 1175.

23. Jan Balzarini and Lut Van Damme, "Microbicide Drug Candidates to Prevent HIV Infection," *The Lancet* 369, no. 9563 (March 3, 2007), 787.

24. Lite, "New Push for Woman-Controlled AIDS Prevention."

25. Lori Heise, "Topical Microbicides: Missing Link for HIV Prevention," *Sexual Health Exchange* 1 (1999): 3–5.

26. Lori Heise, "In Fighting AIDS, We Cannot Delay," *New York Times*, June 27, 2001.

27. Gottemoeller, "Empowering Women to Prevent HIV," 33; Anna Forbes et al., "In Our Own Hands: A Case Study on Mobilizing Demand for HIV Prevention for Women," 2013, 16, https://path.azureedge.net/media/documents/APP_gcm_hiv_cs.pdf.

28. Altman, "Tests to Begin," A11.

29. Forbes et al., "In Our Own Hands," 10–12.

30. Gottemoeller, "Empowering Women to Prevent HIV," 34.

31. Forbes et al., "In Our Own Hands," 15–16.

32. Zeda F. Rosenberg, ScD, https://www.ipmglobal.org/about/ipm-executive-leadership/zeda-f-rosenberg-ceo.

33. Tina Rosenberg, "When a Pill is Not Enough," *New York Times*, August 6, 2006; Peter C. Engelman, *A History of the Birth Control Movement in America* (Santa Barbara, CA: Praeger, 2011), 76–77.

34. Lerner, "Product to Protect Women from H.I.V. Is Elusive."

35. Microbicide Trial Network, "About Us," https://mtnstopshiv.org/about-us.

36. Lawrence Altman, "A Familiar Pair Urge Greater Attention for AIDS," *New York Times*, August 15, 2006, A12; Lawrence Altman, "Tests of Drugs to Block HIV Infection are Halted over Safety," *New York Times*, February 1, 2007, A3.

37. Malathy Iyer, "City scientists May Crack AIDS Code: Lead Research in the Development of Microbicide Gels to Kill HIV," *Times of India*, February 3, 2007, 9.

38. Altman, "Tests of Drugs to Block HIV Infection are Halted"; Donald McNeil, "AIDS Prevention Gel Fails in Trial, Researchers Say," *New York Times*, December 15, 2009.

39. Gottemoeller, "Empowering Women to Prevent HIV," 33; Lerner, "Product to Protect Women from H.I.V. Is Elusive."

40. Dreifus, "A Conversation with Zeda Rosenberg."

41. International Partnership for Microbicides, "Preparing for Access to Microbicides and the Dapivirine Ring for HIV Prevention," May 2011, 26, https://assets.publishing.service.gov.uk/media/57a08af0ed915d3cfd000a20/IPMAccessStrategy.pdf.

42. Bachi Karkaria, "Science and Ethics Can Be Served in Clinical Trials," *Times of India*, March 7, 2008, 14.

43. Dreifus, "A Conversation with Zeda Rosenberg."

44. Forbes et al., "In Our Own Hands," 14.

45. Centers for Disease Control and Prevention, Atlanta, GA, 1993, NLM, https://stacks.cdc.gov/view/cdc/34804.

46. "Finally, a Safe Gel to Protect Women from AIDS! The Gel Uses the Drug Tenofovir and is Quite Acceptable to Women," *Times of India*, February 27, 2008.

47. Quarraisha Abdool Karim et al., "Effectiveness and Safety of Tenofovir Gel, an Antiretroviral Microbicide, for the Prevention of HIV Infection in Women," *Science* 329, no. 5996 (July 2010): 1168–74.

48. Celia W. Dugger, "African Studies Give Women Hope in H.I.V. Fight," *New York Times*, July 19, 2010.

49. Robert M. Grant et al., "Preexposure Chemoprophylaxis for HIV Prevention in Men Who Have Sex with Men," *New England Journal of Medicine* 363 (December 2010): 2587–99.

50. "CDC statement on FDA Approval of Drug for HIV Prevention," July 16, 2012, https://www.cdc.gov/nchhstp/newsroom/2012/fda-approves drugstatement.html.

51. Donald G. McNeil, Jr., "New Lines of Attack in HIV Prevention," *New York Times*, November 9, 2010, D7.

52. Dugger, "African Studies Give Women Hope."

53. Celia W. Dugger, "H.I.V. Prevention Gel Hits Snag: Money," *New York Times*, September 3, 2010.

54. Gus Cairns, "VOICE Trial: Microbicide Gel may have Stopped Two out of Three HIV Infections—In the Women who Used It," *aidsmap*, February 9, 2015, http://www.aidsmap.com/VOICE-trial-Microbicide-gel-may-have-stopped-two-out-of-three-HIV-infections-in-the-women-who-used-it/page/2943410/.

55. KFF, "Women's Health Insurance Coverage," November 8, 2021, https://www.kff.org/other/fact-sheet/womens-health-insurance-coverage/.

56. Anna Forbes, "Women Deserve to Know About HIV Prevention Medication Too," *Rewire News*, March 10, 2015, https://rewirenewsgroup.com/article/2015/03/10/women-deserve-know-hiv-prevention-medication/.

57. Henry J Kaiser Family Foundation, "AIDS 2010: Study Finds Microbicide Containing HIV Drug Lowers Infection Risk in Women by 39%," *KFF*, July 20, 2010, https://www.kff.org/news-summary/aids-2010-study-finds-microbicide-containing-hiv-drug-lowers-infection-risk-in-women-by-39/.

58. McNeil, Jr., "New Lines of Attack in HIV Prevention."

59. Forbes et al., "In Our Own Hands," 38.

60. Nelson, *More Than Medicine*, 208.

61. Royles, *To Make the Wounded Whole*, 216, 214, 220; McTighe, "Our Relationships Carry the Movement," 189.

62. Brier, *Infectious Ideas*, 153.

63. Warren E. Leary, "Female Condom for Market," *New York Times*, May 11, 1993; Donald McNeil, Jr., "Redesigning a Condom So Women Will Use It," *New York Times*, November 13, 2007; Stoever, "Stories Absent from the Courtroom," 1176.

64. Laura Blumenfeld, "Style Plus: The New Sexual 'Reality' Now, A Condom for Women," *Washington Post*, March 9, 1992, B5.

65. Robert M. Grant et al., "Uptake of Pre-Exposure Prophylaxis, Sexual Practices, and HIV Incidence in Men and Transgender Women Who Have Sex

with Men: A Cohort Study," *The Lancet* 14, no. 9 (July 22, 2014): 820–29, https:// doi.org/10.1016/S1473-3099(14)70847-3.

66. Lut Van Damme, M.D., et al., "Preexposure Prophylaxis for HIV Infection among Africa Women," *New England Journal of Medicine* 367, no. 5 (August 2012): 419–22.

67. Cicatelli Associates Inc. (CAI), "African American Women and PrEP," undated, 1, https://docs.wixstatic.com/ugd/68e4cb_8748d15a45cb453c91ff1d31ad 368a65.pdf.

68. Jared M. Baeten, M.D., et al., "Antiretroviral Prophylaxis for HIV Prevention in Heterosexual Men and Women," *New England Journal of Medicine* 367, no. 5 (August 2012): 399–410; Michael C. Thigpen et al., "Antiretroviral Preexposure Prophylaxis for Heterosexual HIV Transmission in Botswana," *New England Journal of Medicine* 367, no. 5 (August 2012): 423–34; NIH, Sustainable Healthcare Implementation PrEP Pilot Study (SHIPP), clinical trial NCT02074891, February 2016, https://clinicaltrials.gov/ct2/show/NCT 02074891.

69. Ida Susser, *AIDS, Sex, and Culture: Global Politics and Survival in Southern Africa* (Chichester, West Sussex, UK: Wiley-Blackwell, 2009), 55.

70. Rodgers, *The Global Gag Rule and Women's Reproductive Health*, 1–2.

71. Susser, *Imperial Moralities*, 47–49, 51–53.

72. KFF, "The Mexico City Policy: An Explainer," January 28, 2021, https:// www.kff.org/global-health-policy/fact-sheet/ mexico-city-policy-explainer/#footnote-509511-41.

73. Nina Brooks et al., "USA Aid Policy and Induced Abortion in Sub-Saharan Africa: An Analysis of the Mexico City Policy," *The Lancet* 7, no. 8 (August 2019): 1046; Editorial, "The Devastating Impact of Trump's Global Gag Rule," *The Lancet* 393 (June 2019): 2359.

74. UNAIDS, "Global HIV & AIDS statistics—Fact Sheet," 2022, https:// www.unaids.org/en/resources/fact-sheet.

75. CDC, "HIV and Women," March 2022, https://www.cdc.gov/hiv/pdf /group/gender/women/cdc-hiv-women.pdf.

76. KFF, "Black Americans and HIV/AIDS: The Basics," February 7, 2020, https://www.kff.org/hivaids/fact-sheet/black-americans-and-hivaids-the-basics/; March of Dimes, "Population," March 2023, https://www.marchofdimes.org

/peristats/data?reg=99&top=14&stop=127&lev=1&slev=1&obj=3; CDC Fact Sheet, "HIV Among African Americans," July 2019, 1, https://www.cdc.gov/nchhstp/newsroom/docs/factsheets/cdc-hiv-aa-508.pdf.

77. CDC, "Core Indications for Monitoring the Ending the HIV Epidemic Initiative (Preliminary Data): National HIV Surveillance Data Reported through September 2021; and Preexposure Prophylaxis (PrEP) Data Reported through June 2021," *HIV Surveillance Data Tables* 2, no. 5 (December 2021): 18, https://www.cdc.gov/hiv/pdf/library/reports/surveillance-data-tables/vol-2-no-5/cdc-hiv-surveillance-tables-vol-2-no-5.pdf.

78. Forbes, "Women Deserve to Know About HIV Prevention Medication Too"; Betts, "Who Gets to be a TruvadaWhore," 158–59. See Gilead Sciences, Inc., "I Like to Party" video, November 4, 2015, accessed July 2022, https://www.youtube.com/watch?v=FXZcoBsoGBY.

79. Judith Auerbach et al., "Knowledge, Attitudes, and Likelihood of Preexposure Prophylaxis (PrEP) Use among US Women at Risk of Acquiring HIV," *AIDS Patient Care STDS* 29, no. 2 (February 2015): 102–10.

80. Gus Cairns, "At Least 28,000 Women in the United States Have Started PrEP," *aidsmap*, July 4, 2020, https://www.aidsmap.com/news/jul-2020/least-28000-women-united-states-have-started-prep.

81. CDC, "Core Indications for Monitoring the Ending of the HIV Epidemic Initiative," 18.

82. CDC, "HIV Risk Behaviors," 2015, https://www.cdc.gov/hiv/pdf/risk/estimates/cdc-hiv-risk-behaviors.pdf.

83. Michelle Chen, "Trump's Global Gag Rule is Making It Harder to Fight the AIDS Crisis," *The Nation*, March 25, 2019, https://www.thenation.com/article/archive/global-gag-rule-trump-hiv-aids/.

84. Kate Zernike, "They Voted to Repeal Obamacare: Now They are a Target," *New York Times*, May 8, 2017.

85. Kiersten Gillette-Pierce and Jamila Taylor, "The Threat to Title X Family Planning: Why It Matters and What's at Stake for Women," *Center for American Progress*, February 9, 2017, https://www.americanprogress.org/issues/women/reports/2017/02/09/414773/the-threat-to-title-x-family-planning/.

86. "Publicly Supported Family Planning Services in the United States," *Guttmacher Institute*, October 2019, https://www.guttmacher.org/fact-sheet/publicly-

supported-FP-services-US#:~:text=In%202018%2C%20there%20were%20nearly, funded%20clinics%20(3.5%20million).

87. Julie Wittes Schlack, "The Title X 'Gag Rule' Plays Politics by Attacking Women's Health," *wbur news*, March 1, 2019, https://www.wbur.org/cognoscenti /2019/03/01/title-x-gag-rule-julie-wittes-schlack.

88. Kaiser Foundation, "Women's Health Insurance Coverage," November 8, 2021, https://www.kff.org/womens-health-policy/fact-sheet/womens-health-insurance-coverage-fact-sheet/.

89. Planned Parenthood, "Medicaid and Reproductive Health," https:// www.plannedparenthoodaction.org/issues/health-care-equity/medicaid-and-reproductive-health, undated; KFF, "Women and HIV in the United States," March 9, 2020, https://www.kff.org/hivaids/fact-sheet/women-and-hivaids-in-the-united-states/.

90. Vanessa A. White and Christine Brazell, "Family Planning Provides Key in Fight Against HIV," undated, *HIV.gov*, https://www.hiv.gov/blog /family-planning-providers-key-in-fight-against-hiv.

91. C. I. Fowler et al., *Family Planning Annual Report: 2017 National Summary*, August 2018, ES-2, https://opa.hhs.gov/sites/default/files/2020–07/title-x-fpar-2017-national-summary.pdf.

92. Margaret Talbot, "How the Trump Administration is Stigmatizing Abortion," *New Yorker*, August 24, 2019, https://www.newyorker.com/news /daily-comment/how-the-trump-administration-is-stigmatizing-abortion.

93. TC Jatlaoui et al., "Abortion Surveillance—United States, 2015," *MMWR Surveillance Summary 67*, no. SS13 (2018): 1–45.

94. "The GOP's War on Women's Health Gets Results," *New York Times*, September 9, 2019, https://www.nytimes.com/2019/09/09/opinion/planned-parenthood-ohio-title-x.html.

95. Kaiser Family Foundation, "Women's Health Insurance Coverage"; Jocelyn Frye, "On the Frontlines at Work and at Home: The Disproportionate Economic Effects of the Coronavirus Pandemic on Women of Color," *Center for Economic Progress*, April 23, 2020, https://www.americanprogress.org/article /frontlines-work-home/.

96. Zahra Barnes, "8 Health Conditions that Disproportionately Affect Black Women," *Self*, March 30, 2017, https://www.self.com/story/black-women-health-conditions.

97. Joseph E. Potter and Kari White, "Defunding Planned Parenthood was a Disaster in Texas. Congress Shouldn't Do It Nationally," *Washington Post*, February 7, 2017.

98. Miriam Berg, "'Defund' Attacks on Planned Parenthood in Texas," Planned Parenthood blog, March 29, 2021, https://www.plannedparenthoodaction.org/blog/defund-attacks-on-planned-parenthood-in-texas.

99. Mattie Quinn, "Why Texas Is the Most Dangerous U.S. State to Have a Baby," *Governing*, May 2017, https://www.governing.com/topics/health-human-services/gov-maternal-infant-mortality-pregnant-women-texas.html.

100. Planned Parenthood, "The Effects of Defunding: Texas and Indiana," undated, https://www.plannedparenthood.org/uploads/filer_public/9e/71/9e713a00-4844-43aa-adf6-3cc9e6cf30e0/the_effects_of_defunding_texas_and_indiana.pdf.

101. Renfro, *Stranger Danger*.

102. Nadine Strossen and Anthony D. Romero, "Religious Refusals and Reproductive Rights: Accessing Birth Control at the Pharmacy," ACLU, 2007, https://www.aclu.org/files/images/asset_upload_file119_29548.pdf.

103. Dima Mazen Qato et al., "The Availability of Pharmacies in the United States: 2007–2015," *PLoS ONE* 12, no. 8 (August 2017), https://doi.org/10.1371/journal.pone.0183172.

104. Ruth Dawson, "Trump Administration's Domestic Gag Rule Has Slashed the Title X Network's Capacity by Half," *Guttmacher Institute*, February 2020, https://www.guttmacher.org/article/2020/02/trump-administrations-domestic-gag-rule-has-slashed-title-x-networks-capacity-half.

105. Health GAP, "AIDS Activists Disrupt Gilead Shareholder Meeting," May 8, 2019, https://www.facebook.com/healthgap/videos/373025566641540/?v=373025566641540.

106. Matt Sharp, "Three Decades of Treatment Activism," *Achieve* 5, no. 4 (2013): 4.

107. Royles, *To Make the Wounded Whole*, 183.

108. Health GAP, "AIDS Activists Disrupt Gilead Shareholder Meeting."

109. Sony Salzman, "Trump Touted Gilead's Donation of HIV-Prevention Medication, But Doctors Want Generics—Not Charity," *Rewire News*, May 23, 2019, https://rewire.news/article/2019/05/23/trump-touted-gileads-donation-of-hiv-prevention-medication-but-doctors-want-generics-not-charity/.

110. CDC, "PrEP for HIV Prevention in the U.S.," page last reviewed November 23, 2021, https://www.cdc.gov/nchhstp/newsroom/fact-sheets/hiv/PrEP-for-hiv-prevention-in-the-US-factsheet.html.

111. Shefali Luthra and Anna Gorman, "Rising Cost of PrEP to Prevent HIV Infection Pushes It out of Reach for Many," *npr*, June 30, 2018, https://www.npr.org/sections/health-shots/2018/06/30/624045995/rising-cost-of-prep-a-pill-that-prevents-hiv-pushes-it-out-of-reach-for-many?t=1653568805186; Liz Highleyman, "Is High Cost Hindering Access to Truvada for PrEP?" *POZ*, September 18, 2020, https://www.poz.com/article/high-cost-limiting-access-truvada-prep.

112. Watkins-Hayes, *Transforming a Life*, 179.

113. Donna Young, "Gilead CEO Defends HIV Drug Truvada's Price, Insists CDC Patent Invalid," *S&P Global Market Intelligence*, May 16, 2019, https://www.spglobal.com/marketintelligence/en/news-insights/latest-news-headlines/51879834.

114. Hoffman, *Health Care for Some*, x–xi.

115. Aaron S. Kesselheim et al., "The High Cost of Prescription Drugs in the United States," *JAMA* 316, no. 8 (August 23–30, 2016): 860, 862, 863.

116. "H.R.1—108th Congress (2003–2004): Medicare Prescription Drug, Improvement, and Modernization Act of 2003," December 8, 2003, 2098.

117. "H.R.3590—111th Congress (2009–2010): Patient Protection and Affordable Care Act," March 23, 2010, 191.

118. Kesselheim et al., "High Cost of Prescription Drugs," 860.

119. Stuart Silverstein, "This is Why Your Prescriptions Cost So Damn Much," *Mother Jones*, October 21, 2016, https://www.motherjones.com/politics/2016/10/drug-industry-pharmaceutical-lobbyists-medicare-part-d-prices/.

120. Greene, *Generic*, xi–xii.

121. Feldman and Frondorf, *Drug Wars*, 24–25.

122. Kesselheim et al., "High Cost of Prescription Drugs," 863; Thrasher, *Viral Underclass*, 184.

123. David M. Oshinsky, *Polio: An American Story* (New York: Oxford University Press, 2005), 211–12 ; Nathaniel L. Moir, "To Boldly Remember Where We Have Already Been: Revisiting the Cutter Polio Vaccine Incident during Operation Warp Speed," *Journal of Applied History* 2 (2020): 18.

124. Charlotte Jacobs, *Jonas Salk: A Life* (New York: Oxford University Press, 2015), 180–82.

125. James C. Hagerty, "Press Release Statement by the President About the Polio Vaccine Situation," May 31, 1955, 3, accessed May 2022, https://www.eisenhowerlibrary.gov/sites/default/files/research/online-documents/salk/salk-g.pdf.

126. CDC, "Polio Elimination in the US," updated August 3, 2022, https://www.cdc.gov/polio/what-is-polio/polio-us.html.

127. Naomi Rogers, "Race and the Politics of Polio: Warm Springs, Tuskegee, and the March of Dimes," *American Journal of Public Health* (May 1, 2007): 786.

128. The PREP4ALL Collaboration, "A National Action Plan for Universal Access to HIV Pre-Exposure Prophylaxis (PrEP) in the United States," 22nd International AIDS Conference, July 2018, 36–40, https://static1.squarespace.com/static/5e937afbfd7a75746167b39c/t/5ea5ff68ccd2820f98798d1f/1587937130060/A+National+Action+Plan+for+Universal+Access+to+HIV+Pre-Exposure+Prophylaxis+%28PrEP%29.pdf.

129. Christopher Rowland, "An HIV Treatment Cost Taxpayers Millions. The Government Patented It. But a Pharma Giant is Making Billions," *Washington Post*, March 26, 2019.

130. Daniel Reynolds, "Gilead Will Donate Truvada to 200,000 People Annually for 11 Years," *Advocate*, May 9, 2019.

131. David Artavia, "Meet the Organizers from PrEP4ALL," *hivplusmag*, May 14, 2019, https://www.hivplusmag.com/uu/2019/5/14/meet-organizers-prep4all.

132. Gordon, *Pitied but Not Entitled*; Hoffman, *Healthcare for Some*; Salzman, "Trump Touted Gilead's Donation."

133. Joshua M. Sharfstein et al., "Long-Acting Cabotegravir for HIV Prevention: Issues of Access, Cost, and Equity," *JAMA* 327, no. 10 (2022): 921.

134. Andrew Pollack, "Drug Goes from $13.50 a Tablet to $750, Overnight," *New York Times*, September 20, 2015.

135. Andrew Buncombe, "AOC asks Pharma CEO Why $2,000 HIV Drug Costs Just $8 in Australia,'" *The Independent*, May 17, 2019, https://www.independent.co.uk/news/world/americas/us-politics/aoc-hiv-drug-cost-us-australia-ceo-gilead-video-a8919316.html.

136. Thrasher, *Viral Underclass*, 185.

137. Brier, *Infectious Ideas*, 164, 181; Benjamin Ryan, "Living with Lipo," *POZ*, January 15, 2016, https://www.poz.com/article/living-lipo.

138. Peter Staley, *Never Silent: ACT UP and My Life in Activism* (Chicago: Chicago Review Press, 2022).

139. *Peter Staley, et al. v. Gilead Sciences, Inc., et al.*, class-action complaint, Case No. 3:19-cv-2573 (2019), 3–4.

140. Terri Wilder, "Oral Arguments in Antitrust Case against HIV Drug Companies Began Last Week," *TheBodyPro*, January 28, 2020, https://www.thebodypro.com/article/peter-staley-oral-arguments-in-antitrust-case-against-hiv-drug-companies.

141. Letter, PrEP4ALL to Attorney General Merrick Garland and Secretary of HHS Xavier Becerra, undated, 2, https://static1.squarespace.com/static/5e937afbfd7a75746167b39c/t/61dc694cba488b1aa94f51fe/1641834828656/U.S.+v.+Gilead+2+year+anniversary+sign+on+-+CLEAN+FINAL.pdf.

142. FDA Briefing Document, "Meeting of the Antimicrobial Drugs Advisory Committee," August 7, 2019, 30, https://www.fda.gov/media/129607/download; Goldstein and Walensky, "Where Were the Women?" 2492–93.

143. Lawrence O. Gostin and Arti K. Rai, "Expanding Access to Reducing Prices for Drugs to Prevent HIV," *JAMA* 232, no. 9 (March 2020): 821; Blake Brittain, "Ruling Gives Gilead a Boost in Billion-Dollar HIV Drug Patent Fight," *Reuters*, December 1, 2022, https://www.reuters.com/legal/litigation/ruling-gives-gilead-boost-billion-dollar-hiv-drug-patent-fight-2022-12-01/.

144. Letter, PrEP4ALL to Garland and Becerra, 3; Fraiser Kansteiner, "Bristol Myers Settles HIV Antitrust Suit, but J&J, Gilead Still Await Their Day in Court," *Fierce Pharma*, April 15, 2022, https://www.fiercepharma.com/pharma/bristol-myers-settles-hiv-antitrust-suit-jj-gilead-still-await-their-day-court.

145. Gostin and Rai, "Expanding Access," 822.

146. Kesselheim et al., "High Cost of Prescription Drugs," 865–66.

147. Bettina M. Beech, "Poverty, Racism, and the Public Health Crisis in America," *Frontiers in Public Health* (September 2021), https://doi.org/10.3389/fpubh.2021.699049; Robin Bleiweis, Alexandra Cawthorne Gaines, and Diana Boesch, "The Basic Facts about Women in Poverty," *American Progress*, August 3, 2020, https://www.americanprogress.org/article/basic-facts-women-poverty/.

148. WHO statement, "WHO continues to Support Its Conditional Recommendation for the Dapivirine Vaginal Ring as an Additional Prevention Option for Women at Substantial Risk of HIV," December 9, 2021, https://www.who.int

/news/item/09-12-2021-who-continues-to-support-its-conditional-recommendation-for-the-dapivirine-vaginal-ring.

149. Liz Highleyman, "Injectable PrEP Offers a New Option for Women," *San Francisco AIDS Foundation*, December 29, 2020, https://www.sfaf.org/collections/beta/injectable-prep-offers-a-new-option-for-women/.

EPILOGUE

1. Amelia Abraham, "Photographing Black, Female, HIV Positive Power," *Refinery 29*, December 8, 2016, https://uk.style.yahoo.com/photographing-black-female-hiv-positive-070500970.html; Josie Thaddeus-Johns, "Portraits of Love and Loss From an HIV-Positive Childhood," *New York Times*, March 3, 2022, https://www.nytimes.com/2022/03/03/arts/design/kia-labeija-fotografiska.html.

2. CDC, "Epidemiologic Notes and Reports Possible Transfusion-Associated Acquired Immune Deficiency Syndrome (AIDS)—California," *MMWR* 31, no. 48 (December 10, 1982): 652–54; CDC, "Unexplained Immunodeficiency and Opportunistic Infections in Infants," 665–67 (see Introduction, n. 2); CDC, "Current Trends Recommendations for Assisting in the Prevention of Perinatal Transmission of Human T-Lymphotropic Virus Type III/Lymphadenopathy-Associated Virus and Acquired Immunodeficiency Syndrome," 721–76, 731–32 (see Chapter 2, n. 20); Marte and Anastos, "Women—The Missing Persons in the AIDS Epidemic—Part II," 11; Bloche, "Beyond Autonomy," 232.

3. Thaddeus-Johns, "Portraits of Love and Loss."

4. Sarah Sugar et al., "Health Coverage for Women Under the Affordable Care Act," *HHS Issue Brief*, March 21 2022, https://aspe.hhs.gov/sites/default/files/documents/9082fc42757552c429d8b1c3c8949595/aspe-womens-coverage-ib.pdf; CDC, "HIV and Women Fact Sheet," March 2022, https://www.cdc.gov/hiv/pdf/group/gender/women/cdc-hiv-women.pdf.

5. Theodore Kerr, "How to Have an AIDS Memorial in an Epidemic," *C Magazine* 142 (Summer 2019), https://cmagazine.com/issues/142/how-to-have-an-aids-memorial-in-an-epidemic.

6. KFF, "Black Americans and HIV/AIDS: The Basics," February 7, 2020, https://www.kff.org/hivaids/fact-sheet/black-americans-and-hivaids-the-basics/;

March of Dimes, "Population," January 2022, https://www.marchofdimes.org /peristats/data?reg=99&top=14&stop=127&lev=1&slev=1&obj=3; CDC Fact Sheet, "HIV among African Americans," June 2019, 1, https://www.cdc.gov/ nchhstp/newsroom/docs/factsheets/cdc-hiv-aa-508.pdf.

7. Michael A. Scarcella, "Woman with HIV Didn't Seek Care for Baby," *Herald Tribune*, January 11, 2008; HIV Justice Network, "US: Florida Woman Guilty of Mother-to-Child HIV Transmission," undated, https://www.hivjustice.net /cases/us-florida-woman-guilty-of-mother-to-child-hiv-transmission/; The Center for HIV Law Policy, "What HIV Criminalization Means to Women in the U.S.," undated, 3, https://www.hivlawandpolicy.org/sites/default/files/Women%20 and%20HIV%20Criminalization.pdf.

8. Ahmed, "HIV and Women," 39.

9. HIV Justice Network, "US: Florida Woman Guilty of Mother-to-Child HIV Transmission."

10. Margo Kaplan, "Behind Bars for Being Pregnant and HIV-Positive," June 8, 2009, https://www.hivlawandpolicy.org/fine-print-blog/behind-bars-being-pregnant-and-hiv-positive; Ahmed, "HIV and Women," 39.

11. Ordaz, "AIDS Knows No Borders"; Chávez, *Borders of AIDS*.

12. Jacobs, King, and Milkis, "Building a Conservative State," 462–65.

13. 19–1392 *Dobbs v. Jackson Women's Health Organization* (June 24, 2022), 1.

14. Sharon Bernstein, "Louisiana Lawmakers Withdraw Bill Declaring Abortion Homicide," *Reuters*, May 13, 2022, https://www.reuters.com/world /us/louisiana-lawmakers-withdraw-bill-declaring-abortion-homicide-2022-05-13/; "State Legislation Tracker: Major Developments in Sexual & Reproductive Health as of February 28, 2023," *Guttmacher Institute*, https://www.guttmacher .org/state-policy.

15. Jia Tolentino, "We're Not Going Back to the Time Before Roe. We're Going Somewhere Worse," *New Yorker*, June 24, 2022, https://www.newyorker .com/magazine/2022/07/04/we-are-not-going-back-to-the-time-before-roe-we-are-going-somewhere-worse.

16. Sam Levin, "She was Jailed for Losing a Pregnancy. Her Nightmare Could Become More Common," *The Guardian*, June 4, 2022, https://www.theguardian .com/us-news/2022/jun/03/california-stillborn-prosecution-roe-v-wade.

17. Ordaz, "AIDS Knows No Borders."

18. McTighe, "Our Relationships Carry the Movement," 188.

19. Thrasher, *Viral Underclass*, 10–11.

20. Ko Bragg and Kate Sosin, "503: Inside the COVID Unit at the World's Largest Women's Prison," *The 19th*, October 11, 2020, https://19thnews.org/2020/10/503-inside-the-covid-unit-at-the-worlds-largest-womens-prison/; CCWP Press Release, "Advocates Demand Action as Largest Women's Prison Experiences Covid-19 Outbreak," January 5, 2021, http://womenprisoners.org/ccwf-covid-outbreak-demands/.

21. Harmeet Kaur, "The Coronavirus Pandemic has been Catastrophic for House Cleaners and Nannies," *CNN*, April 3, 2020, https://edition.cnn.com/2020/04/03/us/social-distancing-pandemic-domestic-workers-trnd/index.html; Melissa L. St. Hilaire, "I Was Fired Because of the Coronavirus: Domestic Workers Need Your Help. And You Need Ours," *New York Times*, April 13, 2020, https://www.nytimes.com/2020/04/13/opinion/sunday/coronavirus-domestic-workers.html; Amanda Blanco, "Who Benefited From Expanded Paid Sick Leave Policies for Service Workers? And Who Didn't," *Federal Reserve Bank of Boston*, April 5, 2022, https://www.bostonfed.org/news-and-events/news/2022/04/paid-sick-leave-inequalities-during-covid-boston-fed.aspx.

22. Jocelyn Frye, "On the Frontlines at Work and at Home: The Disproportionate Economic Effects of the Coronavirus Pandemic on Women of Color," *Center for Economic Progress*, April 23, 2020, https://www.americanprogress.org/article/frontlines-work-home/; Nikki Fortier, "Covid-19, Gender Inequality, and the Responsibility of the State," *International Journal Wellbeing* 10, no. 3 (2020): 78–90.

23. Sarah Todd, "Everything That's Wrong with Relying on Employers for Abortion Access," *Quartz*, June 28, 2022, https://qz.com/2183079/roe-v-wade-what-happens-when-employers-provide-abortion-access/.

24. Elisabeth Gawthrop, "The Color of Coronavirus: Covid-19 Deaths by Race and Ethnicity in the U.S.," *APM Research Lab*, March 21, 2013, https://www.kff.org/policy-watch/growing-data-underscore-communities-color-harder-hit-covid-19/; Thrasher, *Viral Underclass*.

25. Valerie Strauss, "Florida Law Limiting LGBTQ Discussions Takes Effect—and Rocks Schools," *Washington Post*, July 1, 2022, https://www.washingtonpost.com/education/2022/07/01/dont-say-gay-florida-law/.

26. Chávez, *Borders of AIDS*, 4.

27. Jürgens, "Ten Reasons to Oppose the Criminalization of HIV Exposure or Transmission," 166–67.

28. Center for HIV Law Policy, "What HIV Criminalization Means to Women in the U.S.," 1–5.

Bibliography

PRIMARY SOURCES

Manuscript and Archival Sources

Arthur and Elizabeth Schlesinger Library on the History of
  Women in America, Boston, MA
  Ann P. Meredith Papers
  Boston Women's Health Book Collective Records
  Call Off Your Old Tired Ethics Records
  Linda J. Laubenstein Papers
  Periodicals
    Communiqué: from the frontline. New York: Lesbian
      Avengers.
    LAP notes. Lesbian AIDS Project at GMHC.
    Lesbian Health Issues Newsletter. San Francisco, CA: National
      Center for Lesbian Rights.
GLBT Historical Society Archives and Special Collections,
  San Francisco, CA
  Lesbian Avengers Papers

Lesbian Herstory Archives, New York, NY
  Maxine Wolfe Papers
  Subject File: AIDS
LGBT Community Center National Archive, New York, NY
  Judy Greenspan Papers
Library of Congress, Washington, DC
  Ask Dr. Ruth Videotapes
  Unprocessed PR 13 CN 1991:022.
  Unprocessed PR 13 CN 1992:024.
  Unprocessed PR 13 CN 1992:149.
  Unprocessed PR 13 CN 1994:060.
  Abortion Debate at the National Press Club. January 1983.
National Library of Medicine Archives and Modern Manuscripts,
  Bethesda, MD
  C. Everett Koop Papers
New York Public Library Manuscripts and Archives Division, New
  York, NY
  Gay Men's Health Crisis (GMHC) Records
  Women's Action Coalition (WAC) Records
New York University Library Tamiment Library and Robert F. Wagner
  Labor Archives, New York, NY
  Women's Health Action Mobilization (WHAM!) Records
Ronald Reagan Presidential Library and Museum, Simi Valley, CA
  Beryl Sprinkel Files
  Dee Jepsen Files
  James Warner Files
  John Klenk Files
  K. Kae Rairdin Files
  Kathleen D. Koch Files
  Kenneth T. Cribb, Jr. Files
  Nancy Risque Files
  Office of White House Correspondence
  Richard A. Davis Files
  Robert Sweet Files

San Francisco Public Library James C. Hormel LGBTQIA Center, San Francisco, CA

LGBTQIA Ephemera Collection

University of California San Francisco Archives and Special Collections, San Francisco, CA

Nancy E. Stoller Papers Concerning Prison Inmate Health, 1970s–2000s

Selected Published Primary Sources and Memoirs

Banzhaf, Marion, Cynthia Chris, Kim Christensen, Alexis Danzig, Risa Denenberg, Zoe Leonard, Deb Levine, Rachel Lurie, Monica Pearl, Catherine Saalfield, Polly Thistlethwaite, Judith Walker, and Brigitte Weil. *Women, AIDS, and Activism by the ACT UP/NY Women and AIDS Handbook Group.* Boston: South End Press, 1999.

Boston Women's Health Book Collective. *New Our Bodies, Our Selves: A Book by and for Women.* New York: Simon & Schuster, 1992.

Boston Women's Health Collective. *Women and Their Bodies: A Course.* Boston: New England Free Press, 1971.

Boudin, Kathy, and Judith Clark. "Community of Women Organize Themselves to Cope with the AIDS Crisis: A Case Study from Bedford Hill Correctional Facility." *Social Justice* 17, no. 2 (Summer 1990): 90–109.

Cogswell, Kelly. *Eating Fire: My Life as a Lesbian Avenger.* Minneapolis: University of Minnesota Press, 2014.

Hollibaugh, Amber L. *My Dangerous Desires: A Queer Girl Dreaming Her Way Home.* Durham, NC: Duke University Press, 2000.

Jordan, June. *Some of Us Did Not Die: New and Selected Essays.* New York: Basic Books, 2002.

Koop, C. Everett. *The Memoirs of America's Family Doctor.* Grand Rapids, MI: Zondervan Publishing, 1992.

Lorde, Audre. *Sister Outsider: Essays and Speeches.* Berkeley: Crossing Press, c. 1984, 2007.

Mayersohn, Nettie. "The 'Baby AIDS' Bill." *Fordham Urban Law Journal* 24, no. 4 (1997): 721–28.

Members of the ACE Program at Bedford Hills. *Breaking the Walls of Silence: AIDS and Women in a New York Maximum Security Prison*. New York: Overlook Press, 1998.

Moraga, Chierríe, and Gloria Anzaldúa, eds. *This Bridge Called My Back: Writings by Radical Women of Color*. Albany: State University of New York Press, c. 1981, 2015.

Shange, Ntozake. *for colored girls who have considered suicide/when the rainbow is enuf.* New York: Schribner, c. 1977, 2010.

Staley, Peter. *Never Silent: ACT UP and My Life in Activism*. Chicago: Chicago Review Press, 2022.

Wattleton, Faye. *Life on the Line*. New York: Ballantine Books, 1996.

CDC Surveillance Reports

Accessed online through the CDC Reports Archive: https://www.cdc.gov /hiv/library/reports/hiv-surveillance-archive.html.

Court Cases

Dobbs v. Jackson Women's Health Organization, 597 U.S. (2022): 1–66.

Doe v. Jamaica Hospital, 608 N.Y.S.2d 518 (N.Y.App.Div. 1994).

Estelle v. Gamble, 429 U.S. 97 (1976): 104–5.

Peter Staley v. Gilead Sciences, Inc., Case No. 3:19-cv-2573 (2019): 1–136.

Planned Parenthood of Southeastern Pa. v. Casey, 505 U.S. 883 (1992): 833–1002.

Plata v. Davis, 329 F.3d 1101 (9th Cir. 2003): 2–20.

Roe v. Wade, 410 U.S. 113 (1973): 113–78.

Shumate v. Wilson, 95–619 (E.D. Cal. 1995): 1–21.

United States of America v. Gilead Sciences, Inc. et al., No. 1:2019cv02103— Document 61 (D. Del. 2021): 1–21.

Webster v. Reproductive Health Services, 492 US 490 (1989): 490–572.

Congressional Records

Accessed online through the Congressional Records Archive: https://www .congress.gov.

Oral History

ACT UP Oral History Project. http://www.actuporalhistory.org/index1.html.

Selected Newspapers and Periodicals

Boston Globe
The Independent
Irish Times
Los Angeles Times
Ms. Magazine
National Now Times
New Pittsburgh Courier
New York Amsterdam News
New York Magazine
New York Times
Out/Look
Outweek
Philadelphia Inquirer
Philadelphia Tribune
Richmond Times-Dispatch
San Jose Mercury News
Sinister Wisdom
Times of India
Trouble & Strife
University Wire
Wall Street Journal
Washington Blade
Washington Post

PRINTED SECONDARY WORKS

Ahmed, Aziza. "HIV and Women: Incongruent Policies, Criminal Consequences." *Yale Journal of International Affairs* 6, no. 1 (Winter 2011): 32–42.

Alexander, Michelle. *The New Jim Crow: Mass Incarceration in the Age of Colorblindness.* New York: New Press, 2012.

Austin, Sydney Bryn. "AIDS and Africa: United States Media and Racist Fantasy." *Cultural Critique* 14 (Winter 1989–90): 129–52.

Bailey, Moya. *Misogynoir: Black Women's Digital Resistance*. New York: New York University Press, 2021.

Baird, Karen L. *Beyond Reproduction: Women's Health, Activism, and Public Policy*. Madison, NJ: Fairleigh Dickinson University Press, 2009.

Batza, Katie. *Before AIDS: Gay Health Politics in the 1970s*. Philadelphia: University of Pennsylvania Press, 2018.

———. "From Sperm Runners to Sperm Banks: Lesbians, Assisted Conception, and Challenging the Fertility Industry, 1971–1983." *Journal of Women's History* 23, no. 2 (2016): 82–102.

Beckett, Katherine. "Fetal Rights and 'Crack Moms': Pregnant Women in the War on Drugs." *Contemporary Drug Problems* 22 (Winter 1995): 587–612.

Bell, Jonathan. "Between Private and Public: AIDS, Health Care Capitalism, and the Politics of Respectability in 1980s America." *Journal of American Studies* 54, no. 1 (February 2020): 159–83.

———. "Rethinking the 'Straight State': Welfare Politics, Health Care, and Public Policy in the Shadow of AIDS." *Journal of American History* 104, no. 4 (March 2018): 931–52.

Berger, Dan. *Captive Nation: Black Prison Organizing in the Civil Rights Era*. Chapel Hill: The University of North Carolina Press, 2014.

Berman, William C. *America's Right Turn: From Nixon to Clinton*. Baltimore: Johns Hopkins University Press, 1998.

Berube, Allan. *Coming Out Under Fire: The History of Gay Men and Women in WWII*. Chapel Hill: University of North Carolina Press, 2010.

Betts, Devon. "Who Gets to Be a #TruvadaWhore: Promiscuity, Race, and Queer Politics." *Radical History Review* 140 (May 2021): 157–63.

Booth, Karen M. "'Just Testing': Race, Sex, and the Media in New York's 'Baby AIDS' Debate.'" *Gender and Society* 14, no. 5 (October 2000): 644–61.

Bost, Darius. "Black Lesbian Feminist Intellectuals and the Struggle against HIV/AIDS," *Souls* 21, nos. 2–3 (2019): 169–91.

Bracewell, Lorna Norman. "Beyond Barnard: Liberalism, Antipornography Feminism, and the Sex Wars." *Signs* 42, no. 1 (Autumn 2016): 23–48.

Brandt, Allan M. *No Magic Bullet: A Social History of Venereal Disease in the United States Since 1880*. New York: Oxford University Press, 1987.

Braukman, Stacy. "'Nothing Else Matters but Sex': Cold War Narratives of Deviance and the Search for Lesbian Teachers in Florida, 1959–1963." *Feminist Studies* 27, no. 3 (Autumn 2001): 553–75.

Braxton, Joanna M., and Trimiko Melancon. *Black Female Sexualities*. New Brunswick, NJ: Rutgers University Press, 2015.

Brier, Jennifer. "'I'm Still Surviving': Oral Histories of Women Living with HIV/AIDS in Chicago." *The Oral History Review* 45 (2018): 68–83.

———. *Infectious Ideas: U.S. Political Responses to the AIDS Crisis*. Chapel Hill: University of North Carolina Press, 2009.

———. "'Save Our Kids, Keep AIDS out': Anti-AIDS Activism and the Legacy of Community Control in Queen's New York." *Journal of Social History* 39, no. 4 (Summer, 2006): 965–87.

Brier, Jennifer, Jonathan Bell, Julio Capó, Jih-Fei Cheng, Daniel M. Fox, Christina Hanhardt, Emily K. Hobson, and Dan Royles. "Interchange: HIV/AIDS and U.S. History." *Journal of American History* 104, Issue 2 (September 2017): 431–60.

Briggs, Laura. *Reproducing Empire: Race, Sex, Science, and U.S. Imperialism in Puerto Rico*. Berkeley: University of California Press, 2002.

———. *Taking Children: A History of American Terror*. Oakland: University of California Press, 2020.

Brownlee, W. Elliot, and Hugh David Graham, eds. *The Reagan Presidency: Pragmatic Conservatism and Its Legacies*. Lawrence: University Press of Kansas, 2003.

Caldwell, John C., and Pat Quiggin. "The Social Context of AIDS in Sub-Saharan Africa." *Population and Development Review* 15, no. 2 (June 1989): 185–234.

Canaday, Margot. *Queer Career: Sexuality and Work in Modern America*. Princeton, NJ: Princeton University Press, 2022.

———. *The Straight State: Sexuality and Citizenship in Twentieth-Century America*. Princeton, NJ: Princeton University Press, 2009.

Capo, Beth Widmaier. *Textual Contraception: Birth Control and Modern American Fiction*. Columbus: Ohio State University Press, 2021.

Carroll, Tamar W. *Mobilizing New York: AIDS, Antipoverty, and Feminist Activism*. Chapel Hill: University of North Carolina Press, 2015.

Chappell, Marisa. *The War on Welfare: Family, Poverty, and Politics in Modern America*. Philadelphia: University of Pennsylvania Press, 2010.

Chase, Marilyn. *The Barbary Plague: The Black Death in Victorian San Francisco.* New York: Random House, 2003.

Chávez, Karma R. *The Borders of AIDS: Race, Quarantine, and Resistance.* Seattle: University of Washington Press, 2021.

Christiansen, Adrienne E., and Jeremy J. Hanson, "Comedy as Cure for Tragedy: ACT UP and the Rhetoric of AIDS." *Quarterly Journal of Speech* 82, no. 2 (1996): 157–70.

Cobble, Dorothy Sue, Linda Gordon, and Astrid Henry. *Feminism Unfinished: A Short, Surprising History of American Women's Movements.* New York: Liveright Publishing, 2014.

Cogswell, Kelly. *Eating Fire: My Life as a Lesbian Avenger.* Minneapolis: University of Minnesota Press, 2014.

Cohen, Cathy J. *The Boundaries of Blackness: AIDS and the Breakdown of Black Politics.* Chicago: University of Chicago Press, 1999.

———. "Punks, Bulldaggers, and Welfare Queens: The Radical Potential of Queer Politics?" *GLQ* 3 (1997): 427–65.

Cohen, Peter F. "'All They Needed': AIDS, Consumption, and the Politics of Class." *Journal of the History of Sexuality* 8, no. 1 (July 1997): 86–115.

———. *Love and Anger: Essays on AIDS, Activism, and Politics.* New York: Routledge, c. 1993, 2013.

Coker Burks, Ruth. *All the Young Men.* London: Trapeze, 2021.

Collins, Patricia Hill. *Black Feminist Thought: Knowledge, Consciousness, and the Politics of Empowerment.* New York: Routledge, 1991.

Colter, Ephen G. *Public Sex: Queer Politics and the Future of AIDS Activism.* Boston: South End Press, 1996.

Cooper, Melinda. *Family Values: Between Neoliberalism and the New Social Conservatism.* New York: Zone Books, 2017.

Corbman, Rachel. "Remediating Disability Activism in the Lesbian Feminist Archive." *Continuum: Journal of Media & Cultural Studies* 32, no. 1 (2017): 18–28.

Corea, Gena. *The Invisible Epidemic: The Story of Women with AIDS.* New York: HarperCollins, 1992.

Crimp, Douglas. "How to Have Promiscuity in an Epidemic." In "AIDS: Cultural Analysis/Cultural Activism." Special issue, *October* 43 (Winter 1987): 237–71.

———. *Melancholia and Moralism: Essays on AIDS and Queer Politics.* Cambridge, MA: MIT Press, 2002.

Critchlow, Donald T. *Phyllis Schlafly and Grassroots Conservatism*. Princeton, NJ: Princeton University Press, 2005.

Cvetkovich, Ann. *An Archive of Feelings: Trauma, Sexuality, and Lesbian Public Cultures*. Durham, NC: Duke University Press, 2003.

Davis, Angela Y. *Are Prisons Obsolete?* New York: Seven Stories Press, 2003.

Davis, Angela Y., and Cassandra Shaylor. "Race, Gender, and the Prison Industrial Complex: California and Beyond." *Meridians* 2, no. 1 (2001): 1–25.

D'Emilio, John, and Estelle B. Freedman. *Intimate Matters: A History of Sexuality in America*. 3rd ed. Chicago: University of Chicago Press, 2012.

D'Emilio, John, and William B. Turner, eds. *Creating Change: Sexuality, Public Policy, and Civil Rights*. New York: St. Martin's Press, 2000.

De Orio, Scott. "The Invention of Bad Gay Sex: Texas and the Creation of a Criminal Underclass of Gay People." *Journal of the History of Sexuality* 26, no. 1 (January 2017): 53–87.

Diaz-Cotto, Juanita. *Chicana Lives and Criminal Justice: Voices from El Barrio*. Austin: University of Texas Press, 2006.

Downs, Jim. *Stand by Me: The Forgotten History of Gay Liberation*. New York: Basic Books, 2016.

Dubow, Sara. *Ourselves Unborn: A History of the Fetus in Modern America*. New York: Oxford University Press, 2011.

Engel, Johnathan. *Poor People's Medicine: Medicaid and American Charity Care Since 1965*. Durham, NC: Duke University Press, 2006.

Engelman, Peter C. *A History of the Birth Control Movement in America*. Santa Barbara, CA: Praeger, 2011.

English, Deirdre, Amber Hollibaugh, and Gayle Rubin. "Talking Sex: A Conversation on Sexuality and Feminism," *Feminist Review* 11 (Summer 1982): 40–52.

Engs, Ruth C. *The Progressive Era's Health Reform Movement: A Historical Dictionary*. Westport, CT: Praeger, 2003.

Epstein, Steven. *Impure Science: AIDS, Activism, and the Politics of Knowledge*. Berkeley: University of California Press, 1996.

Esterberg, Kristin G. "From Accommodation to Liberation: A Social Movement Analysis of Lesbians in the Homophile Movement." *Gender and Society* 8, no. 3 (September 1994): 442–443.

Evans, Sara M. *Tidal Wave: How Women Changed America at Century's End*. New York: Free Press, 2003.

Faderman, Lillian. *Odd Girls and Twilight Lovers: A History of Lesbian Life in 20th-Century America*. New York: Columbia University Press, 1991.

———. *Surpassing the Love of Men: Romantic Friendship and Love Between Women from the Renaissance to the Present*. New York: Morrow, 1981.

Faith, Karlene. *Unruly Women: The Politics of Confinement and Resistance*. Vancouver: Press Gang Publishers, 1993.

Fateman, Johanna, and Amy Scholder. *Last Days at Hot Slit: The Radical Feminism of Andrea Dworkin*. Cambridge, MA: MIT Press, 2019.

Fee, Elizabeth, and Daniel M. Fox, eds. *AIDS: The Burdens of History*. Berkeley: University of California Press, 1988.

Feldman, Robin, and Evan Frondorf. *Drug Wars: How Big Pharma Raises Prices and Keeps Generics Off the Market*. Cambridge: Cambridge University Press, 2017.

Ferguson, Ann. "Sex War: The Debate between Radical and Libertarian Feminists." *Signs* 10, no. 1 (Autumn 1984): 106–12.

Flint, Adrian, and Vernon Hewitt. "Colonial Tropes and HIV/AIDS in Africa: Sex, Disease, and Race." *Commonwealth and Comparative Politics* 53, no. 3 (2015): 294–314.

Flowers, Prudence. "'Voodoo Biology': The Right-to-Life Campaign against Family Planning Programs in the United States in the 1980s." *Women's History Review* 29, no. 2 (2020): 331–56.

Frank, Gillian. "'The Civil Rights of Parents': Race and Conservative Politics in Anita Bryant's Campaign against Gay Rights in 1970s Florida." *Journal of the History of Sexuality* 22, no. 1 (January 2013): 126–60.

Freedman, Estelle B., "The Prison Lesbian: Race, Class and the Construction of the Aggressive Female Homosexual." *Feminist Studies* 22, no. 2 (Summer 1996): 397–415.

Gabriel, Joseph M. *Medical Monopoly: Intellectual Property Rights and the Origins of the Modern Pharmaceutical Industry*. Chicago: University of Chicago Press, 2014.

Genter, Alix. "Appearances Can be Deceiving: Butch-Femme Fashion and Queer Legibility in New York City, 1945–1969." *Feminist Studies* 42, no. 3 (2016): 604–31.

Gerstle, Gary. *The Rise and Fall of the Neoliberal Order*. New York: Oxford University Press, 2022.

Ghaziani, Amin. *The Dividends of Dissent: How Conflict and Culture Work in Lesbian and Gay Marches on Washington.* Chicago: University of Chicago Press, 2008.

Gilman, Sander L. "AIDS and Syphilis: The Iconography of Disease." *October* 43 (Winter 1987): 87–107.

Gilmore, Ruth W. *Golden Gulag: Prisons, Surplus, Crisis, and Opposition In Globalizing California.* Berkeley: University of California Press, 2006.

Glick, Elisa. "Sex Positive: Feminism, Queer Theory, and the Politics of Transformation." *Feminist Review* 64 (Spring 2000): 19–45.

Golden, Janet. "'An Argument that Goes Back to the Womb': The Demedicalization of Fetal Alcohol Syndrome, 1973–1992." *Journal of Social History* 33, no. 2 (Winter 1999): 269–98.

Goldstein, Nancy, and Jennifer L. Manlowe. *The Gender Politics of HIV/AIDS in Women.* New York: New York University Press, 1997.

Goodwin, Michele. "How the Criminalization of Pregnancy Robs Women of Reproductive Autonomy." *The Hastings Center Report* 47 (2017): S19-S27.

Gordon, Linda. *Pitied but Not Entitled: Single Mothers and the History of Welfare, 1890–1935.* New York: Free Press, 1994.

Gould, Deborah B. *Moving Politics: Emotion and ACT UP's Fight Against AIDS.* Chicago: University of Chicago Press, 2009.

Grant, Judith. "Andrea Dworkin and the Social Construction of Gender: A Retrospective." *Signs* 31, no. 4 (Summer 2006): 967–93.

Greene, Jeremy A. *Generic: The Unbranding of Modern Medicine.* Baltimore: Johns Hopkins University Press, 2014.

Greenspan, Judy. "Struggle for Compassion: The Fight for Quality Care for Women with AIDS at Central California Women's Facility." *Yale Journal of Law & Feminism* 6 Issue. 2 (1993): 393–95.

Hall, Simon. "Americanism, Un-Americanism, and the Gay Rights Movement." *Journal of American Studies* 47 (November 2013): 1109–30.

Hammonds, Evelynn. "Missing Persons: African American Women, AIDS, and the History of Disease," *Radical America* 21, no. 2 (1990): 17–18.

———. "Race, Sex, AIDS: The Construction of 'Other.'" *Radical America* 20, no. 6 (September 1987): 28–39.

Hanhardt, Christina B. *Safe Space: Gay Neighborhood History and the Politics of Violence.* Durham, NC: Duke University Press, 2013.

Hansen, Randall, and Desmond King. *Sterilized by the State: Eugenics, Race, and the Population Scare in Twentieth-Century North America*. Cambridge: Cambridge University Press, 2013.

Hewitt, Nancy, ed. *A Companion to American Women's History*. Malden, MA: Blackwell Publishing, 2002.

Higginbotham, Evelyn Brooks. *Righteous Discontent: The Women's Movement in the Black Baptist Church*. Cambridge, MA: Harvard University Press, 1993.

Hill, Amy Pétre. "Death through Administrative Indifference: The Prison Litigation Reform Act Allows Women to Die in California's Substandard Prison Health Care System." *Hastings Women's Law Journal* 13, no. 2 (Summer 2002): 231–60.

Hilliman, Betty Luther. "'The Most Profoundly Revolutionary Act a Homosexual Can Engage In': Drag and the Politics of Gender Presentation in San Francisco Gay Liberation Movement." *Journal of the History of Sexuality* 20, no. 1 (January 2011): 153–81.

Hinton, Elizabeth. *From the War on Poverty to the War on Crime*. Cambridge, MA: Harvard University Press, 2016.

Hobson, Emily. *Lavender and Red: Liberation and Solidarity in the Gay and Lesbian Left*. Berkeley: University of California Press, 2016.

Hoffman, Beatrix. *Healthcare for Some: Rights and Rationing in the United States Since 1930*. Chicago: University of Chicago Press, 2012.

———. "Healthcare Reform and Social Movements in the US." *American Journal of Public Health* 93, no. 1 (2003): 75–85.

Hollibaugh, Amber L. *My Dangerous Desires: A Queer Girl Dreaming Her Way Home*. Durham, NC: Duke University Press, 2000.

Hoppe, Trevor. *Punishing Disease: HIV and the Criminalization of Sickness*. Oakland: University of California Press, 2018.

Irvine, Janet M. *Talk About Sex: The Battles over Sex Education in the United States*. Berkeley: University of California Press, 2002.

Jacobs, Charlotte. *Jonas Salk: A Life*. New York: Oxford University Press, 2015.

Jacobs, Nicholas F., Desmond King, and Sidney M. Milkis. "Building a Conservative State: Partisan Polarization and the Redeployment of Administrative Power." *American Political Science Association* 17, no. 2 (June 2019): 453–69.

Jeffries, Charlie. "Adolescent Women and the Antiabortion Politics in the Reagan Administration." *Journal of American Studies* 52, no. 1 (2018): 193–213.

Johns, Andrew L. *A Companion to Ronald Reagan.* Malden, MA: Wiley Blackwell, 2015.

Johnson, David K. *The Lavender Scare: The Cold War Prosecution of Gays and Lesbians in the Federal Government.* Chicago: University of Chicago Press, 2004.

Johnson, Haynes. *Sleepwalking through History: America in the Reagan Years.* New York: W. W. Norton, 2003.

Johnston, Jill. *Lesbian Nation: The Feminist Solution.* New York: Bantam, 1973.

Jones, James J. *Bad Blood: The Tuskegee Syphilis Experiment.* New York: Free Press, 1981.

Jonsen, Albert R., and Jeff Strikes, eds. *The Social Impact of AIDS in the United States.* Washington, DC: National Academies Press, 1993.

Kalman, Laura. *Right Star Rising: A New Politics, 1974–1980.* New York: W. W. Norton, Inc., 2010.

Kennedy, Elizabeth Lapovsky, and Madeline D. Davis. *Boots of Leather, Slippers of Gold: The History of a Lesbian Community.* New York: Routledge, 1993.

Klein, Jennifer. "The Business of Health Security: Employee Health Benefits, Commercial Insurers, and the Reconstruction of Welfare Capitalism, 1945–1960." *International Labor and Working Class History* 58 (Fall 2000): 293–313.

Kline, Wendy. *Bodies of Knowledge: Sexuality, Reproduction, and Women's Health in the Second Wave.* Chicago: University of Chicago Press, 2010.

——. *Coming Home: How Midwives Changed Birth.* Oxford: Oxford University Press, 2019.

Kohler-Hausmann, Julilly. *Getting Tough: Welfare and Imprisonment in 1970s.* Princeton, NJ: University of Princeton Press, 2017.

Kunzel, Regina. *Criminal Intimacy: Prison and the Uneven History of Modern American Sexuality.* Chicago: University of Chicago Press, 2008.

Law, Victoria. *Resistance behind Bars: The Struggles of Incarcerated Women.* Oakland, CA: PM Press, 2009.

Lee, Ellie. *Abortion, Motherhood, and Mental Health: Medicalizing Reproduction in the United States and Great Britain* (Hawthorne, NY: Aldine de Gruyter, 2003).

Logan, Enid. "The Wrong Race, Committing Crime, Doing Drugs, and Maladjusted for Motherhood: The Nation's Fury over 'Crack Babies.'" *Social Justice* 26, no. 1 (Spring 1999): 115–38.

Loyd, Jenna M., and Alison Mountz, *Boats, Borders, and Bases: Race, the Cold War, and the Rise of Migration Detention in the United States*. Oakland: University of California Press, 2018.

Manne, Kate. *Down Girl: The Logic of Misogyny*. New York: Oxford University Press, 2018.

Martin, William. *With God on Our Side: The Rise of the Religious Right in America*. New York: Broadway Books, 1996.

Mason, Carol. *Killing for Life: The Apocalyptic Narrative of Pro-Life Politics*. Ithaca, NY: Cornell University Press, 2018.

Mason, Robert. *The Republican Party and American Politics from Hoover to Reagan*. Cambridge: Cambridge University Press, 2011.

Matthiesen, Sara. "Equality versus Reproductive Risk: Women-and-AIDS Activism and False Choice in the Clinical Trials Debate." *Signs* 41, no. 3 (2016): 579–601.

McAndrews, Lawrence J. *What They Wished For: American Catholics and American Presidents, 1960–2004*. Athens: University of Georgia Press, 2014.

McGirr, Lisa. *Suburban Warriors: The Origins of the New American Right*. Princeton, NJ: Princeton University Press, 2001.

McGovern, Theresa. "S. P. v. Sullivan: The Effort to Broaden the Social Security Administration's Definition of AIDS." *Fordham Urban Law Journal* 21, no. 4 (1994): 1083–96.

McGuire, Danielle L. *At The Dark End of the Street: Black Women, Rape, and Resistance; A New History of the Civil Rights Movement from Rosa Parks to the Rise of Black Power*. New York: Alfred A. Knopf, 2010.

McKay, Richard A. *Patient Zero and the Making of the AIDS Epidemic*. Chicago: University of Chicago Press, 2017.

McTighe, Laura. "Our Relationships Carry the Movement." *Radical History Review* 140 (May 2021): 186–96.

Meulen Rodgers, Yana van der. *The Global Gag Rule and Women's Reproductive Health: Rhetoric Versus Reality*. New York: Oxford University Press, 2018.

Miley, William M. *The Psychology of Well Being*. Westport, CT: Greenwood Publishing, 1999.

Moir, Nathaniel L. "To Boldly Remember Where We Have Already Been: Revisiting the Cutter Polio Vaccine Incident during Operation Warp Speed." *Journal of Applied History* 2 (2020): 17–35.

Moran, Rachel Louise. "A Woman's Health Issue? Framing Post-Abortion Syndrome in the 1980s." *Gender & History* 33, no. 3 (2021): 790–804.

Morgen, Sandra. *Into Our Own Hands: The Women's Health Movement in the United States, 1969–1990.* New Brunswick, NJ: Rutgers University Press, 2002.

Mukherjee, Siddhartha. *The Emperor of All Maladies: A Biography of Cancer.* London: Fourth Estate, 2011.

Mumford, Kevin J. *Not Straight, Not White: Black Gay Men from the March on Washington to the AIDS Crisis.* Chapel Hill: University of North Carolina Press, 2016.

Murakawa, Naomi. *The First Civil Right: How Liberals Built Prison America.* Oxford: Oxford University Press, 2014.

Musser, Amber Jamilla. "From Our Body to Yourselves: The Boston Women's Health Book Collective and Changing Notions of Subjectivity, 1969–1973." *Women's Studies Quarterly* 35, nos. 1–2 (2007): 93–109.

Nelson, Alondra. *Body and Soul: The Black Panther Party and the Fight against Medical Discrimination.* Minneapolis: University of Minnesota Press, 2011.

Nelson, Jennifer M. *More Than Medicine: A History of the Feminist Women's Health Movement.* New York: New York University Press, 2015.

———. *Women of Color and the Reproductive Rights Movement.* New York: New York University Press, 2003.

Newman, Karen. *Fetal Position: Individualism, Science, Visuality.* Stanford, CA: Stanford University Press, 1996.

Noe, Victoria. *Fag Hags, Divas, and Moms: The Legacy of Straight Women in the AIDS Community.* Chicago: King Company Publishing, 2019.

O'Connor, John. "Us Social Welfare Policy: The Reagan Record and Legacy." *Journal of Social Policy* 7, no.1 (1998): 37–61.

Odem, Mary E. *Delinquent Daughters: Protecting and Policing Adolescent Female Sexuality in the United States, 1885–1920.* Chapel Hill: University of North Carolina Press, 2000.

Olivarius, Kathryn. *Necropolis: Disease, Power, and Capitalism in the Cotton Kingdom.* Cambridge, MA: Harvard University Press, 2022.

Ordaz, Jessica. "AIDS Knows No Borders." *Radical History Review* 140 (2021): 175–85.

Oshinsky, David M. *Polio: An American Story.* New York: Oxford University Press, 2005.

Owens, Deidre Cooper. *Medical Bondage: Race, Gender, and the Origins of American Gynecology*. Athens: University of Georgia Press, 2017.

Patterson, James T. *Restless Giant: The United States from Watergate to Bush v. Gore*. New York: Oxford University Press, 2005.

Patton, Cindy. *Inventing AIDS*. New York: Routledge, 1990.

———. *Last Served? Gendering the HIV Pandemic*. London: Taylor & Francis, 1994.

Petro, Anthony M. *After the Wrath of God: AIDS, Sexuality, and American Religion*. New York: Oxford University Press, 2015.

Reagan, Leslie J. "Crossing the Border for Abortions: California Activists, Mexican Clinics, and the Creation of a Feminist Health Agency in the 1960s." *Feminist Studies* 26, no. 2 (Summer 2000): 323–48.

———. *Dangerous Pregnancies: Mothers, Disabilities, and Abortion in Modern America*. Berkeley: University of California Press, 2010.

———. *When Abortion was a Crime: Women, Medicine, and Law in the United States, 1867–1973*. Berkeley: University of California Press, 1997.

Redick, Alison, Eva Pendleton, Ephen Glenn Colter, and Wayne Hoffman, eds. *Policing Public Sex: Queer Politics and the Future of AIDS Activism*. (Boston: South End Press, 1996).

Renfro, Paul. *Stranger Danger: Family Values, Childhood, and the American Carceral State*. New York: Oxford University Press, 2020.

Rich, Adrienne. "Compulsory Heterosexuality and Lesbian Existence." *Signs* 5, no. 4 (Summer 1980): 631–60.

Richie, Beth E. *Arrested Justice: Black Women, Violence, and America's Prison Nation*. New York: New York University Press, 2012.

Roberts, Dorothy E. *Killing The Black Body: Race, Reproduction, and the Meaning of Liberty*. New York: Vintage Books, 1999.

———. *Shattered Bonds: The Color of Child Welfare*. New York: Basic Books, 2002.

Rogers, Naomi. "'Caution: The AMA May be Dangerous to Your Health': The Student Health Organizations (SHO) and American Medicine, 1965–1970." *Radical History Review* 80 (Spring 2001): 5–34.

———. "Race and the Politics of Polio: Warm Springs, Tuskegee, and the March of Dimes." *American Journal of Public Health* (May 1, 2007): 784–95.

Rosenberg, Charles. *The Cholera Years: The United States in 1832, 1849, and 1866*. Chicago: University of Chicago Press, 1962.

Rossinow, Doug. *The Reagan Era: A History of the 1980s.* New York: Oxford University Press, 2015.

Roth, Nancy L., and Katie Hogan. *Gendered Epidemic: Representations of Women in the Age of AIDS.* New York: Routledge, 1998.

Roth, Rachel. *Making Women Pay: The Hidden Costs of Fetal Rights.* Ithaca, NY: Cornell University Press, 2000.

Royles, Daniel. *To Make the Wounded Whole: The African American Struggle against HIV/AIDS.* Chapel Hill: University of North Carolina Press, 2021.

Ruzek, Sheryl B. *The Women's Health Movement: Feminist Alternatives to Medical Control.* New York: Praeger, 1978.

Schaller, Michael. *Right Turn: American Life in the Reagan-Bush Era, 1980–1992.* New York: Oxford University Press, 2007.

Scheffler, Judith A., ed. *Wall Tappings: An International Anthology of Women's Prison Writings, 200 to the Present.* New York: Feminist Press at CUNY, 2002.

Schneider, Beth E., and Nancy E. Stoller, *Women Resisting AIDS: Feminist Strategies of Empowerment.* Philadelphia: Temple University Press, 1995.

Schoen, Johanna. *Abortion after Roe.* Chapel Hill: University of North Carolina Press, 2015.

Schulman, Sarah. *Let the Record Show: A Political History of ACT UP New York, 1987–1993.* New York: Farrar, Straus and Giroux, 2021.

Self, Robert O. *All in the Family: The Realignment of American Democracy Since the 1960s.* New York: Hill and Wang, 2012.

Shilts, Randy. *And the Band Played On: Politics, People, and the AIDS Epidemic.* New York: Penguin, 1988.

Shotwell, Alexis. "'Women Don't Get AIDS, They Just Die From It': Memory, Classification, and the Campaign to Change the Definition of AIDS." *Hypatia* 29, no. 2 (Spring 2014): 509–25.

Silliman, Jael Miriam, Marlene Gerber, and Loretta Ross. *Undivided Rights: Women of Color Organize for Reproductive Rights.* Chicago: Haymarket Books, 2016.

Skocpol, Theda. *Protecting Soldiers and Mothers: The Political Origins of Social Policy in the United States.* Cambridge, MA: Belknap Press of Harvard University Press, 1992.

Solinger, Rickie, ed. *Abortion Wars: A Half Century of Struggle, 1950–2000.* Berkeley: University of California Press, 1998.

—————. *Beggars and Choosers: How the Politics of Choice Shapes Adoption, Abortion, and Welfare in the United States*. New York: Farrar, Straus and Giroux, 2002.

—————. *Pregnancy and Power: A Short History of Reproductive Politics in America*. New York: New York University Press, c. 2005, 2019.

—————. *Wake Up Little Susie*. New York: Routledge, 2000.

Sontag, Susan. *Illness as Metaphor and AIDS and Its Metaphors*. New York: Anchor Books, 1989.

Staggenborg, Suzanne. "The Survival of the Pro-Choice Movement." *Journal of Policy History* 7, no. 1 (1995): 160–76.

Stern, Scott W. *The Trials of Nina McCall: Sex, Surveillance, and the Decades-Long Government Plan to Imprison "Promiscuous" Women*. Boston: Beacon Press, 2019.

Stillwaggon, Eileen. "Racial Metaphors: Interpreting Sex and AIDS in Africa." *Development and Change* 34, no. 5 (2003): 809–32.

Stoever, Jane K. "Stories Absent from the Courtroom: Responding to Domestic Violence in the Context of HIV and AIDS." *North Carolina Law Review* 87, 1157 (May 2009): 1157–1229.

Stoller, Nancy E. *Lessons from the Damned: Queers, Whores, and Junkies Respond to AIDS*. New York: Routledge, 1998.

Strongman, SaraEllen. "'Creating Justice Between Us': Audre Lorde's Theory of the Erotic as Coalitional Politics in the Women's Movement." *Feminist Theory* 19, no. 1 (2017): 41–59.

Susser, Ida. *AIDS, Sex, and Culture: Global Politics and Survival in Southern Africa*. Chichester, West Sussex, UK: Wiley-Blackwell, 2009.

Taylor, Keeanga-Yamahtta. *Race for Profit: How Banks and the Real Estate Industry Undermined Black Homeownership*. Chapel Hill: University of North Carolina Press, 2019.

Taylor, Verta, and Leila J. Rupp. "Women's Culture and Lesbian Feminist Activism: a Reconsideration of Cultural Feminism." *Signs* (1993): 32–61.

Theoharis, Jeanne, Komozi Woodard, and Dayo F. Gore, eds. *Want to Start to a Revolution? Radical Women in the Black Freedom Struggle*. New York: New York University Press, 2009.

Thompson, Becky. "Multiracial Feminism: Recasting the Chronology of Second Wave Feminism." *Feminist Studies* (Summer 2002): 336–60.

Thompson, Heather Ann. *Blood in the Water: The Attica Prison Uprising of 1971 and Its Legacy*. New York: Pantheon Books, 2016.

———. "Why Mass Incarceration Matters: Rethinking Crisis, Decline, and Transformation in Postwar American History." *Journal of American History* 97, no. 3 (December 1, 2010): 703–34.

Thrasher, Steven W. *The Viral Underclass: The Human Toll When Inequality and Disease Collide*. New York: Macmillan, 2022.

Thuma, Emily L. *All Our Trials: Prisons, Policing, and the Feminist Fight to End Violence*. Urbana: University of Illinois Press, 2019.

Treichler, Paula A. "AIDS, Homophobia, and Biomedical Discourse: An Epidemic of Signification." *October* 43 (Winter 1987): 31–70.

———. *How to Have Theory in an Epidemic: Cultural Chronicles of AIDS*. Durham, NC: Duke University Press, 1999.

Turner, William B. "'Adolph Reagan?' Ronald Reagan, AIDS, and Lesbian/Gay Civil Rights." (July 13, 2009): 15–16. Available at SSRN: https://ssrn.com/abstract=1433567.

Wacquant, Loïc. *Punishing the Poor: The Neoliberal Government of Social Insecurity*. Durham, NC: Duke University Press, 2009.

Warshaw, Robin. *I Never Called It Rape: The Ms. Report on Recognizing, Fighting, and Surviving Date and Acquaintance Rape* (New York: Harper and Row, 1988).

Washington, Harriet A. *Medical Apartheid: The Dark History of Medical Experimentation on Black Americans from Colonial Times to the Present*. New York: Doubleday, 2006.

Watkins-Hayes, Celeste. *Remaking a Life: How Women Living with HIV-AIDS Confront Inequality*. Oakland: University of California Press, 2019.

Weil, Brian. *Every Seventeen Seconds: A Global Perspective on the AIDS Crisis*. New York: Aperture, 1992.

Wexler, Alice. *The Woman Who Walked into the Sea: Huntington's and the Making of a Genetic Disease*. New Haven: Yale University Press, 2008.

Wilentz, Sean. *The Age of Reagan: A History, 1974–2008*. New York: HarperCollins, 2008.

Winnow, Jackie. "Lesbians Evolving Health Care: Cancer and AIDS." *Feminist Review* 41 (Summer 1992): 68–76.

Young, Neil J. *We Gather Together: The Religious Right and the Problem of Interfatih Politics.* New York: Oxford University Press, 2016.

Ziegler, Mary. *Abortion and the Law in America: Roe v. Wade to the Present.* Cambridge: Cambridge fader

——. *After Roe: The Lost History of the Abortion Debate.* Cambridge, MA: Harvard University Press, 2015.

Index

antiabortion activism *(continued)*
murder, 204; Title X (Public Health
Service Act), "domestic gag-rule"
amendment, 81; *Whatever Happened to
the Human Race?* (film), 77; white
women's pregnancies as priority of,
71. *See also* abortion; family values
politics; fetal rights; Koop's abortion
report (never published); Planned
Parenthood and other nonprofit
health services—Trump administration's political assault on
antiretroviral therapy (ART, "drug
cocktail"): announcement of (1996),
130; and change from "dying with
AIDS" to "living with HIV," 13, 170,
200; cost of, as prohibitive, 170; the
epidemic as ongoing after the advent
of, 13–14; lesbian activists working to
secure access, 130; prevalence of AIDS
rising after introduction of, 171; prison
cases of HIV/AIDS, costs of treatment
leading to neglect, 138–39; side effects
as severe, 170
anti-welfare agenda of neoliberalism: the
CDC's definition of AIDS deliberately
limited to avoid expenditures, 27;
Clinton administration welfare
reform, 67, 121–22, 146; cuts to welfare
services, and likelihood of HIV-positive children entering foster care, 88;
pressure to terminate pregnancies by
HIV-positive women to avoid the
costs of sick children, 60, 66–68, 71,
94–95; racial and gender prejudices
attributing poverty and social unrest
to perceived "pathology," 8; the
shrinking of the welfare state and

redeployment of state power to
expand the carceral state, 8, 146;
"small state" rhetoric of, 67; and
structural inequalities, refusal to
address, 8, 146; vilification of people
reliant on state aid as justification of,
3, 67, 121–22; women's health care and
social support funding slashed, 43, 53,
60–61, 66–67, 80. *See also* carceral
state, expansion of; family values
politics; neoliberalism; Planned
Parenthood and other nonprofit
health services—Trump administration's political assault on
Archer, David, 152–53
Arkansas, 94
artificial insemination, 100, 129
artists: documenting growing up an
HIV-positive woman of color,
199–202; on the fear and isolation of
HIV/AIDS women, 87; on the
guilty-innocent binary of HIV/AIDS,
92, 93; on intimate partner violence in
response to women's HIV/AIDS
disclosure, 49; protesting diagnosis
discrimination, 32. See also *Safer Sex
Handbook for Lesbians* (LAP)
ART. *See* antiretroviral therapy (ART,
"drug cocktail")
Asian and Pacific Islander Coalition on
HIV/AIDS, 200
Atlanta, Georgia, 32
Atwood, Margaret J., 80
AZT (azidothymidine): approval by FDA
(1987), 34; approval for prevention of
perinatal transmission (1994), 38,
93–94; criticism of high price of, 35;
drug trial in pregnant women (076),

and controversies, 35–38; drug trials, original, 34; found to cause cancers in animals, 35, 37, 87; international trials of, 37–38; the moral panic over mother-to-child transmission as eased by approval of, 15, 38, 42, 93, 96, 101; prison cases of HIV/AIDS, cost of treatment leading to neglect, 139–40; side effects and toxicity of, 37. *See also* antiretroviral therapy (ART, "drug cocktail")

bacterial pneumonia, 33, 143
Bailey, Moya, 137
Baker, Joan, 4–5, 109–10, *110*
Banzhaf, Marion, 30, 36–37, 49–50, 51, 105
Barry, Ellen, 156
Bauer, Gary L., 72, 75–76, 83
Bayh-Dole Act (1980), 192
Beal v. Doe, 72
Bedford Hills Correctional Facility (Westchester County, NY): ACT UP/New York Women's Caucus members as formerly incarcerated in, 30; AIDS Counseling and Education (ACE) program, 11–12, 135, 143, 144; education of guards and other inmates, 143–44; isolation of HIV-positive women and unnecessary use of PPE, 143–44; medical mistreatment of women in, 163, 165. *See also* women's prisons
Bennett, Kwan, 200
Bennett, William, 75–76
Betts, Devon, 182
Bill and Melinda Gates Foundation, 174
bisexual women: heterosexist biases and marginalization in health care system, 129; intravenous drug use

among, 108; prevalence of HIV infection among, 108–9. *See also* gay and lesbian (LGBTQI+) rights, attacks on; women who have sex with women
Black communities: criminalization of HIV as disproportionately affecting, 207–8; expansion of the carceral state and increase in HIV/AIDS rates, 146; historic exploitation by medical researchers, 36–37, 42–43; historic failure of public health agencies to address STDs in, 26; racial stereotypes linking Blackness with criminality, 90. *See also* crack cocaine
Black feminists: critiquing failure of lesbian separatism to address intersectional oppressions, 103; and queer politics, development of, 5–6; and the radical feminist stance against pornography and sadomasochism, 103
Black gay men: race excluded in initial PCP reports, 23. *See also* men who have sex with men (MSM)
Black women: collaboration on *New Our Bodies, Ourselves* with BWHBC, 49–50; criminalization of HIV and disproportionate prosecution of, 69, 70–72, 95, 204; drug and HIV testing and reporting of pregnant women, 7, 69, 70–71, 87–88, 95; forced sterilization of, 42, 53; and HIV drug trials, controversies surrounding, 36–37; and mandatory HIV testing of pregnant women, activists' concerns about, 42–43; maternal mortality rates as steeply increasing, 186; misdiagnosis

California Department of Corrections and Rehabilitation (CDCR): *Brown v. Plata* requiring the reduction of prison population, 164; class-action suit for medical mistreatment of women with HIV/AIDS (see *Shumate v. Wilson*); co-pay for sick call visits, 148; guards as Medical Technician Assistants (MTAs), as gatekeepers of women's access to health care, 137, 141–42, 147–48, 151, 152–53, 155, 157, 161, 163; policies of, as punitive and inefficient, 142, 148; rules used to forbid HIV support groups, 145; suits for men's prison conditions, 164. *See also* CCWF

California Institution for Women (CIW, Frontera), 144. See also *Shumate v. Wilson*

Call Off Your Old Tired Ethics (COYOTE), 42–43

Campbell, Catherine, 151, 156

Canaday, Margot, 64, 117

capitalist health-care system (US): overview, 179; charity from private companies, limitations on, 193; employment disparities and, 206; on health care as a right and not a privilege, 6, 57; only the insured benefit from medical advances, 140; private retail clinics, 186–87; and universal health care, need for, 130, 198, 206. *See also* health insurance, lack of; pharmaceutical industry profiteering; universal health care

carceral state, expansion of: aging of the prison population and, 146; Clinton administration and, 146; and increase in HIV/AIDS rates, 146; mandatory sentencing laws and, 146–47; misogyny of, and intersection of multiple forms of discrimination, 16, 137–38; and the neoliberal punitive turn, 7–8, 11, 133, 136, 137, 138, 142, 146, 148, 163–64; power imbalance of, and inability of women in prison to improve health facilities, 11; Prison Litigation Reform Act (1996), as narrowing ability to petition for improvements, 161; racism and, 137–38; and shrinking of the welfare state, 8, 146; systemic violence against women and, 136, 160; the US has the highest proportion of population incarcerated in the world, 136. *See also* men's prisons; tough-on-crime politics (reliance on punishment to address social issues); women's prisons

Carlomusto, Jean, 30

Carlson, Margaret, 73, 74

Caruso, Gina Marie, 150

Catholic Charities' HIV/AIDS in Prison Project, 151

Catholic church: abstinence-only sex education promoted by, 123–24; opposition to tiny segment on gay families in Rainbow Curriculum (NYC), 122–23; private AIDS house for HIV-positive children, 91

CCWF (Central California Women's Facility, Chowchilla): building and size of facility, 133, 147; co-payment system, 137–38, 148, 160; Covid-19 and, 205; deaths due to medical negligence, 145–46, 148–49, 155, 162–64; guards

CCWF *(continued)*

(MTAs), abuse of women by, 152–53; guards (MTAs) as gatekeepers for access to health care, 137, 141–42, 147–48, 151, 155, 157, 161, 163; punitive ideology and inefficiencies of, 142, 148; sick call system as abusive, 142–43, 147–49; typical crimes and sentences given, 133. *See also* women's prisons

—ACTIVISM OF WOMEN IN: overview, 138, 165–66; Black women as leaders of, 134; guards actively blocking, 135, 145, 150, 152; persistence of, 165; petition demanding a guard/MTA be fired, 152–53; protests by women, 134; punitive measures taken against, 135, 145, 153, 160, 164, 165, 205; support groups providing critical information, 149–50, 152

—ALLIANCES BETWEEN INSIDE AND OUTSIDE ACTIVISTS: overview, 132, 138, 205; California legislative hearing on women's prison medical mistreatment, 161–62; Coalition to Support Women Prisoners at Chowchilla (CSWPC), 151, 153, 154, 156; compassionate releases successfully supported, 153–54, 155; deaths of women inside, public attention to, 155, 163; demands for investigations of medical mistreatment, 153, 155–56, 163; demonstration held outside the prison gates (1994), 132, 154–55; demonstrations in support of *Shumate v. Wilson*, 158–60, *159*; DOJ investigation of disability discrimination, 155–56; Judy Greenspan (ACT UP/San Francisco), advocacy and networking

of, 151–53, 154, 155–56, 158, 160; guards blocking, 150, 152; help with peer education program approval, 152; independent investigation into health care (Campbell and Weinstein), 151, 156; letters and complaints sent to activists and professionals outside, 150–51, 153; media contacts, 153, 154, 155, 156, 160; networking of outside activists, 151–52, 154; retaliatory treatment of women inside by prison officials, 160. *See also* litigation—to improve prison conditions; *Shumate v. Wilson* (1995 class action against CDCR)

CDC (US Centers for Disease Control and Prevention): first notices of AIDS defined by white gay men, 23; guidelines encouraging HIV-positive women to avoid or terminate pregnancy, 65–66, 200; hierarchy of exposure categories used for men but not women, 113; "men to have sex with men" (MSM) as term adopted by, 111; notice of heterosexual transmission and infection of women (1983), 25; notice of opportunistic infections in infants (1982), 25, 200; number of people who could benefit from PrEP but cannot access it, 188; on prevention as key (2000), 171; protests at headquarters of (Atlanta), 32; recommendation for testing of all pregnant women unless they declined (opt-out approach), 94; woman-to-woman transmission data not collected by, 112–13. *See also* CDC's definition of AIDS; "risk group" concept of AIDS; woman-to-woman transmission denied by the CDC; woman-to-woman transmission recognized by the CDC

CDC's definition of AIDS: austerity cited by CDC as excuse for constricting the definition, 27; the discovery of HIV virus and (1985), 25; expansions of, and sharp increases of reported cases in women and other understudied populations, 27, 33; financial and other patient supports as dependent on receiving diagnosis, 26–27, 31–32, 56; first (1982), as formerly rare diseases in otherwise healthy gay white men (GRID: gay-related immunodeficiency), 23–24, 26; first, structured to ignore convergence with existing health problems of women, and people living in poverty, 24, 32; HIV antibody testing and expansion of (1987), 27; list of recognized symptoms, 27; and women's AIDS diagnoses viewed as anomaly, 20–21; women-specific conditions excluded from, 25–27, 148; women-specific conditions included through "joint strategy" activism (1993), 21, 22, 31–33, 52, 54, 56–57, 143, 169. See also deaths from HIV/AIDS; HIV/AIDS statistics; misdiagnosis of women

censorship: of HIV/AIDS educational materials for women in prison, 150, 153; of pornography, 103–4, 116. See also Safer Sex Handbook for Lesbians— censorship by the political right

Center for Constitutional Rights (CCR), 63–64

Center for Health and Gender Equality, 171

cervical cancer, 26, 33, 141, 149

cervical secretions, 112, 113–14

Charen, Mona, 125

Chávez, Karma R., 39

the child as symbol: evoked in opposition to Rainbow Curriculum due to tiny lesbian and gay section (NYC), 122–23; evoked to shore up white, male, heterosexual power ("family values politics"), 120–21, 206–7; and moral panic over gay "recruitment," 120–21, 122, 126–28; the Safer Sex Handbook for Lesbians (LAP) framed by the political right as dangerous homosexual propaganda endangering children, 101, 120, 125–28; the state as responding more readily to women's needs involving, 9–10, 22, 57, 89, 101

children. See child as symbol, the; infant mortality and disability; mothers and motherhood; mother-to-child (perinatal) transmission; pediatric HIV/AIDS; pregnant women who are HIV positive; reproductive justice; state removal of children from HIV-positive women

Children's Hospital of Philadelphia, 90

children's welfare services: hospitals testing infants and women of color and reporting to, 69, 70–71. See also state removal of children from HIV-positive women

Chowchilla. See CCWF (Central California Women's Facility, Chowchilla)

Christensen, Kimberly, 29, 56–57

chronic fatigue, 108

Chu, Susan Y., 129

citizenship and residency applicants, mandatory HIV testing proposals for, 40

Clark, Judith, 143

classism: arrests of ACT UP women leveraging class privilege, 32; as blunting the state response to HIV/AIDS, 3; disproportionate drug testing of women in public hospitals, 71; and the "guilty-innocent" binary of illness, 2–3, 28, 92–93, *93*, 112–13. *See also* systemic barriers to health care and social services

Clinton, Bill, and administration: blocking generic versions of HIV medicines manufactured outside the US, 188; Defense of Marriage Act (1996), 121; "domestic gag-rule" rescinded by, 81; "Don't Ask, Don't Tell," lesbians and gay men in the military, 121; Elementary and Secondary School Act reauthorization (1994), 127–28; firing of Joycelyn Elders (surgeon general), 124; neoliberalism advanced under, 99, 121–22; pharmaceutical industry deregulation, 168; "third way" sought by, 121; universal health care, failure to implement, 130, 146; Violent Crime Control and Law Enforcement Act (1994), 146; welfare reform, 67, 121–22, 146

Clit Club, 118

coalitions, power of, 57

coalitions of women and men working together: and class-action suit against SSA for discrimination (*S. P. v.*

Sullivan), 31–33; intimate relationships between lesbian-identified women and gay-identified men within, 104–5, 131; mandatory testing proposals, response to, 39; and queer politics, development of, 6, 131

Coalition to Support Women Prisoners at Chowchilla (CSWPC), 151, 153, 154, 156

Cohen, Cathy, 5–6

Cohens, Hattie Mae, 97–98, 99

Collins, Paul, 150

Combahee River Collective Statement, 103

Committee for Abortion Rights and Against Sterilization Abuse, 88

Community Health project, 118

conceptual prophylaxis, 61

condoms (female), as disappointment, 45, 172, 179–80

condoms: *Cosmopolitan* magazine recommending use of, 30; intimate partner violence against women who request the use of, 48, 172; Charles Everett Koop endorsing, 62, 75, 77, 82; *Listen Up!* (GMHC pamphlet), 124, 128; men's prisons and distribution of, 138–39, 140; nonoxynol-9 additive increases women's risk of HIV infection, 168, 207; public health and corporate campaigns telling women to require men to use condoms or to refuse to have sex, 45, 46–47, 115, 176, 207; public health campaigns placing emphasis on use of, 45; public high school distribution of, 122; sexual violence and inability to avail, 46, 50, 172; stealthing, 172; women's lack of control in use of, 45, 46–47, 172, 176, 182; women's prisons and failure to provide, 140. *See also* condoms (female); safer sex

conference activism, 52–54

Conference of Peer Education for HIV (NYU), 124–25

Congress, US: Abandoned Infants Assistance (AIA) Act, 91, 92–93; Americans with Disabilities Act (1990), 156; attempts to establish that life begins at conception, 7; Bayh-Dole Act (1980), 192; Defense of Marriage Act (1996), 121; Elementary and Secondary School Act reauthorization, amendment blocking funding for schools representing gay men and lesbians positively (1994), 126–28; Hatch-Waxman Act (1984), 190–91; hearing to inquire about Gilead profiteering, 193–94; Microbicide Development Act (proposed), 173–74; NIH Revitalization Act (1993), 54–55; Office of Women's Health established by (1994), 55; Polio Vaccination Assistance Act (1955), 191; Prison Litigation Reform Act (1996), 161; prohibition on government negotiation of drug prices, 189; Ryan White CARE Act (1990), 70; Violent Crime Control and Law Enforcement Act (1994), 146; welfare reform (1996), 121–22

Connecticut, 144, 158

contact tracing, calls for, 39

contraception: coercion of Native American women to use long-acting hormonal forms of, 42, 53; constitutional right to, 187; the female condom, 179–80; IUDs, problems with, 33–34; microbicides to be available in noncontraceptive or contraceptive forms, 171, 178; and the need for greater information for HIV-positive women, 53–54; the pill, exploitation of Puerto Rican women for drug trials of, 36, 42; the pill, profitability for drug companies, 173; private retail clinics and the power to refuse to sell, 186–87

Cooke, Pandora M., 80

Copelon, Rhonda, 64

Cortines, Ramon C., 124–25

Cosmopolitan magazine, 28–29, 30–31

Covid-19 pandemic, 205–6

crack cocaine: coded as Black, 3, 90; disproportionate targeting of women of color for prosecution and removal of children, 70–71, 87; drug prosecutions and women's prison growth, 146–47

Crimp, Douglas, 93, 115

Crisis Pregnancy Center, 62

Crowe, Felicia, 144

Cummins, Mary A., 122–23, 126, 127, 131

Curran, James, 66–67, 128

Cytomegalovirus retinitis, 153

D'Adesky, Anne-Christine, 98

Daily, Bishop Thomas V., 122

Daraprim pills, 193

Daughters of Bilitis, 107

Davidson, Felicia, 140

Davis, Angela, 136

Davis, Gray, 163

deaths from HIV/AIDS: and activist demonstrations protesting CDC

deaths from HIV/AIDS (continued)
denial of woman-to-woman transmission, 109–11, 110; early deaths of women due to late diagnosis, 26; as leading cause of death among women aged 25 to 34 (1988, NYC), 29; mortality rates of pediatric AIDS, 67; prior to acknowledgment of woman-to-woman transmission, without a diagnosis, 113–14, 129; prior to acknowledgment of women's HIV during the first decade of the epidemic, without a diagnosis, 26, 143; prior to official discovery, in poor women and men, 24; systemic barriers to health care as directly and indirectly causing, 130. See also HIV/AIDS statistics
deaths in women's prisons due to medical negligence, 145–46, 148–49, 155, 162–64
DeBerry, Dee, 98
Defense of Marriage Act (1996), 121
De La Cruz, Iris, 30, 32
Della Femina, Jerry, 46
dementia, 27, 153
Democratic Party: and bipartisan commitment to inhumane punishment, 163; and bipartisan commitment to tough-on-crime politics, 138; and Clinton's "third way," 121; global gag rule overturned by every administration of, 181. See also Clinton, Bill, and administration
Denenberg, Risa, 26, 49–51
Department of Health and Human Services (HHS): guidelines for women's sterilization, 42; women's

action against discrimination in SSA benefits, 32
Department of Justice (DOJ): investigation of medical discrimination in women's prisons, 155–56; lawsuit against Gilead for infringement of HHS's patents on PrEP, 192, 195–96
Depo-Provera, 42
DES (diethylstilbestrol), 33–34
DeSantis, Ron, 206
Descovy, 194–95
developing countries: foreign aid by the US, global gag rule enforcing antiabortion agenda, 181–82, 183, 197; and the global reach of neoliberalism, 9, 179; and microbicides as women's HIV prevention method, 168
DeWine, Mike, 185
diabetes, 145–46
diagnosis of AIDS. See CDC's definition of AIDS; misdiagnosis of women
Diallo, Dázon Dixon, 32, 114, 130, 179
Diamond, Jan, 139
Diaz-Cotto, Juanita, 138
diethylstilbestrol (DES), 33–34
Discover, 28
discrimination: class-action lawsuit (S. P. v. Sullivan) for denial of SSA benefits, 31–33; medical mistreatment of women with HIV/AIDS as, 156; in prisons, as deterrent to HIV testing, 149
Dobbs v. Jackson Women's Health Organization (2022), 203–4
Doe, Carol, 62–63
domestic violence. See intimate partner violence
Dominican Republic, AZT trials in, 37–38

Evans, Linda, 144

Evotaz, 195

Eye Photography Gallery (San Francisco), 87

families, gay. *See* gay and lesbian (LGBTQI+) rights, attacks on

family values politics (upholding white, patriarchal, middle-class heteronormativity): overview, 8, 203; assumptions about who is deserving of government-funded supported as rooted in, 17; as backlash against social justice movements of the 1960s and 1970s, 99, 120–21, 203; criminal penalties and abortion restrictions as advancing, 62; designation as the "general population," 38; mandatory premarital HIV testing as symbolic protection for, 41; and nineteenth- and twentieth-century debates over race, 120, 121; and pressure to penalize nonnormative and anti-normative sexual and gender behaviors, 40, 101; Republican use of funding to implement agenda of, 181–82; the *Safer Sex Handbook for Lesbians* produced against backdrop of, 100, 116, 121, 131–32; as silencing the articulation of lesbian sexuality, 131–32; the state as "protector" of "innocent" citizens from the "immoral" lifestyles of those who fall outside the norms of, 8, 38, 70–71, 201–3, 207–8; state laws restricting teachers' speech to, 206–7; Trump administration as culmination of forty-year campaign, 203; and violence against lesbians and gay

men, 99. *See also* antiabortion activism; child as symbol, the; classism; eugenics and eugenics laws; gay and lesbian (LGBTQI+) rights, attacks on; homophobia; moral panics; racism; sexism

Fauci, Anthony, 74

Federal Correctional Institution (Pleasanton, CA), 144

Fedlman, Robin, 191

feminist organizing: ACT UP's successes attributed to learning the feminist theory of self-advocacy, 30; HIV/AIDS organizing as modeled on, 11–12, 29–30, 48, 50, 56–57, 106; prison organizing as based in, 135–36, 144; self-advocacy theory in, 12, 30. *See also* Black feminists; international activism; lesbian feminists

feminist public health publicity: overview, 22, 54, 56; and the false distinction between a woman's health and that of her fetus, countering of, 47–48; as inspired by public health and commercial campaigns placing the burden of prevention on women, 47; multiply marginalized women's rights as centered in, 47–48, 50–52; *Safer Sex Handbook for Lesbians* (LAP) as meant to differ from tone of, 116. See also *Our Bodies, Ourselves* (BWHBC); *Safer Sex Handbook for Lesbians* (LAP)

Fernandez, Joseph A., 122–23

fetal alcohol syndrome, 42, 71

fetal rights: overview and definition of, 7, 202; criminalization and prosecution of women for miscarriage and other pregnancy losses, 204; drug "war" and punitive treatment of (mostly) women of color, 7, 69, 71, 87–88, 95; false distinction between a woman's health and that of her fetus, 33, 45, 47–48, 52, 202; federal legislative attempts to establish, 7; HIV/AIDS and punitive treatment of women, 7, 69, 71, 73, 95, 202; identification of the fetus as a "child" separate from a woman, 72–73, 78, 86, 95, 202; Charles Everett Koop and rhetoric of, 62, 78, 85–86, 94–95; language used to oppose a compassionate public health response to AIDS, 84; "life begins at conception" idea, 62, 78, 86, 204; state legislation and language of, 204; state proposals to equate abortion with murder, 204; and "unblinding" anonymous testing of infants, 69; women's bodies as harmful hosts, 78, 95, 202. *See also* antiabortion activism

Fitzwater, Marlin, 72

Florida: HIV criminalization laws, 69–70, 201–2; HIV testing laws, 68; Parental Rights in Education Law (2022), 206–7; quarantine law, 40; repeal of gay civil rights ordinance (1977), 121; sex workers targeted in, 40; violence against gay men and lesbians, 98; women's prison health care policy, 142

Food and Drug Administration (FDA): AZT approval (1987), 34; burden of responsibility placed on individual women to assess the risks of drug trial participation, 55, 57; citizen petition charging gender discrimination by, 54; exclusion of women from drug trials, 34; female condom approval (1993), 45; inclusion of women (1993), and failure to enforce, 34, 54, 55, 169; Office of Women's Health (1994), 55

Forbes, Anna, 179, 182

foreign aid by the US, global gag rule enforcing antiabortion agenda, 181–82, 183, 197

foster care: anti-welfare politics and likelihood of children entering, 88; and HIV-positive children, difficulty placing in, 90, 91; HIV-positive children entering, 88, 89; privatization of, 88, 89

Fox, Harold E., 35

Freiberg, Charles N., 156

Friedman-Kien, Alvin E., 23

Fried, Marlene Gerber, 89

Frondorf, Evan, 191

fungal meningitis, 155

Gasper, Jo Ann, 81

gay and lesbian (LGBTQI+) rights, attacks on: Defense of Marriage Act (1996), 121; "Don't Ask, Don't Tell" military policy, 121; Elementary and Secondary School Act reauthorization, amendment blocking funding for schools representing gay men and lesbians positively (1994), 126–28; and moral panic over gay "recruitment"/ the child as symbol, 120–21, 122, 126–28; opposition to tiny segment on gay families in Rainbow Curriculum (NYC), 122–23; punitive proposals for HIV testing, quarantining, and tattooing, 39; repealing gay civil

gay and lesbian (LGBTQI+) rights,
attacks on *(continued)*
rights ordinances, 121; safer sex
materials produced by gay men,
federal funding blocked for (1987), 127;
state initiatives proposed to prohibit
gay teachers, 121; on transgender
community, 18. *See also* family values
politics; homophobia

gay men: Black, excluded from first PCP
reports, 23; federal government's focus
on regulating, 117; lesbian work as
caregivers for, 107–8; safer sex materials
produced by, federal funding blocked
for (1987), 127; safer sex pamphlets
created by, as explicit, 115; vibrant
mobilization of resistance by, 18. *See
also* coalitions of women and men
working together; men who have sex
with men (MSM); white gay men

Gay Men's Health Crisis (GMHC, NYC):
and LAP's *Safer Sex Handbook for
Lesbians*, 100, 118–20, 124–25; *Listen Up!*
pamphlet, 124, 128

gender: and the "guilty-innocent" binary
of illness, 92–93, *93*; state laws
restricting teachers' speech about,
206–7; twentieth-century policing of
women judged to have transgressed
norms of, 116–17. *See also* systemic
barriers to health care and social
services

generic HIV medicines: brokered deals
to delay generic entry, 191, 192, 194–95;
Clinton administration blocking
manufacture outside the US, 188; and
lower prices, 190–91, 193

genetic diseases: and abortion pressure
by medical and social authorities, 65;
eugenics laws and, 64–65

Georgia, 32, 69–70

Gerald, Gil, 76

Gilead Sciences Inc.: class-action
antitrust lawsuit against, 194–95;
Congressional inquiry into profiteering, 193–94; Descovy, 194–95; DOJ
lawsuit seeking damages for infringement of HHS's patents on PrEP, 192,
195–96; programs to assist access, 188,
192–93; protests of high cost of their
drugs, 187–88, 192; Stribild, 188. *See
also* PrEP; tenofovir; Truvada

Gingrich, Newt, 99, 126

Global Campaign for Microbicides
(GCM), 173–74, 178

global context of neoliberalism, 9, 179

Gomez, James, 153, 155, 157

Gonzales, Awilda, 143

Goodrow, Brenda, 194

Gottemoeller, Megan, 171, 174, 175

Gottlieb, Michael, 23

Gould, Deborah, 105

Gould, Robert, *Cosmopolitan* article,
28–29, 30–31

Grandma's House (Washington, DC),
91–93, *92*

Gran Fury (art/activist collective):
"Control," 92, *93*; "Women Don't Get
AIDS, They Just Die From It," 32

Greenspan, Judy, advocacy and networking of, 6, 151–53, 154, 155–56, 158, 160

GRID (gay-related immunodeficiency),
24. *See also* CDC's definition of
AIDS

HIV/AIDS statistics: Black women, 29, 182; as leading cause of death among women aged 25 to 34 (1988, NYC), 29; low prevalence among sex workers, 40, 112; mortality rates, 29, 67; new infections (2012–2016), 188; new infections (2015–2019), 200; pediatric HIV/AIDS mortality rates, 67; pediatric HIV/AIDS rates of infection, 38, 60; prisoner rates of infection as higher in women, 134; rising rates in women and children (1987), 60; women and girls living with HIV, 182; women of color mortality rates, 29; women who have sex with women, elevated HIV/AIDS risk of, 108–9

HIV disclosure: criminalization of nondisclosure, 69–70, 94, 201–2, 204; intimate partner violence in response to, 49, 201–2

HIV Law Project (HLP), 31–33, 54

HIV testing: activists' calls for voluntary, anonymous, or confidential, 68; activists' criticism of infant test results used against women, 68, 69; AZT approval and increased risk of coerced testing and criminalization, 93–94; CDC recommendation for testing of pregnant women unless they declined (opt-out approach), 94; criminalization of HIV-positive women's pregnancies and use of, 69, 70–71, 94, 95; criminalization of pregnancy as deterrent to women seeking, 95; discrimination in prisons as deterrent to women seeking, 149; ELISA test licensed for blood screening (1985), 38; and expansion of CDC's definition of AIDS, 27; false negatives, 41; infant and maternal testing used to remove infants from mothers at birth, 69, 70–71; infant testing reveals only the mother's HIV status, 68; infant testing used as proxy for HIV rates of infection in women, 68–69; introduction of (1987), 27; mandatory mass testing, calls for, 39; mandatory or routine testing of pregnant women, and activist concerns about reproductive rights abuses, 42–43, 50–51, 53; mass testing of infants, 68–69; mass testing of women proposed, to advise against having children, 60, 67–68, 200; in prisons, 40, 139–40, 148–49; state laws, as lacking uniformity, 68–69; as tool to exclude and confine, 39. See also marriage licenses, mandatory blood testing for

Hobson, Emily K., 52

Hoffman, Beatrix, 6, 57

Hollibaugh, Amber: background and working life of, 106–7; on behaviors vs. lesbian identity and HIV/AIDS risk, 102, 104, 130–31; at the CDC's Lesbian HIV Issues meeting (1995), 128–29; on the censoring campaign against the handbook, 131; as commissioning the *Safer Sex Handbook for Lesbians*, 100, 116, 117; on the division of the lesbian community about HIV risk, 131; goal of providing resources to low-income women of color, 106–7; and lesbians with HIV as "the disappeared," 107; "Seducing Women into a 'Lifestyle of Vaginal Fisting'," 131; on the variety of lesbian self-identification, 106. *See also* Lesbian AIDS Project (LAP); *Safer Sex Handbook for Lesbians* (LAP)

homophobia: as blunting the state response to HIV/AIDS, 3; in censorship campaign of *Safer Sex Handbook for Lesbians* (LAP), 126–27; and marginalization of lesbians within the health-care system, 111–12; men with relative class and race privilege encountering the debilitation of, 5; in public health campaigns, 46; statewide homophobic initiatives, 97, 98; violence against gay men and lesbians, 97–99. *See also* gay and lesbian (LGBTQI+) rights, attacks on

Honan, Marie, 98

Hoppe, Trevor, 38, 69

hospitals: "boarder babies with AIDS" and, 90–91; cuts to Medicaid and dumping of patients, 90; mandatory HIV testing proposals for patients, 40; testing infants and women of color and reporting to children's welfare services, 69, 70–71

housing: local benefits for, CDC-defined AIDS diagnosis required to receive, 27; neoliberal avoidance of investment in, 61

Hubbard, Jim, 30, 57

Hubbard, Lynette "Cookie," 112

Hudson, Rock, 28

Human Rights Watch, 154

Huntington's chorea, 65, 66

Hyde Amendment (1976), 7, 72, 82, 88–89, 181, 185

Idaho, 69–70

Illinois, 41–42

immigrants: ban on HIV-positive (1987), 39; eugenics laws placed on, 64–65; mistreatment of people with HIV/AIDS in detention centers, 204–5; xenophobic panic about, 202

Incarnation Children's Center (NYC), 91

Indiana, 186

infant mortality and disability: cultural anxiety about, 60, 67–68; eugenics laws in the early to mid-twentieth century, 60; expenses for unwell and disabled children, avoidance of, 60. *See also* children; pediatric HIV/AIDS

informed consent: abortion done without, 63; antiabortion activists and appropriation of language and tactics of the women's health movement, 79, 80; and opt-out approach to universal HIV testing of women, 94; for sterilization, 42

international activism: conference activism, 52–54; distribution of the *Safer Sex Handbook for Lesbians*, 118; drug trials, 37–38; reproductive rights, 53–54; and third-world feminism as influence, 52; and woman-controlled prevention tools, call for, 171

International Conference(s) on AIDS, 52–54, 130, 167, 170, 173, 177

International Partnership for Microbicides (IPM), 174–75, 197

International Working Group on Women and AIDS, 52–53

internment. *See* quarantining

intimate partner violence against women: and HIV/AIDS disclosure, 49, 201–2, 207; and request for condom use by men, 48, 172; as systemic barrier to health care, 29; and use of the female condom, 180

intravenous drug use: Black women demonized as "carrying" HIV to the larger community, 28; clean needles advocacy, 77, 114; and hierarchy of exposure categories assigned by CDC for men but not women, 113; in prisons, and clean needle policies, 139, 140; right wing rhetorical and legislative attacks on, 39; as "risk group," 2, 24–25; *Safer Sex Handbook for Lesbians* (LAP) covering, 117; by women who have sex with women, 100, 102, 105, 107, 108, 129

IUD (intrauterine devices), 33–34

Ivy, Brenda Lee, 150

JAMA (Journal of the American Medical Association), 65

Jamaica Hospital (NYC), 62–63

Janssen Pharmaceuticals, 194–95

Jenkins, Jackie, 155

Jordan, June, 108

Journal of the American Medical Women's Association, 129

Kaposi's sarcoma (KS), 23, 24, 25, 26

Kasich, John, 185

Kennedy, Edward, 128

Kenya, 180

King County Hospital (NYC), 63

Kohler-Hausmann, Julilly, 136

Koop, Charles Everett (US surgeon general): overview of approach to the office, 73–74; abortion as viable option for HIV-positive pregnant women, 59–60, 61–62, 71–72, 77–78, 185; abortion, refusal to affirm the safety of, 78, 85; advancing the view of women's bodies as harmful hosts, 78, 95; "Children with HIV and Their Families" workshop, 90–91; confirmation in office by Congress, and opposition to, 73, 77; end of term in office, 85; endorsement of clean needles, 77; endorsement of condoms and sex education in public schools for HIV prevention, 62, 75–76, 77, 82–83; fetal rights rhetoric and, 62, 78, 85–86, 94–95; National Press Club speech (1987), 59–60, 61, 72; personal opposition to abortion, 59, 73, 77, 79; pragmatic public health agenda of, 74–78, 79, 82–83, 84, 85; Republican denouncements of, 77. *See also* Koop's abortion report (never published); Koop's AIDS report

Koop's abortion report (never published): antiabortion activists as frustrated with, 78, 79, 83–85; input of diverse organizations invited for, 82; Planned Parenthood and activists' worries in advance of, 78–79; Reagan ordering preparation of, 79–80, 81–82, 83, 85, 94; refusal of Koop to publish any report or to legitimize the antiabortion concept of post-abortion syndrome (PAS), 62, 77, 79, 82, 83, 85, 94

Koop's AIDS report: overview of
  pragmatic public health approach to,
  74; condoms endorsed in, 62, 75, 77, 82;
  dispelling the rumor of transmission
  through nonsexual, casual contact, 75;
  distribution of 22 million copies of, 75;
  distribution of condensed version to
  all 107 million US households, 84;
  frank language used to describe
  transmission, 75; input of diverse
  organizations invited for, 74–75, 76;
  mandatory blood testing denounced
  in, 75; positive reception of, 76–77,
  82–83; quarantining denounced in, 75;
  Reagan ordering preparation of, 74;
  Republicans offended by, 75–76, 79,
  83–84; sex education in public schools
  endorsed, 62, 75–76, 77, 82–83, 124;
  silence and misinformation, condem-
  nation of, 75

LaBeija, Kia, 199–201
Lancet, 23
Langone, John, 28
LAP. See Lesbian AIDS Project; Safer Sex
  Handbook for Lesbians (LAP)
Latina women: historic exploitation by
  medical researchers, 36, 42–43; and
  HIV drug trials, controversies
  surrounding, 36; and mandatory HIV
  testing of pregnant women, activists'
  concerns about, 42–43; mortality rates
  of, 29; rate of HIV infection, 184; and
  the stereotypes and stigma of HIV/
  AIDS, 2–3; and use of nonprofit health
  care services, 184; and women's
  prisons, medical negligence in,
  145–46. See also single mothers of color

Laubenstein, Linda, 23
law enforcement: drug and HIV testing
  of pregnant women and reporting to,
  7, 69, 70–71, 95; increased targeting of
  low-level offenses, 147; twentieth-
  century policing of women's gender
  norms, 116–17. See also tough-on-crime
  politics
Law, Victoria, 135, 136
Lee, Barbara, 150–51
Legal Services for Prisoners with
  Children (LSPC), 150, 154, 160–61, 164
Leigh, Carol, 42–43
Leonard, Zoe, 47, 105, 114
lesbian(s): and AIDS as intersectional
  women's health issue, 107–8; as
  central figures in debate over women
  and AIDS, 95–96; excluded from drug
  trials, 34; as founders of ACT UP/New
  York Women's Caucus, 29–30;
  heterosexist biases as marginalizing
  in the health care system, 129; work as
  caregivers of gay men, 107–8. See also
  gay and lesbian (LGBTQI+) rights,
  attacks on; lesbian feminists; lesbian
  identities; lesbian immunity from
  HIV/AIDS, myth of; women who
  have sex with women
Lesbian AIDS Project (LAP): and AIDS
  as intersectional women's health
  issue, 107–8; founding by Amber
  Hollibaugh, 100, 107; LAP Notes
  (newsletter), 102; and message of
  behaviors vs. lesbian identity as HIV/
  AIDS risk, 102, 104–7, 130–31; previous
  organizing as model for, 11–12, 101,
  106–7, 114; refusal to "degay" identity
  to seem less threatening, 101, 107;

Lesbian AIDS Project (continued)
sexual and empowerment workshops,
114–15. See also Hollibaugh, Amber;
Safer Sex Handbook for Lesbians
Lesbian and Gay Community Center, 118
Lesbian Avengers/New York: action in
support of the Rainbow Curriculum
(1992), 123; "Dyke March" (1993,
Washington, DC), 98; fire eating as
trademark of, 98; founding of, 98,
242n8; previous organizing as model
for, 11–12, 98, 99, 101, 106; refusal to
"degay" identity, 101
Lesbian Avengers/San Francisco:
activism for women prisoners, 132;
demands to the CDC to study
woman-to-woman transmission, 111;
leaflets and demonstrations protesting CDC denial of woman-to-woman
transmission, 110–11; political funeral
for Joan Baker, 109–10, 110
lesbian feminists: Black feminists and
intersectional oppressions, 103;
debates on the nature and meaning of
lesbian identity, 103; definition of,
102–3; as divided about lesbian risk of
HIV infection, 105, 131; as political
project vs. erotic identity, 103; radical
feminists (anti-pornography and
anti-sadomasochism), 103–4, 116; and
resentment of energy of lesbians
given to AIDS, 108; separatist lesbians,
103, 108; "sex wars" debates, 103–4. See
also lesbian feminists, pro-sex
lesbian feminists, pro-sex: critique of
anti-pornography, anti-sadomasochism
radical feminists, 103–4, 116; critique
of "real" lesbian prescriptive ideas

of identity, 104; Safer Sex Handbook
for Lesbians as coming from, 116. See
also Lesbian AIDS Project (LAP);
women who have sex with women
(WSW)
lesbian identities: butch/femme, 102, 104;
romantic friendships (early twentieth
century), 102; white, middle-class
lesbians downplaying nonnormative
and sexual aspects of relationships as
political strategy, 101, 107, 114. See also
lesbian feminists; lesbian immunity
from HIV/AIDS, myth of—lesbian
identities and
lesbian immunity from HIV/AIDS,
myth of: overview, 99–100; coining
of term, 99; perpetuated by the
CDC denial of woman-to-woman
transmission, 99, 113, 130, 140; in
prisons, 140. See also woman-to-
woman transmission denied by
the CDC
—LESBIAN IDENTITIES AND: overview,
99–100, 102; definition of, 99; division
within the lesbian community about
HIV risk, 105, 131; prescriptive ideas of
"real" lesbian identity as producing,
104, 107, 130; shaming of or hiding
behaviors not prescribed for "real"
lesbians, 104–5; and the silence,
invisibility, and isolation of lesbians
with HIV/AIDS, 106, 107
LGBTQI+ rights. See gay and lesbian
(LGBTQI+) rights, attacks on
litigation: for coerced abortion in
HIV-positive woman, 62–63; DOJ
lawsuit against Gilead seeking
damages for infringement of HHS's

media: "boarder babies with AIDS" coverage, 89–90, 91–93, 92; as bolstering the censorship campaign against the *Safer Sex Handbook for Lesbians*, 125–27; calls for punitive disease control as fueled by, 39–40; and crack cocaine, disproportionate targeting of Black women, 71; fetal alcohol syndrome framed as "Indian problem" by, 71; HIV-positive infants represented as poor and Black in, 88; and "joint strategy" of ACT UP, 30, 32, 57; Koop's AIDS report and positive reception in, 76–77, 82–83; misinformation about the vagina, 28, 29, 127; misinformation claiming AIDS not a threat to women, 27–29, 30–31; misinformation in, women's activism to counteract, 29–31; and the myth of first world uniqueness, 29; on prevention as byword, 170–71; on prison mistreatment of women, 154–55, 158; sex workers constructed as malicious actors by, 40; Sonia Sherman's sexual and class status and differential treatment by, 20–21; simultaneous objectification and marginalization of women in, and the CDC's refusal to acknowledge HIV in women, 3; stereotyping of Black women in, 2, 21, 88; "stop having sex outside marriage" message in, 39; structural inequalities as ignored by, 88; vilifying HIV-positive women who become pregnant, 67; on violence against lesbians and gay men, 97–98; on woman-controlled prevention methods, 171, 173; women's prison advocates and contacts in, 153, 154, 155, 156, 160; xenophobic portrayals of heterosexual transmission in Africa and Haiti, 28, 29

Medicaid: anti-welfare politics and federal budget cuts to, 67; and CDC's expansion of AIDS definition to include women, 33; cuts to, and dumping of AIDS patients from emergency rooms, 90; drug price negotiation power of, 189; expansion of, proposed, 196; Hyde Amendment banning use of funds for abortion, 7, 72, 88–89, 185; Planned Parenthood and other nonprofit health services banned from receiving funds for nonabortion preventative services, 182–83; state funding of abortion, bans on, 89; Title X sites and coverage from, 184

medical journals: claim that women are not threatened by AIDS, 28; first reports as strengthening the association with white gay men, 23; on nonexistence of post-abortion syndrome (PAS) as a medical syndrome, 85; pressure to terminate pregnancies of HIV-positive women, 65; woman-to-woman transmission, CDC-funded special issue on (1995), 129

medical research: history of exploitation of Black, Latinx, and Native American communities, 36, 42–43; history of gender bias in, 34. *See also* drug clinical trials; pharmaceutical research

Medicare, 33, 189, 196

Meese, Edwin, 104

men. *See* coalitions of women and men working together; gay men; heterosexual transmission; men's prisons; men who have sex with men (MSM)

men's prisons: condoms, drug treatments, and needle-cleaning solutions made available in some systems, 138–39, 140; cost of drug therapies, as leading to neglect, 139–40; HIV/AIDS cases in, as usual focus of attention, 134, 136–37; HIV testing, 139–40; litigation for rights of prisoners, 156–57, 158; segregation of HIV-positive men, 139

menstrual blood, 105, 113–14

men who have sex with men (MSM): Black women's partners, stereotypes of, 28, 46; hierarchy of exposure categories used by the CDC to collect data, 113; term used by the CDC to separate men's sexual behaviors from their identities, 111

Meredith, Ann P., 87, 107

Mexico City Policy (global gag rule), 181–82, 183

Michigan, 68, 69–70, 130

Microbicides 2000 (international conference), 174

microbicides as HIV prevention method for women: overview, 167; CAPRISA 004 trial (South Africa), 177–78; context for use addressed with, 171–72, 176, 178; in contraceptive and noncontraceptive forms, 171, 178; dapivirine vaginal ring withdrawn from approval process, 197; definition of, 167, 171; developing countries and need for, 168, 173, 178; Global Campaign for Microbicides (GCM), 173–74, 178; International Partnership for Microbicides (IPM), 174–75, 197; intersectional feminist perspective on need for, 178, 179, 197–98, 207; low-cost as important feature of, 167, 168, 175, 178; male consent not required for use, 172, 176; Microbicide Development Act (proposed), 173–74; Microbicides 2000 (international conference), 174; Microbicide Trials Network (MTN), 174; NIH budget for (1999), 173, 174; nonoxynol-9 found to increase women's rate of infection, 167–68, 207; nonprofit and governmental support needed for research, 173–74; pharmaceutical companies' disinterest in researching, 168, 172–73, 175–76; research and development, 174–75, 176–78, 207; the rise of PrEP as marking the decline of, 176, 177; tenofovir gel, 176–78. *See also* prevention methods, woman-controlled

Microbicide Trials Network (MTN), 174

military servicemembers: "Don't Ask, Don't Tell" policy (lesbians and gay men), 121; federal policing of women's same-sex relationships, 117; mandatory HIV testing proposals for, 40

Miller, Meredith, 87

Minkoff, Howard L., 65

misdiagnosis of women: and exclusion of women in CDC's AIDS definition, 26; later diagnosis and early deaths of women, 26; racial inequities and, 26; the "risk group" concept and, 25; and

misdiagnosis of women (continued)
woman-to-woman transmission
denied by CDC, 113–14; in women's
prisons, 147–48, 155

misogyny: anti-Black (misogynoir), 137;
expansion of the carceral state and
intersectional oppressions, 16, 137–38;
Republican censorship of the *Safer Sex
Handbook for Lesbians* and, 126;
Republican use of funding to
implement agenda of, 181–82; as
Trump administration agenda, 16. *See
also* intimate partner violence; sexual
violence

Missouri, 10, 69–70, 127, 131

Mitchell, Janet, 36, 37, 49–50, 93

Mobilization Against AIDS, 153

Mock, Brian H., 97–98, 99

Moices, Doris, 143

Montefiore Hospital (NYC), 108

moral panics: about "crack cocaine
epidemic," 70–71, 146–47; about gay
"recruitment," 120–21, 122, 126–28;
about mother-to-child transmission,
and criminalization of pregnancy,
202; about mother-to-child transmission, as eased by approval of AZT, 15,
38, 42, 93, 96, 101

Morbidity and Mortality Weekly Report
(MMWR), 23, 33

Morella, Connie, 173–74

Morgan, Tracy, 37, 51

mothers and motherhood: assumption
that HIV-positive women should not
have children, 3, 86; and childcare
during Covid-19 pandemic, 206; early
medical neglect of women and bias
toward seeing women as, 21; exclu-

sion of women from drug trials as
reinforcing heteronormative roles, 34;
historic treatment of pregnant
women as vectors of disease in men
and children, 21, 61; visibility of
women to the CDC as, 25; of white,
heterosexual, middle- and upper-class
women, as valued, 10; women
leveraging, to gain political traction,
9–11; of women of color, as devalued,
10. *See also* mother-to-child (perinatal)
transmission; pregnant women and
pregnancy; single mothers of color

mother-to-child (perinatal) transmission:
advocacy to ensure women's rights
not undermined in measures taken to
reduce, 35, 36–38, 42–43, 50–52; AZT
approval and easing of moral panic
over, 15, 38, 42, 93, 96, 101; AZT
approval to block perinatal transmission, 38, 93–94; AZT drug trial (076),
35–38; breastfeeding and, 200;
mandatory premarital HIV testing
proposed to reduce, 41, 42–43;
percentage chances of transmission,
38, 43, 60; and visibility of women to
the CDC, 25; women represented as
vectors of transmission, 25, 52;
women's access to clinical trials to
prevent, 10, 21, 33, 35, 169. *See also*
abortion, medical and public health
pressure for HIV-positive women to
terminate pregnancies; pediatric
HIV/AIDS; pregnant women who are
HIV positive

multiply marginalized HIV-positive
women: definition of, 3; and focus on
transformative justice vs. specific

gains, 6; and the "injury of inequality," 3; and the politics of respectability, rejection of, 5–6. *See also* reproductive rights of multiply marginalized women; women who have sex with women

Mycobacterium avium complex, 153

myth of first world uniqueness, 29

myth of lesbian immunity. *See* lesbian immunity from HIV/AIDS, myth of

National Advocates for Pregnant Women, 204

National Black Women's Health Project, 88

National Coalition of Black Lesbians and Gays, 74, 76

National Educational Association, 74

National Gay and Lesbian Health Association, 128

National Hemophilia Foundation, 74

National Institute of Allergy and Infectious Diseases, AZT trial (076), 35

National Institutes of Health (NIH): activism for inclusion of women, 54; exclusion of women from HIV drug trials, 34; inclusion of women (1986), and failure to enforce, 34, 169; and microbicide research, 173, 174, 176–77; NIH Revitalization Act requiring clinical trials to include women and racial and ethnic minorities (1993), 54–55; Truvada patents owned by, and ability to break Gilead's patent on the drug, 192, 195–96; and vaccine research, 173

nationalized health systems, drug prices, 189

National Minority AIDS Council, 74

National Organization for Women (NOW), 73, 88

National Women's Health Network, 179–80

Native American women: coerced into using long-acting hormonal contraceptives, 42, 53; criminalization of HIV and disproportionate punishment of, 69, 70–72; drug and HIV testing and reporting of pregnant women, 7, 69, 70–71; fetal alcohol syndrome framed as problem of, 71; forced sterilization of, 42, 50–51, 53; historic exploitation by medical researchers, 36, 42–43; and HIV drug trials, controversies surrounding, 36; and mandatory HIV testing of pregnant women, activists' concerns about, 42–43; state removal of children of, 71

Nelson, Jennifer, 11, 66

neoliberalism: the Clinton administration advancing, 99, 121–22; deregulation of the pharmaceutical industry, 9, 168; global context of, 9, 179

neoliberalism, as shifting responsibility for addressing social problems from the state to private families and organizations: overview, 7–8; and the disconnect between rhetoric and action, 60–61, 80, 88, 93; drug trials, burden of risk assessment placed on individual women for participation in, 55, 57; foster care privatization, 88, 89; and mandatory marriage-license HIV testing as failure, 22, 43; nonprofit health care services neoliberalism, as shifting responsibility for addressing social problems (*continued*)

Oklahoma, *44*, 45, 69–70

opportunistic infections, 23–24, 25. *See also* CDC's definition of AIDS

Ordaz, Jessica, 204–5

Oregon, 68, 97

Oregon Citizens Alliance, 97

Otto, Brenda, 162–63

Our Bodies, Ourselves (BWHBC), 48, 49–50, 51, 54, 116. *See also* Boston Women's Health Book Collective

Out of Control, 154

Parents for the Restoration of Values in Education, 124

Paris, France, discovery of HIV virus, 25

Parran, Thomas, 40–41

patents on drugs: federally funded research and assertion of consequent patent rights by the government, 192, 195–96; the polio vaccine precedent (Eisenhower), 191–92; and profiteering, 190–91. *See also* pharmaceutical industry profiteering

Patton, Cindy, 2–3, 39, 105

Paul, Deborah, 152

Pearson, Cynthia A., 179–80

pediatric HIV/AIDS: as "abandoned" children, 10, 90–91; claims that "babies with AIDS have no parents," 67; cost of, and institutionalized AIDS houses, 90–91; cost of, and state pressure on multiply marginalized HIV-positive women to terminate pregnancies, 60, 66–68, 71, 94–95; cost of, and the neoliberal gap between rhetoric and reality, 88; and the "guilty-innocent" binary of illness, 92–93, *92*, 201; health care as a

privilege and not a right, and desire to limit the reproductive freedom of HIV-positive poor women of color, 60; infection rates, 60; mortality rates, 67; private AIDS houses for children without parents or legal guardians ("boarder AIDS babies"), 88, 89–93, *92*; the structural inequalities hampering women's ability to provide care, as denied or ignored, 88, 90–91; and vilification of HIV-positive mothers, 91–93; and women becoming visible to the CDC as mothers, 25; women's ability to contract the virus realized due to occurrences of, 9–10. *See also* foster care; mother-to-child (perinatal) transmission

Pelosi, Nancy, 173–74

pelvic inflammatory disease, 26, 31

Pence, Mike, 186

Penney, Jamie, 49–50, 53–54, 173

Pennsylvania, 158

People with AIDS Coalition New York, 155

Peter Staley, et al. v. Gilead Sciences, In., et al., 194–95

Petro, Anthony, 51, 62

pharmaceutical industry profiteering: brokered deals to delay generic entry, 191, 192, 194–95; charity programs, 192–93; the Clinton administration as facilitating, 168; and disparities in access to drugs, 188–89; dividends to shareholders, 191; generic drugs and lower prices, 190–91, 193; Hatch-Waxman Act (1984), 190–91; neoliberal deregulation and, 9, 168; as particular to the US, 168, 189; patents and period

pharmaceutical industry profiteering
(continued)
of market exclusivity, 190–91;
prohibition on the government
negotiating cheaper prices, 189;
secondary patents, 191
—ACTIVISM AND GOVERNMENT ACTIONS
TO LIMIT: class-action antitrust
lawsuit, 194–95; Congressional
inquiry, 193–94; demonstrations
against high prices, 187–88, 192; the
Eisenhower administration and the
polio precedent, 191–92; federally
funded research and assertion of
consequent patent rights by the
government, 192, 195–96; negotiation
of prices by the government, 196
pharmaceutical marketing, marginalizing women, 168, 169
pharmaceutical research: high prices
claimed to be necessary to finance,
191; and microbicides, disinterest in,
168, 172–73, 175–76. See also drug
clinical trials, exclusion of women
from; drug clinical trials, inclusion of
women in; vaccine for HIV
Piot, Peter, 175
Planned Parenthood: in coalition to
protect women's right to abortion, 88;
fear of Charles Everett Koop's
abortion report, 78–79; Republican
women and support for, 78, 80;
support for Koop's AIDS report,
82–83; Faye Wattleton as the first
Black president of, 78–79, 80, 82–83,
86. See also Planned Parenthood and
other nonprofit health services—

Trump administration's political
assault on
Planned Parenthood and other nonprofit
health services—Trump administration's political assault on: overview, 9,
16, 182–83; clinics leaving the Title X
program in order to continue offering
comprehensive care, 187, 196–97;
closures of clinics, 185, 186; demonstrations in protest of, 183; and lack of
access to PrEP, 168; Medicaid
reimbursement banned for other
preventative services offered, 183;
private retail clinics opening, 186–87;
state funding cuts, 185, 186; Title X
policy changes that effectively defund
all nonabortion services, 183–86
Planned Parenthood v. Casey, 86, 131
Plumb, Marj, 128–29
Pneumocystis carinii pneumonia (PCP),
23, 24
Polanco, Richard, 161–62
polio vaccine, 191–92
pornography, censorship of, 103–4, 116
Porter, Katie, 185
poverty: the CDC's definition of AIDS as
failing to account for the already
compromised health of people living
in, 24, 32; and deaths from HIV/AIDS
prior to official discovery, 24; and
denial of SSA benefits due to lack of
CDC-defined AIDS diagnosis, 27, 31;
and need for woman-controlled
prevention methods, 172, 175, 178, 180;
as women's health issue, 108. See also
anti-welfare agenda of neoliberalism;
carceral state, expansion of; family

prevention methods, woman-controlled *(continued)*
   important feature of, 172, 175, 178, 180; male consent not required, importance of, 172, 176; marginalization of women's sexual and reproductive health needs and need for, 175–76; undetectability as important feature for, 180. *See also* microbicides as HIV prevention method for women

prevention of HIV infection: overview, 43, 45; abstinence, 43, 207; with intersectional awareness, as goal, 170; limiting sexual partners, 43; and systemic inequalities, the need to address, 169–70. *See also* condoms; PrEP (pre-exposure prophylaxis); prevention methods, woman-controlled; public health campaigns—placing the burden of prevention on women

Prison Litigation Reform Act (1996), 161

prisons. *See* litigation—to improve prison conditions; men's prisons; women's prisons

private sector. *See* neoliberalism, as shifting responsibility for addressing social problems from the state to private families and organizations

Progressive era: premarital blood testing for STDs, 40–41, 64; respectability politics and, 5. *See also* eugenics and eugenics laws

pro-sex lesbian feminists. *See* lesbian feminists, pro-sex

protease inhibitors, 13, 130, 170. *See also* antiretroviral therapy (ART, "drug cocktail")

public health campaigns: framing women as vectors of disease in infants, 45; women encouraged to seek treatment and services on behalf of their fetuses and not for themselves, 38, 43, 45, 115. *See also* feminist public health publicity; Koop, Charles Everett (US surgeon general)
   —PLACING THE BURDEN OF PREVENTION ON WOMEN: overview, 21–22, 43, 57–58, 60–61, 207; as absolving the state and men of responsibility, 45; and Black women, 45–46; and gender power imbalance in condom use, 45, 46–47, 172; neoliberal politics and, 22, 43, 45; "No Time Bombs for Your Baby" (Oklahoma campaign), 44, 45; and simultaneous state attacks on women's health care and social services, 43, 60–61

Public Health Service (PHS), 38

Public Health Service Act. *See* Title X (Public Health Service Act)

public schools: Elementary and Secondary School Act reauthorization, amendment blocking funding for schools representing gay men and lesbians positively (1994), 126–28; integration of, 120, 121; neoliberal avoidance of investment in, 61; Rainbow Curriculum controversy due to lesbian and gay families section (NYC), 122–23; state laws proposed to prohibit gay teachers, 121; state laws restricting teachers' speech to "family values," 206–7. *See also* sex education in public schools

Puerto Rican women: exploitation for drug trials of birth control pills, 36, 42; forced sterilization of, 50–51, 53 pulmonary tuberculosis, 33

punitive disease control: overview, 38–39; criminalization of HIV, 69–70, 94; criminalization of pregnancy in HIV-positive women, 61, 69–72, 94, 95, 201–3, 204, 207–8; definition of, 38; extreme proposals making other punitive measures seem more reasonable, 39; and HIV testing as tool to exclude and confine, 39; the media as fueling, 39–40; sex workers singled out for, 39–40

Purdy, Matthew, 139

QLT (immigrant from Cameroon), 202

quarantining of HIV-positive people: calls for, 39; Florida law, 40; Koop's AIDS report denouncing as unnecessary and harmful, 75; in prisons, 139

queer politics, development of: Black feminist scholars and, 5–6; coalitions of women and men and, 6, 131; definition of, 6; lesbian feminist AIDS activism and, 5–6, 100, 106, 115

racism: as blunting the state response to HIV/AIDS, 3; the CDC's definition of AIDS as failing to account for the already compromised health of people due to, 24; and the CDC's exclusion of women-specific conditions from AIDS definition, 26; criminality stereotype in, 90; disproportionate punitive drug and HIV testing of women, 69, 70–71, 95; feminist public health publicity as centering, 50–51; forced sterilization and coerced family planning

decisions, 42, 50–51, 53, 64–65; and the "guilty-innocent" binary of illness, 2–3, 28, 92–93, 93, 112–13; historic medical exploitation of people of color in clinical research, 36, 42–43; state laws restricting teachers' speech about, 206–7; stereotypes and stigma of HIV/AIDS and, 2–3, 28, 29, 46, 182; and twentieth-century policing of women judged to have transgressed gender norms, 116–17; women's prisons as environment of, 137–38. See also anti-welfare agenda of neoliberalism; eugenics and eugenics laws; family values politics; respectability politics; stereotypes and stigmas of Black women; systemic barriers to health care and social services

Ramspacher, Karen, 51

Reagan, Ronald, and administration: overview, 3, 99, 203; and the antiabortion movement, 79–81, 85, 86; and the anti-pornography movement, 104; Black women maligned as "welfare queens," 3; block grants to states, 66–67; Domestic Policy Council (DPC), 76, 78, 83; global gag rule, 181; gutting of women's health care and social services, 8–9, 27, 43, 53, 60–61, 66–67, 80; mandatory premarital testing for HIV supported by, 41; "small government" rhetoric of, 67. See also anti-welfare agenda; carceral state, expansion of; family values politics; Koop, Charles Everett; Koop's abortion report (never published); Koop's AIDS report; neoliberalism; tough-on-crime politics

Rehabilitation Act of 1973 (Section 504), 63, 156, 164

religious grounds, retail clinics refusing to sell birth control, 187

reproductive justice: abortion rights, mobilization for, 88; advocacy against discriminatory HIV testing, 68; advocacy to ensure women's rights not undermined in drug trials, 35, 36–38, 56; conference activism for, 53–54; health and welfare as requirement of, 53, 55; the right of HIV-positive women to have children if they so desire, 51, 88. *See also* prevention methods, woman-controlled

reproductive justice, assaults on: overview, 7–9; Republican use of federal funding to advance, 8–9; women of color disproportionately affected by, 9; women's health care and social supports, 43, 53, 60–61, 66–67, 80. *See also* antiabortion activism; anti-welfare agenda; fetal rights; neoliberalism; Planned Parenthood and other nonprofit health services—Trump administration's political assault on

reproductive rights of multiply marginalized women: abuses, federal and state history of, 42–43, 50–51, 53; desire to avoid paying costs for HIV-positive children and restrictions on, 60, 66–67, 71, 95; feminist public health publicity as centering, 47–48, 50–52; punitive HIV and drug testing disproportionately used against, 69, 70–71, 95; and woman-controlled prevention methods, need for, 175–76.

See also abortion, medical and public health pressure for HIV-positive women to terminate pregnancies

Reproductive Rights National Network, 88

Republican Party: denouncements of Charles Everett Koop, 75; extreme right-wing faction gaining prominence in, 10, 99, 121; global gag rule reinstated by every administration of, 181; HIV criminalization laws, 69–70; offended by Koop's AIDS report, 75–76, 79, 83–84; support for Planned Parenthood and abortion by women in, 78, 80; use of federal funding to advance the assault on reproductive justice, 8–9. *See also* anti-welfare agenda; carceral state, expansion of; child as symbol, the; family values politics; neoliberalism; Reagan, Ronald, and administration; tough-on-crime politics; Trump, Donald, and administration

respectability politics, 5–6, 28

retail clinics, 186–87

Reyes, Dianna, 145–46

Reyes, Molly, 155

Rhode Island, 68

Ricci, Judy, 162, 166

Rich, Adrienne, 103

Richardson, Lynda, 125

Richie, Beth E., 136

"risk group" concept of AIDS: as "4-H" club, 2, 24; "deviant behavior" of the individual as focus of, 2, 3, 24–25, 29; the "general population" as distinguished from, 38; hierarchy of exposure categories used for men but not women, 113; as identity based, 2, 24–25; mistreatment and misdiagnosis of AIDS in women as fueled by, 25; opportunistic infections in people who did not report male homosexuality as leading to, 24; as stigmatized "other" and "foreign," 2, 24–25, 39; the systemic barriers to health care and social services ignored in, 2, 29; "unknown" category (for those whose risk fell outside the designated groups), 24

Risque, Nancy, 83, 84, 85

Riva, Debra Johnes, 201

Rivera, Ada, 143

Rockefeller Foundation, 172

Roe v. Wade (1973), 7, 86; reversal of, 203–4. See also antiabortion activism; reproductive justice

Rome, Esther R., 46

Rosenberg, Zeda Fran, 171, 174, 175

Ross, Betty Jo, 153–54

Royles, Dan, 179

rubella, 45, 65, 66

Rubin, Gayle, 103–4

Rust v. Sullivan, 81

Ryan White CARE Act (1990), 70

Saag, Michael, 193

Saalfield, Catherine, 106

sadomasochism, radical feminist opposition to, 103

safer sex: education alone cannot end the epidemic, 130; feminist public health publicity covering, 50; gay men creating explicit pamphlets on, 115; intimate partner violence in response to women's demand for, 48, 172; in

women's prisons, ad hoc improvisations for, 140. See also condoms; feminist public health publicity; Koop's AIDS report; public health campaigns; Safer Sex Handbook for Lesbians (LAP); sex education in public schools

Safer Sex Handbook for Lesbians (LAP, authored by Madansky and Tolentino Wood): overview, 100; children or family use not the intended audience for, 115–16; distribution of brochure, 118; pro-sex lesbian feminist basis of, 116; and queer politics, development of, 100; reception by the lesbian community, 118, 120; respectability politics rejected in, 5; uncensored and explicit tone and visuals of, 116, 117–20, 119, 125; women's sexual agency promoted in, 117. See also Lesbian AIDS Project (LAP)

—CENSORSHIP BY THE POLITICAL RIGHT: overview, 10, 100–101, 115, 207; accidental placement of the brochure at the 1994 Conference of Peer Education and subsequent censure by the Board of Education, 124–26; family values politics and, 100, 116, 121, 131–32; framing lesbian sexuality as fatal and sadistic, 125–27; framing the handbook as dangerous homosexual propaganda endangering children, 101, 120, 125–28; media coverage bolstering the censorship campaign, 125–27; as political backlash to the visibility of lesbian sexual behaviors, 116–17, 128; as silencing the articulation of lesbian sexuality, 131–32; used

Shubb, William B., 161

Shumate, Charisse, 149–50, 157, 160, 162, 163

Shumate v. Wilson (1995 class action against CDCR): overview, 135–36, 165–66, 205; CCWF and CIW women's prisons represented in, 157, 158; demonstrations held in support of, 158–60, *159*; filing and complaints, 156, 157–58, 160; legacy of, 164–65; media commentary on, 158; motion to reopen discovery denied and case dismissed, 161; plaintiffs threatened with retaliation by prison officials, 160; preliminary investigations for, 151, 156; publicity/media work in support of, 160, 165; retaliatory threats by prison officials against plaintiffs, 160; settlement terms and monitoring (1997), 136, 160–61, 163

sickle cell anemia, 141–42, 149, 151, 160

Siegal, Nina, 141, 158

Silverberg, Lisa, 128–29

Simo, Ana María, 98

single mothers of color: the anti-welfare agenda of neoliberalism as focused on, 3, 8, 21; blame of, and racist drug and HIV prosecution policies, 70–71; Covid-19 pandemic disparities and, 206; and Trump-era loss of low-income health clinics, 185–86

SisterLove (Atlanta), 32, 179

Sisters of Perpetual Indulgence, 115

Sliker, Cecelia Ann, 201–2

Smith, Barbara and Beverly, 103

Smith, Bob (senator), 127–28

social factors determining health. *See* systemic barriers to health care and social services

Social Security Administration (SSA): amendment of criteria to include women-specific conditions (1993), 33; CDC-defined AIDS diagnosis required to receive benefits, 27, 31; class-action lawsuit for denial of benefits (*S. P. v. Sullivan*), 31–33

Social Security Disability Benefits, CDC-defined AIDS diagnosis required to receive benefits, 27

Sorella, Naja, 108

South Africa: microbicide research (CAPRISA 004 trial), 177–78; PrEP trial in cisgender women, 180; and price differentials on HIV drugs, 193

South Carolina, HIV criminalization laws, 69–70

South End Press, 48

Southern Baptist Convention, Christian Life Council, 74

Southern Poverty Law Center, 42

Specter, Michael, 85

spina bifida, 67

S. P. v. Sullivan (SSA discrimination), 31–33

Staley, Peter, 194

Staples, Sonja, 153, 155

the state as "protector" of "innocent" citizens from those who fall outside the "family values" norms: overview, 8, 38; and criminalization of HIV, 70–71, 201–3, 207–8

state neglect coexisting with state interference: overview, 1–2, 3; activism of women and constant risk of, 18–19, 61; as central contradiction of neoliberalism, 8; and discriminatory denial of SSA benefits for women, 31–32; visibility of lesbian

state neglect coexisting with state interference *(continued)*
sexual practices and, 116–17, 128; of women who foregrounded sexual activity and practice instead of childbearing potential, 10–11. *See also* neoliberalism, as shifting responsibility for addressing social problems from the state to private families and organizations; public health campaigns— placing the burden of prevention on women; women's prisons, co-occurring neglect and intervention obstructing health-care access

state removal of children from HIV-positive women: and denial of SSA benefits due to CDC AIDS-definition exclusions, 31–32; fear and isolation of women under threat of, 87–88; private organizations caring for children, 61; testing infants and women for drugs and HIV and, 69, 70–71; vilification of mothers, 91. *See also* foster care

states: benefits provided by, CDC-defined AIDS diagnosis required to receive, 27; following CDC guidelines advising HIV-positive women to avoid pregnancy, 66; legislatures debating the equation of abortion with murder, 204; prison health care policies as varying between, 138–39; Reagan administration block grants to, 66

states, laws of: abortion restrictions, 72, 85–86, 89; abortion restrictions, fetal rights language in, 7, 72; compulsory sterilization eugenics laws, 42; criminalization of HIV, 69–72, 201–3,

207–8; gay rights limitations, proposed, 121; mandatory premarital HIV testing, 41–42; restricting teachers' speech to "family values," 206–7; "three-strikes" laws, 146, 256n63. *See also* eugenics and eugenics laws

STDs (sexually transmitted diseases): and the Black community, historic failure of public health agencies to address, 26; and historic exploitation of the Black community by medical researchers, 36; and historic treatment of women under normative assumptions about sex and gender, 112–13; and lack of AIDS diagnoses for Black women, 26. *See also* marriage licenses, mandatory blood testing for

Stein, Zena, 171

stereotypes and stigma of HIV/AIDS: Black men who have sex with men on the "down low," 28, 46; Black promiscuity and hypersexuality, 182; Black women as "vectors" of HIV, 2–3, 28; and criminalization of pregnancy as deterrent to seeking health care, 95, 208; as deterring HIV testing and treatment, 29; heterosexual transmission in Africa, 28, 29; intravenous drug users, 28; Latina women as "vectors" of HIV, 2–3; right wing capitalization on, 39; "risk group" concept of AIDS and, 24–25; white, middle-class women as excused from, 2–3, 28; woman-controlled prevention methods and need to address, 178

stereotypes and stigmas of Black women: deriving from enslavement, 2;

devaluing of caregiving by Black mothers, 88; respectability politics as counter to, 5–6

sterilization: coercive and compulsory, 42, 50–51, 53, 64–65; HHS rules requiring informed consent and minimum age, 42; increases in, in the absence of legal abortion, 66; offered to HIV-positive women as alternative to abortion, 64

Stoever, Jane K., 172

Stoller, Nancy, 151

Stribild, 188

structural inequalities. *See* systemic barriers to health care and social services

Sununu, John H., 41

Supplementary Security Income (SSI), CDC-defined AIDS diagnosis required to receive benefits, 27, 31

Supreme Court, US: the "domestic gag-rule" upheld by, 81; obligation of jails and prisons to provide health care affirmed by, 157; order for California to reduce its prison population upheld by, 164; refusal of federal funding for abortions upheld by, 72; *Roe v. Wade*, abortion rights, 7, 86; *Roe v. Wade*, reversal of, 203–4; upholding state restrictions on abortion upheld by, 85–86, 131

Sweet, Robert "Bob," 75–76, 78, 83, 83–85

syphilis, 36, 66. *See also* STDs

systemic barriers to health care and social services: overview, 18–19, 29, 130; the anti-welfare agenda and refusal to address, 8, 146; anti-welfare

attacks on women's care and services, 43, 53, 60–61, 66–67, 80, 146; the CDC's definition of AIDS as structured to ignore, 24; the Covid-19 pandemic and, 205–6; criminalization of HIV-positive women's pregnancies, 61, 69–72, 94, 95, 201–3, 204, 207–8; and the global effects of neoliberalism, 179; media and public discussions as ignoring, 88; prevention of HIV/AIDS and need to address, 170–71, 196–98; qualification for financial and other supports as dependent on CDC AIDS-defined diagnosis, 26–27, 31–32, 56; "risk group" concept of AIDS as ignoring, 2, 29; social positionality and types of activism available to women, 11, 57; and woman-controlled HIV prevention methods, need for, 178, 179, 197–98, 207; women who have sex with women as marginalized from the health care system, 111–12, 129. *See also* classism; gender; homophobia; misogyny; pharmaceutical industry profiteering; Planned Parenthood and other nonprofit health services—Trump administration's political assault on; poverty; racism; reproductive justice, assaults on; sexism

Tanzania, 180

Tate, Debbie, 91

tattooing, calls for, 39

Taylor, Keeanga-Yamahtta, 9

Temporary Assistance for Needy Families (TANF), 121–22

tenofovir alafenamide (TAF), 194–95

tenofovir disoproxil fumarate (TDF), 177, 194; microbicide gel, 176–78. *See also* PrEP; Truvada

Terson, Alice, 102

Teva Pharmaceutical Industries Ltd., 192

Texas, 142, 186

Thailand, AZT trials in, 37–38

thalidomide, 33, 34

Thistlethwaite, Polly, 47

Thrasher, Steven W., 61, 146, 191, 194, 205

"three-strikes" laws, 146, 256n63

thrush, 148

Thuma, Emily L., 135, 163

Title X (1970, Public Health Service Act): "domestic gag-rule" antiabortion amendment, 81; Trump administration policy gutting, 183–86, 187, 196–97

Tolentino Wood, Julie: as author of *Safer Sex Handbook for Lesbians*, 100, 116, 117–18; as owner of the Clit Club, 118

tough-on-crime politics (reliance on punishment to address social issues): overview, 203; as bipartisan commitment, 138; Black women maligned as "welfare queens" to justify, 3; building prisons, 133, 137; criminalization of HIV, 69–70, 94; criminalization of miscarriages and other pregnancy losses, 204; criminalization of pregnancies of HIV-positive women, 61, 69–72, 94, 95, 201–3, 204, 207–8; "drug war" expansion, 146–47; increased targeting of low-level offenses, 147; as jobs source, 146; and pressure to penalize nonnormative and anti-normative sexual and gender behaviors, 40, 101; "three-strikes" laws, 146, 256n63; Truth in Sentencing

programs (mandatory sentencing), 146, 147; women in prison, typical crimes and sentences of, 133, 146–47, 149. *See also* carceral state, expansion of; men's prisons; women's prisons

Traditional Values Coalition, 126

transmission of HIV. *See* heterosexual transmission; mother-to-child (perinatal) transmission; "risk group" concept of AIDS; woman-to-woman transmission

trans women: overview of inclusion of, 17–18; elevated HIV/AIDS risk among women who have sex with women, 109; political attacks on the transgender community, 18; in PrEP trials, 177, 180. *See also* gay and lesbian (LGBTQI+) rights, attacks on

Treatment Action Group (TAG), 194–95

treatment of HIV: biomedical solutions alone cannot end AIDS, 169–70, 188. *See also* antiretroviral therapy (ART, "drug cocktail"); AZT

Treichler, Paula, 2–3

Trump, Donald, and administration: attempts to repeal the ACA, 183; as culmination of forty-year campaign for "family values," 203; global gag rule reinstated by (foreign aid may not be used for abortion, abortion counseling, or abortion rights advocacy), 181–82, 183, 197; *Roe v. Wade* reversal (*Dobbs*), 203–4. *See also* Planned Parenthood and other nonprofit health services—Trump administration's political assault on

Truvada: clinical trials and approval, 177; generic version, 195; high cost of, 178,

187–88, 193–94; NIH funding of, and HHS patents owned, 192, 195–96; regular lab tests required with, 178. *See also* PrEP

tuberculosis, 152

Turing Pharmaceuticals, 193

Tuskegee Syphilis Study, 36, 37

UC Los Angeles, 23

Uganda, 178

United Nation's AIDS Program, 175

universal health care: the Clinton administration and failure to implement, 130, 146; drug price negotiations and bulk buying, 189; and multiply marginalized women's fight for transformative justice, 6; need for, 130, 198, 206

University of Medicine and Dentistry of New Jersey, 35

urinary tract infections, persistent, 32

Vacaville State Prison (CA), 139

vaccine for HIV: failures in research for, 170; NIH budget for, 173; preference of pharmaceutical industry for research on, vs. microbicides, 175

vaccines, polio precedent, 191–92

vaginal secretions, 112, 113–14

vaginal yeast infections, persistent, 32

Valley State Prison for Women (Chowchilla, CA), 147

Veterans Administration (VA), drug price negotiation power of, 189

violence: against lesbians and gay men, 97–99; systemic, and expansion of the carceral state, 136, 160; in women's

prisons, 144. *See also* intimate partner violence; sexual violence

Violent Crime Control and Law Enforcement Act (1994), 146

WAC/San Francisco, 109–10

Walker, Alice, 103

Walker, Joann, 133–34, 148–49, 150, 151–55, 163

Wallace, Twillah, 150–51, 155, 163

Washington, 69–70, 108

Washington, DC, 98, 140; Grandma's House, 91–93, 92

wasting syndrome, 27

Watkins-Hayes, Celeste, 3, 95, 169, 171–72, 174

Wattleton, Faye, 78–79, 80, 82–83, 86

Weather Underground, 143

Webster v. Reproductive Health Services, 85–86

Weinstein, Corey, 141, 151, 156

WHAM! (NYC), 54; "Stop the Church" protest (1989), 123–24

white blood cell count (below 200), 33

white gay men: AIDS as initially defined in terms of, 23–24; as AZT trial participants, 34; as downplaying gay identity to make AIDS more politically palatable, 101; PrEP as marketed to, 168, 182

white hegemony, preservation of. *See* family values politics (upholding white, patriarchal, middle-class heteronormativity)

Whitehorn, Laura, 144

white, middle-class, heterosexual women: cocaine use by, 71; excused from stereotypes and stigma of HIV/

white, middle-class heterosexual women *(continued)*

AIDS, 2–3, 28; motherhood of, as valued, 10; respectability politics seeking acceptance into ideals of, 5; rubella perceived as mostly afflicting, and liberalization of attitudes to abortion, 65

white, middle-class lesbian activists: arrests of ACT UP women leveraging their white privilege, 32; as downplaying nonnormative and sexual aspects of relationships for credibility, 101, 107, 114

White, Ryan, 87

Wilhoite, Michael, *Daddy's Roommate*, 122, 128

Wilson, Pete, 157

Windom, Robert E., 81

Winnow, Jackie, 108

Wofford, Carrie, 37

Wolfe, Maxine, 30, 37, 98, 105, 242n8

woman-to-woman transmission denied by the CDC: overview, 99; activist demonstrations to protest, 109–11, *110*, 129; definition of "lesbian" used by CDC as erasing the diversity of women's sexual lives, 111, 112, 129; failure to collect data on woman-to-woman transmission, 112–13; failure to study HIV-viral behavior in women's bodies, 112, 113–14; and lesbian community divisions about lesbian risk, 105, 131; menstrual blood treated as "nonissue," 105; misconception that lesbians don't have much sex, 114; and misdiagnosis of women, 113–14; the "myth of lesbian immunity" perpetuated by, 99, 113, 130, 140;

studies showing elevated HIV/AIDS risk among women who have sex with women, 208–9. *See also* woman-to-woman transmission recognized by the CDC; women who have sex with women

woman-to-woman transmission recognized by the CDC: adoption of the term "women who have sex with women," 129–30; CDC-funded special issue of medical journal on HIV in women (1995), 129; internal working group to review literature (1994), 128; Lesbian HIV Issues (1995 meeting in Decatur, GA), 128–29; prevention interventions recommended, 129

Women, AIDS, and Activism (ACT UP/ New York Women's Caucus), 48–49, 50–51, 54

Women and AIDS Resource Network (WARN), 47

women, as inclusive category, 17–18. *See also* trans women

Women PrEP Working Group, 179, 180

women's activism against HIV/AIDS: overview, 4–6, 12–19; and the epidemic as ongoing, 13–14; motherhood leveraged in, 9–11; previous feminist organizing as model for, 11–12, 29–30, 48, 50, 98, 99, 101; self-advocacy as precedent for, 12, 30; social positionality and difference types of activism available, 11, 57; white privilege leveraged in, 32. *See also* ACT UP; CDC's definition of AIDS; feminist organizing; feminist public health publicity; Lesbian AIDS Project (LAP); Lesbian Avengers;

women's prisons—co-occurring neglect and intervention *(continued)* to health care" by virtue of incarceration, 132, 134; guards (MTAs) as gatekeepers for women's access to care, 137, 141–42, 147–48, 151, 152–53, 155, 157, 161, 163; guards (MTAs), misdiagnosis and incorrect treatments given, 147–48, 155; health complications and requests for services occurring at higher rates than for men, 142; HIV testing, 139, 148–49; HIV testing refused by inmates due to discrimination against HIV-positive women, 149; HIV transmission, 140; isolation of HIV-positive women and unnecessary PPE use, 143–44; misogyny and, 16, 137–38; multiple health needs of women, refusal to address, 136, 137, 142–43, 148; preventative care as nonexistent, 141–42; and "protection" of society from prisoners, 133; racism and, 137–38; reproductive and chronic illnesses not properly addressed, 140–42, 145–46, 147–49; sanitary products not provided, 148; sick call system as abusive, 141–43, 145–46, 147–49, 162–64; systems set up for healthy young males as model prisoners, 137, 140–41, 143; women's pain denied, 137. *See also* litigation—to improve prison conditions

Women's Project (Little Rock, AR), 140
women who have sex with women (WSW): and behavior (not identity) as HIV risk, 100, 102, 105, 114, 129; CDC's adoption of the term, 129–30; CDC's failure to acknowledge the need to use the term, 111; elevated HIV/AIDS risk of, 108–9; intravenous drug use as possible activity of, 100, 102, 105, 107, 108, 129; lack of disclosure of sexuality to health-care providers by, 111–12; marginalization within the health-care system, 111–12, 129; multiply marginalized women and, 106–8; and the need to expand the conception of lesbian identity to include alternative lives and techniques, 104–7; in prison, 140; sex with men as possible activity of, 100, 102, 105, 107, 109, 129. *See also* Lesbian AIDS Project (LAP); *Safer Sex Handbook for Lesbians* (LAP); woman-to-woman transmission
Wong, Toby, 154–55
Woodcock, John, 202, 205
Wright, Cathie, 162

York Correctional Institution (CT), 144

Zeh, John, 139–40
Zimbabwe, 178

Founded in 1893,
UNIVERSITY OF CALIFORNIA PRESS
publishes bold, progressive books and journals
on topics in the arts, humanities, social sciences,
and natural sciences—with a focus on social
justice issues—that inspire thought and action
among readers worldwide.

The UC PRESS FOUNDATION
raises funds to uphold the press's vital role
as an independent, nonprofit publisher, and
receives philanthropic support from a wide
range of individuals and institutions—and from
committed readers like you. To learn more, visit
ucpress.edu/supportus.